Radiology
for dental auxiliaries

Radiology
for dental auxiliaries

Herbert H. Frommer, A.B., D.D.S.

Professor and Director of Radiology
New York University College of Dentistry
New York, New York
Diplomate of the American Board of Oral and
Maxillofacial Radiology

Sixth Edition

with 543 illustrations

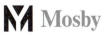 Mosby

St. Louis   Baltimore   Boston   Carlsbad   Chicago   Naples   New York   Philadelphia   Portland
London   Madrid   Mexico City   Singapore   Sydney   Tokyo   Toronto   Wiesbaden

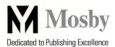

Mosby

Dedicated to Publishing Excellence

A Times Mirror
Company

Publisher: Don Ladig
Editor: Linda L. Duncan
Developmental Editor: Jo Salway
Project Manager: Deborah Vogel
Production Editor: Mamata Reddy
Editing/Production: Carlisle Publishers Services
Manufacturing Supervisor: Linda Ierardi
Designer: Pati Pye

SIXTH EDITION

Printed in the United States of America
Composition by Carlisle Communications, Ltd.
Printing/binding by R. R. Donnelley & Sons Company

Mosby-Year Book, Inc.
11830 Westline Industrial Drive
St. Louis, Missouri 63146

International Standard Book Number 0-8016-1701-4

NWST
IAHT 9493

For My Family—
Both
Immediate and Expanded

Preface

It is very difficult for this author to believe that the sixth edition of this textbook represents more than 21 years of my career as a dental radiologist. As I look back, I realize how much the field of dental radiology has changed and my hope is that this book has reflected and will continue to reflect these changes. Instead of the title Radiology, we might be more correct in using Dental Maxillofacial Imaging to more accurately describe the scope of our ever-expanding field.

Through the changes in these six editions, I have tried to keep current with the fields of dental radiology, dental practice and the concerns of government regulations and our patients. It still remains a textbook that applies basic principles to the practice of a clinical discipline.

I am truly grateful for the support of and continued response for this text. The constructive criticism and helpful suggestions that I have received from colleagues have motivated me to continually strive to improve this book.

A major change to this edition is the availability of a corresponding study guide. Each chapter of the study guide corresponds to a chapter in the textbook. The study questions that, in previous editions, had appeared at the end of the chapter or in an appendix are now found in the study guide. I hope this new approach will benefit students and faculty who use this text. For this edition, the section that deals with radiographic interpretation and diagnosis has been expanded to reflect the growing emphasis on and interest in this area by dental hygienists and assistants. The new emerging digital imaging techniques also are covered in greater detail than in previous editions.

As always, some words of credit and thanks for colleagues, family and friends who helped and encouraged me in my work in preparing this sixth edition: in the Radiology Department of The New York University College of Dentistry: Dr. Rajinder Jain, Dr. Allan Friedman, and Dr. Stanley Gibbs; President of New York University, Dr. L. Jay Oliva; and Dr. Edward G. Kaufman, Dean of the College of Dentistry, for encouraging and supporting faculty scholarship; and once again Carol Robson for her wonderful illustrations. Of course, this project could not have been completed without the encouragement, support and understanding from my wife Eleanor and my sons Ross and Dan.

Herbert H. Frommer

Contents

Radiology

for dental auxiliaries

Chapter

one

Ionizing Radiation and Basic Principles of X-Ray Generation

A preliminary understanding of x-rays and x-ray generation can be acquired simply by visualizing the everyday office procedure of taking a radiograph of a patient. The patient is seated in the dental chair and draped with a lead apron. Following the infection control protocol, which will be described in Chapter 5, a film packet in a film-holding device is positioned in the patient's mouth. An activating switch already has turned on the dental x-ray machine (Figure 1-1). The open-ended, rectangular, position-indicating device then is aimed at the film packet in the patient's mouth. Radiation is produced, and the film is exposed by pressing a button attached to an electric cord leading to the x-ray machine. The film then is processed and interpreted by the dentist.

From this description we can make some important observations on the properties of x-rays. X-rays are produced by a machine whose source of energy is electricity; x-rays are produced by pushing a button that completes an electric circuit. Because no sign of x-ray production is apparent during the interval of exposure, x-rays must be invisible. The x-ray beam is directed at the film packet, so x-rays must travel in straight lines.

The ability of x-rays to produce an image on the film packet inside the patient's mouth by a machine positioned outside the mouth, indicates that x-rays can penetrate an opaque structure such as skin or teeth.

After penetrating the dense tissue, x-rays can produce an effect on an imaging system such as the dental film placed in the patient's mouth. This effect becomes visible by processing the film in the darkroom so that an image of the penetrated structures appears on the film.

Because x-rays produce undesirable effects, the patient is draped with a lead apron for protection, and the operator either leaves the room or stands 6 feet away from the machine or behind a suitable barrier when the exposure is made.

In summary, we have observed these properties of x-rays:

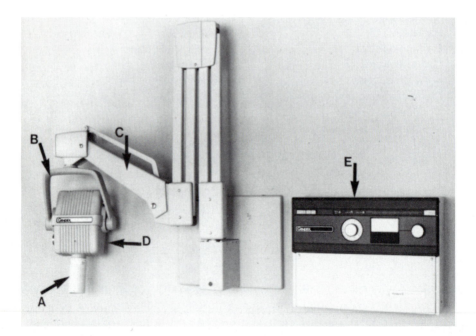

FIGURE 1-1   Dental x-ray machine. **A,** Position indicating device; **B,** Yoke; **C,** Arm; **D,** Tube head; **E,** Control panel. *Courtesy Gendex Corp. Milwaukee, Wis.*

1   X-rays are produced by the conversion of electric energy into radiation.
2   X-rays are invisible.
3   X-rays travel in straight lines.
4   X-rays can penetrate opaque tissues and structures.
5   X-rays can affect a photographic emulsion which, when processed, produces a visible image.
6   X-rays can adversely affect living tissue.

HISTORY

The x-ray was discovered in November 1895 by Wilhelm Conrad Roentgen, a professor of physics at the University of Wurzberg in Germany. He was working with a vacuum tube called a Crookes tube, through which an electric current was passed (Figure 1-2). Roentgen, like many of his colleagues, was interested in the cathode ray and the type of light produced across a vacuum tube when an electric current was applied. Since he was concerned with light, he was working in a darkened room with black cardboard covering the Crookes tube, and there were many fluorescent plates in his laboratory. Thus the stage was set for one of the most important discoveries that would aid medical and dental science.

One evening while working in his darkened laboratory, Roentgen noticed that one of the fluorescent plates at the far side of the room was glowing. He quickly realized that something coming from the Crookes tube was striking the fluorescent plate and causing it to glow. Since he did not know what it was, he called the phenomenon x-ray, *x* being the algebraic designation for the unknown. By placing various objects in the path of the x-ray beam, he could produce images on the screen. He inadvertently placed his hand between the tube and the screen and saw the faint outline of the bones of his hand. He went on to expose and produce images on photographic plates. Some of the first radiographs Roentgen took were of his wife Bertha's hand and his shotgun. Thus, we see the first medical and industrial use of x-radiation. It is interesting to note how closely the essential parts of Roentgen's tube and the modern day x-ray tube resemble each other. They both are highly exhausted vacuum tubes with an anode and a cathode through which an electrical current passes. Roentgen's tube had a fixed amount of electrons available, in contrast to the present variable source (milliamperage), and the potential across his tube was fixed, whereas today it is variable (kilovoltage).

Roentgen presented a paper on his discovery in late December, and in January 1896 Dr. Otto Walkhoff, a dentist in Braunschweig, Germany, made the first dental use of an x-ray, a radiograph of a lower premolar. He used a small glass photographic plate wrapped in black paper and covered with rubber. The exposure time was 25 minutes. Today, for comparable exposure, we would use about ¹⁄₁₀ second (6 impulses). For his work in the discovery of x-rays, Roentgen was awarded the first Nobel Prize in physics in 1901. For many years, the science of imaging with the use of x-ray was called roentgenology. We still use his name today, expressing the units of x-ray exposure in *roentgens.*

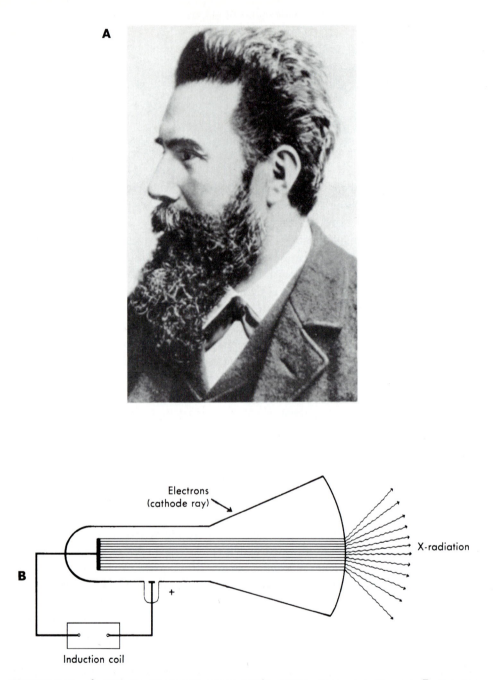

FIGURE 1-2, A, Wilhelm Conrad Roentgen (1845–1925), discoverer of x-rays. B, Crookes tube, which Roentgen worked with at the time of the discovery of x-rays in 1895.

C. Edmond Kells, a New Orleans dentist, is credited with taking the first intraoral radiographs in 1896. Other early workers with intraoral radiographs were W. J. Morton and William Rollins. Rollins developed the first dental x-ray unit in 1896.

Many of the early workers with dental x-rays suffered from effects of their work. Rollins reported burns to the skin on his hands, and Kells, before his death, had three fingers, his hand, and finally his arm amputated. Kells used a technique called "setting the tube" to adjust the x-ray beam before radiographing patients. He held his hand between the tube and a fluoroscope and adjusted the beam quality until the bones of his hand were seen clearly.

In 1913 William D. Coolidge invented the hot cathode x-ray tube, which is the prototype of x-ray tubes used today. The hot filament provided a variable source of electrons in the tube and eliminated the need for residual gas as a source for ionization in the tube.

Also in 1913 the first American dental x-ray machine was manufactured. In 1923 the Victor X-ray Corporation, which later became General Electric X-ray Corporation and now Gendex Corporation, introduced a dental x-ray machine with a Coolidge tube in the head of the unit cooled by oil immersion.

The x-rays were produced in Roentgen's vacuum tube by the electric current applied to the tube, which caused ionization of the gas molecules in the tube. That is, the neutral molecules were broken into negative ions and positive ions. Because of the difference in electric potential, the negative particles (electrons) were attracted to the positive side of the tube where they collided with the tube wall, and x-rays were produced. Modern dental x-ray tubes employ the same principle with some modifications, the most significant being a higher voltage, or difference in potential across the tube, and a variable source of electrons (hot filament). Today's tubes also have radiation safety features and cooling devices.

ATOMIC STRUCTURE

To understand x-ray production and the effect of radiation on tissue, we must understand the basic structure of matter. All matter is made of molecules. A molecule is the smallest particle of a substance that retains the property of the substance. Molecules are in turn composed of atoms (Figure 1-3). An atom contains a relatively heavy inner core, or nucleus, that possesses a positive electric charge and a number of light, negatively charged subatomic particles called *electrons* that orbit around the nucleus (Figure 1-4). The nucleus of an atom is composed of positively charged subatomic particles, called *protons,* and particles that have no charge, called *neutrons.* The number of protons in the nucleus of an element is specific for each element, determines its atomic number, and is designated by the symbol Z. The total number of protons and neutrons in the nucleus of an atom is the mass number and is designated by the letter A. An atom of an element that has the required number of protons but a different number of neutrons in the nucleus is said to be an *isotope* of the element. Isotopes of an element have the same atomic number (number of protons) but a different atomic mass number (number of neutrons) of the element (e.g., carbon-14). They may be stable or unstable, and the unstable isotopes may give off gamma rays. Many isotopes are used as tracer elements in diagnosis or for treatment of malignancies.

In the neutral or stable atom, the number of orbiting electrons (−) equals the number of protons (+) in the nucleus; hence, the atom is electrically neutral.

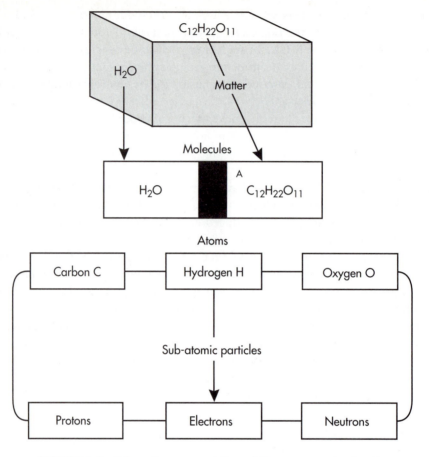

FIGURE 1-3   Schematic representation of the components of matter.

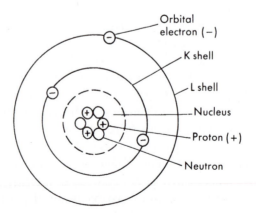

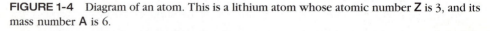

FIGURE 1-4   Diagram of an atom. This is a lithium atom whose atomic number **Z** is 3, and its mass number **A** is 6.

Electrons travel around the nucleus in definite orbits called *shells.* There is a maximum number of electrons that can occupy each shell and a definite energy level that binds the electrons in each shell to the nucleus. The shells farthest from the nucleus have less binding energy than the inner shells. The shell closest to the nucleus is called the *K shell,* the next outer shell the *L shell,* and then successively the *M, N,* and *O shells.* More energy is needed to remove an electron from the K shell than from the outer shells, because the binding energy is greater.

IONIZATION

When an orbiting electron is ejected from its shell in an electrically stable or neutral atom, the process is called *ionization* (Figure 1-5). The electrically neutral atom will then be changed into two ions, one positively charged and one negatively. The remainder of the atom has a positive charge, and the ejected electron has a negative charge. Electrons can be removed from atoms by heating or interaction with x-ray photons. In all cases, however, the energy must be greater than the binding energy that holds the electron in orbit around the nucleus of the atom. Thus the inner shell electrons can be dislodged only by high-energy photons such as x-rays, gamma rays, or particulate radiations, while the loosely bound electrons of the outer shell can be dislodged by low-energy photons such as in ultraviolet light. The new ions do not have all the same properties of the former neutral atom. Since x-rays, gamma rays, and

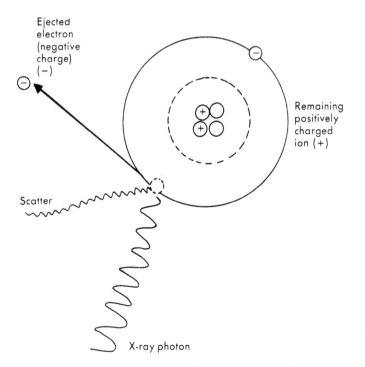

FIGURE 1-5   Diagram of ionization. The x-ray photon interacts with a neutral atom to form negatively and positively charged ions.

some particulate radiation can cause this type of reaction, they are classified as ionizing radiations. The ionizing potential of certain radiations accounts for their harmful biologic effects. A simple illustration is the water molecule, H_2O. If it is ionized, as it can be by radiation, two hydrogen ions and one oxygen ion are formed. The two ions may recombine to form water or they may in certain instances recombine as H_2O_2, which is hydrogen peroxide, a tissue poison.

RADIATION

Radiation is the emission and propagation of energy through space or a substance in the form of waves or particles. Particulate radiation consists of atoms or subatomic particles that have mass and travel at high speeds to transmit their kinetic energy. Some examples of particulate radiation are electrons, sometimes called *beta particles,* protons, neutrons, and alpha particles. Particulate radiations most commonly are emitted from radioactive substances called *radionuclides.* Another type of radiation is the wave form. We are most concerned with the wave form of radiation, since x-rays are energy waves with no mass and are part of a grouping called *electromagnetic radiation.*

ELECTROMAGNETIC SPECTRUM

The electromagnetic spectrum is a grouping of energy waves that has in common the weightlessness of the waves and the speed at which they travel (186,000 miles per second). The individual radiations of the spectrum differ in their wavelengths and frequencies and thus in many of their properties. Those with shorter wavelengths and higher frequencies have more photon energy. Looking at Figure 1-6, we immediately recognize energy waves that we encounter every day.

It is not known whether these electromagnetic radiations are actually waves of energy or the individual units of energy called photons. Some phenomena can be best explained using the wave theory and some by considering the theory of discrete units of energy. If the radiation is considered a wave, it is measured by its length. If it is considered a bundle of photon energy, it can be measured in ergs. We will use both forms in this text, sometimes referring to waves of energy and at other times to photons of energy.

Let us consider the concept of an energy wave. An energy wave travels in the same way that a ripple crosses a body of still water. The height of the wave is called the crest, and the depth of the wave is called the trough. The distance from one crest to another is called the wavelength and is usually abbreviated with the Greek letter lambda (λ). The frequency of a wave is the number of oscillations per unit of time (Figure 1-7). The wavelength of x-rays is very short and is measured in Angstrom units, which are $\frac{1}{100,000,000}$ of a centimeter and can be expressed as 10^{-8} cm. The difference in the electromagnetic spectrum between visible light and x-rays is their wavelengths; x-rays have shorter wavelengths. The shorter the wavelength and the greater the

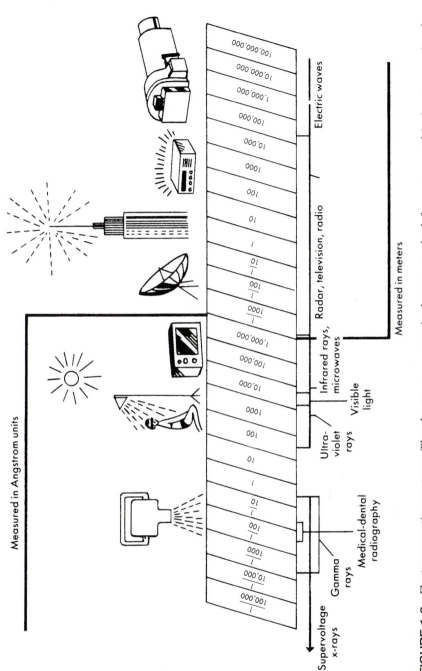

FIGURE 1-6 Electromagnetic spectrum. The shorter more energized waves to the left are measured in Angstrom units, the longer waves are measured in meters.

frequency, the more energy it bears. This energy gives the x-ray the ability to penetrate matter—specifically, the teeth, bones, and gingivae of the dental patient. Light waves cannot penetrate teeth and bone because the wavelength is too long and does not have sufficient energy.

The effect of electromagnetic radiation on living organisms varies depending on the wavelength. Television and radio waves, which are ever present in the atmosphere, have no effect on human tissue. Microwaves, which are low-energy radiations, can produce heat within organic tissues and are so employed in microwave ovens. Microwaves do not have enough energy to be ionizing and therefore do not have the same effects on living tissue as x-rays, gamma rays, or particulate radiations. Electromagnetic radiations that are too low in energy to cause ionization are employed in magnetic resonance imaging (MRI) for diagnostic purposes. These radiations are located in Figure 1-6 near the radio waves.

Figure 1-6 also shows that there is an overlap between gamma rays and the x-rays used for diagnostic purposes in medicine and dentistry, because both have identical wavelengths. Gamma rays and x-rays have identical properties if their wavelengths are the same; they differ only in their source. X-rays are the result of electron and atomic interactions within an x-ray tube, whereas gamma rays originate within the nucleus of radioactive materials.

Ultrasonic radiation is another type of radiation used in medicine, and dental patients often question dentists about its use and relationship to dental x-rays. Ultrasound is a nonelectromagnetic, nonionizing radiation that can be used to image

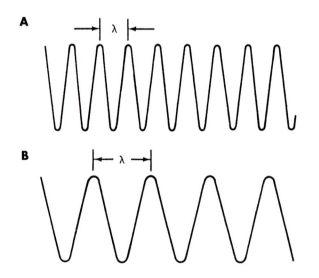

FIGURE 1-7   Diagram of x-ray energy wave. The distance between the two crests is the wavelength lambda (λ) and the number of oscillations is the frequency. Wave "A" has a shorter wavelength and a higher frequency than does "B."

internal structures. The fact that it is nonionizing makes its use acceptable in cases in which ionizing radiation might prove harmful (e.g., fetal imaging in pregnant women).

To understand the energy aspect of radiation, let us use the example of throwing a ball. We impart energy to the ball, which is expressed by the speed with which the ball travels. As this energy is lost, the ball falls, hits the ground, and rolls to a stop. The total energy is lost when the ball stops. This is also true of radiation. As x-rays travel over a distance, they lose their energy. For this reason, in the dental office the operator stands a safe distance (6 feet) away from the patient being exposed to x-rays to avoid unnecessary exposure.

If the ball is caught in midair, the energy can be felt by the impact on the hand catching the moving ball. The impact of the ball is in part a product of the weight of the ball and the speed with which it was thrown. X-rays and other radiations have no weight; they have only speed and energy, but their effect is as tangible as the sting of the ball on the hand. This effect is produced by interaction with the basic unit of matter, the atom, and the resultant ionization.

X-RAY PRODUCTION

X-rays used in dentistry are produced in an x-ray tube. With modifications the modern tube resembles the cathode ray tube used by Roentgen, and the principles of high-speed electrons being attracted to and colliding with a positively charged target to produce x-rays and heat are still valid. Figures 1-8 through 1-10 are schematic drawings of the production of x-rays in the dental x-ray tube.

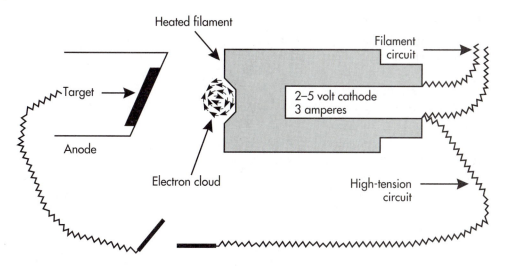

FIGURE 1-8 An x-ray tube illustrating formation of an electron cloud at the cathode as filament circuit is activated. Note the exposure switch is open.

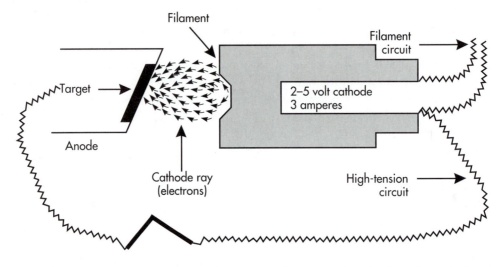

FIGURE 1-9   An x-ray tube showing electrons traveling across the tube from the cathode to anode (target) as high-tension circuit (exposure switch) is activated.

When a dental x-ray machine is turned on and the indicator light is glowing, it is ready to produce x-rays. Turning on the machine closes the filament circuit and heats the tungsten filament, causing electrons to "boil off" in what is called the *thermionic emission effect.* The electrons stay at the filament and are referred to as an *electron cloud* (Figure 1-8). The electrons are attracted across the tube only when there is a difference in electric potential across the tube or, stated another way, when the high-voltage circuit is closed or completed. This high-voltage circuit is activated by the exposure switch and remains active for the length of time for which a timer is set.

With the high-voltage circuit completed by closing the exposure switch, the electrons produced by the thermionic emission effect at the cathode are attracted to the positively charged anode, which contains a tungsten target (Figure 1-9). This stream of electrons crossing the tube is called the *cathode ray.*

Federal regulations require that on new dental x-ray machines an audible signal be sounded when an exposure is being made, in addition to the signal lights in the control panel.[1]

X-rays and heat are produced in the tube when the high-speed electrons strike the tungsten target (Figure 1-10). This is a transference of energy. The kinetic energy of the moving electron is converted into the energy-laden x-ray photon and heat energy. The faster the electrons travel across the tube, the more energized and penetrating are the x-rays produced. The speed of the electrons across the tube is determined by the kilovoltage.

As illustrated in Figure 1-17, the tungsten target is angled and the x-rays produced are directed to an exit point (porte) in the tube. The rest of the x-ray tube is lead lined, and x-rays can leave the tube only through the porte. If x-rays leave the tube in any area other than the porte, the machine is said to have head leakage. This is a safety hazard to both patient and operator, and a radiation safety code violation.

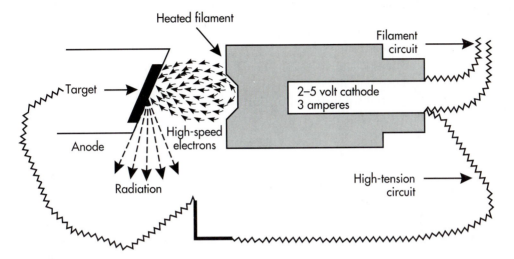

FIGURE 1-10   An x-ray tube showing production of x-rays as high-speed electrons collide with target.

BREMSSTRAHLUNG AND CHARACTERISTIC X-RAYS

Let us now examine the formation of x-rays at the level of the atom. That is, what is the atomic mechanism of the formation of x-rays when the high-speed electrons strike the tungsten target?

The phenomenon of x-ray production can be best understood by considering the tungsten atom and the possibilities that arise when a high-speed electron enters its orbit, as it would at the target of a dental x-ray machine (Figure 1-11). The tungsten target consists of an infinite number of tungsten atoms. We will consider only one surface atom that will serve as a representative example for the rest of the atoms in the tungsten target.

The first possibility, which rarely occurs, is that the high-speed electron might hit the nucleus of the tungsten atom and give up all its energy. The second possibility, represented by entering electron A in Figure 1-11, is that the entering high-speed electron might be slowed down and bent off its course by the positive pull of the nucleus. This slowing down represents a loss of energy that is given off as x-rays and heat. This is the major source of x-ray production in the dental x-ray tube. The slowing down and veering off course of the entering high-speed electron with its loss of energy expressed in x-rays and heat is called *bremsstrahlung,* the German word for "breaking radiation."

Since the tungsten target is not just one atom thick, this bremsstrahlung is repeated an infinite number of times. The exiting electron A′ (Figure 1-11) will enter another tungsten atom, and the reaction will be repeated with the production of more x-rays. A′ and the succeeding A″, A‴, and so forth each will have less energy than the original entering electron A; hence the x-rays produced at each succeeding bremsstrahlung will have less energy or longer wavelengths. Because of the multiple bremsstrahlung reactions, all the x-rays produced do not have the same energy content (wavelength). A heterogeneous x-ray spectrum is produced. The later bremsstrahlung reactions produce x-rays whose energy is not sufficient to penetrate teeth and bone and, as we will see, are removed by filtration.

The third possibility, represented by entering electron B, is that the high-speed electron might hit and dislodge one of the orbiting electrons of the tungsten atom. This can happen only when the entering electrons possess more energy than that binding the orbiting electrons to the nucleus. In the dental machine, this means it can happen only at settings of 70 kVp (70,000 volts) and above, because the binding energy of the K shell of electrons is 69,000 electron volts. If an orbiting electron is dislodged, a rearrangement or cascading of electrons inward fills up the electron vacancies in the inner shells. This rearrangement produces a loss of energy that is expressed in x-ray energy. The x-rays thus produced are called characteristic x-rays and account for a very small part of the x-rays produced in the dental machine and only in those machines operating at 70 kVp and above.

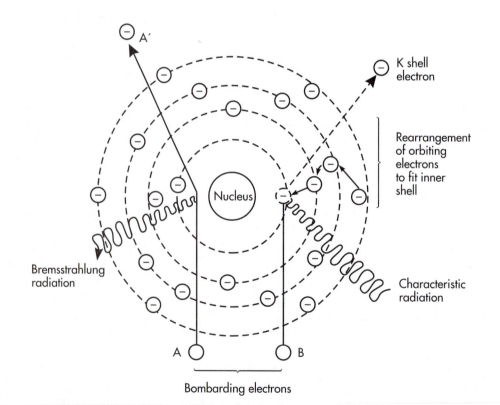

FIGURE 1-11   Electrons colliding with a simulated tungsten atom, forming **A,** bremsstrahlung radiation and **B,** characteristic radiation.

THE DENTAL X-RAY MACHINE

Electricity

Since the primary source of energy for the x-ray machine is electricity, it is necessary to learn or review some basic concepts of electricity.

Electric current is the flow of electricity through a circuit; it can either be alternating (AC) or direct (DC). By direct current we mean current that flows in only one direction in an electric circuit, whereas alternating current flows in one direction and then flows in the opposite direction in the circuit (Figure 1-12). In the dental x-ray tube this means that the tungsten filament is only the negative pole half the time because of the reversal of the direction of the current. During this part of current flow, no x-rays are produced.

The term *cycle* in alternating current refers to the flow of current in one direction and then the reversal and flowing of the current in the opposite direction. There are usually 60 cycles per second in most alternating current circuits.

Rectification. Since the dental x-ray machine is operating on alternating current, this means that in the x-ray tube itself the polarity is reversed 60 times per second. When the direction of the current flow is reversed, the tungsten target becomes the negative pole, or cathode, and the tungsten filament becomes the positive pole, or anode. During the alternating $\frac{1}{120}$ second (half of a cycle) when the current is reversed, no x-rays are produced, because no electrons are available at the target to travel across the tube and strike the target; thus the current is blocked from traveling across the tube. This blocking of the reversal is called *rectification* and since the dental x-ray tube is designed to produce this effect, it is said to be self or half-wave rectified (Figure 1-13).

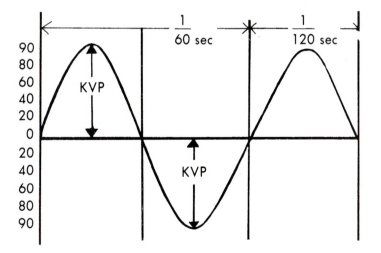

FIGURE 1-12   Sine wave of 60-cycle alternating electric current operating at 90,000 volts (90 kVp).

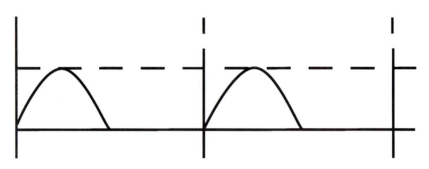

FIGURE 1-13   Half-wave rectification.

We can see that x-rays are not produced in a steady stream but in spurts or pulses, and these pulses take place only during one half of the alternating current cycle. Since most alternating current is 60 cycles, the dental x-ray machines will express exposure units in pulses or sixtieths of a second instead of the usual ½ second or ³⁄₁₀ second. A ½-second exposure is equal to 30 pulses. It should be obvious that exposure time of ¹⁄₇ second is not possible, since it is not divisible into 60, and it is impossible to get a fraction of a cycle of alternating current. Some newer model dental x-ray machines are designed to supply full-wave rectification. In this circuitry, the negative portion of the alternating current cycle is reversed. If currents then are superimposed, there is less of a drop in voltage between cycles. These machines do not produce pulses of x-radiation but rather a constant stream of x-rays. Thus exposure time can be reduced by one half since x-rays are not being produced half the time, as they are in the self-rectified circuit, but all the time. The radiation exposure to the patient is the same; it just requires one half the time.

Voltage is the term used to describe the electric potential or force that drives an electric current through a circuit. The unit of measurement is the volt. The kilovolt (kV) is 1000 volts. In an alternating current, where the direction of the current is constantly changing, the voltage is also changing, and the term *kilovolt peak (kVp)* is used to denote the maximum or peak voltage that is described by the sine wave that plots the alternation of the current (see Figure 1-12). A dental x-ray machine that is set for a potential of 90 kVp will only reach 90 kVp at the peak of the alternating current during exposure. As seen in the diagram of the exposure's sine wave, other voltage levels also occur during the exposure. This has great clinical significance, because these differences in voltage contribute to the heterogeneity of the x-ray beam and the need for filtration.

Ampere is the unit of measurement used to describe the amount of electric current flowing through a circuit. The milliampere (mA) is equal to ¹⁄₁₀₀₀ of an ampere.

A *transformer* is a device that can either increase or decrease the voltage in an electric circuit. It is composed of two coils of electric wire insulated from one another. The magnetic field from one coil induces an electric current in the second coil. The number of turns in the induction coil in relation to the number of turns in the second coil will determine what the action of the transformer will be (Figure 1-14).

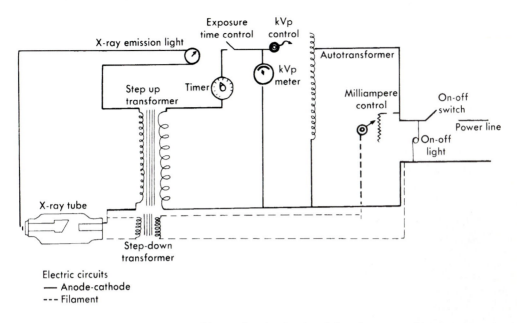

FIGURE 1-14 Diagram of basic electric circuits of dental x-ray machine.

The dental x-ray machine also has an autotransformer, which utilizes only one coil and can be used only for making minor changes in voltage. If the transformer increases the voltage, it is referred to as a "step-up" transformer, and if it decreases the voltage, it is referred to as a "step-down" transformer. The dental x-ray machine utilizes both types in taking ordinary line or house voltage of 110 volts and stepping it up to a range of 65,000 to 100,000 volts (65 to 100 kVp) in the high-voltage circuit or stepping line voltage down to 3 to 5 volts in the filament circuit, these being the two basic circuits in the dental x-ray machine.

Circuitry

Dental x-ray machines use 110-volt alternating current (Figure 1-14). The two major circuits in the x-ray machine are the filament circuit and the high-voltage circuit. Each circuit utilizes a transformer to convert the line voltage and current. The filament circuit uses 3 to 5 volts, so the 110-volt line current is reduced by means of a step-down transformer. The heating of the cathode filament by the electric current is controlled by a rheostat in the circuit and is a function of the milliamperage selector on the control panel of the machine. The high-voltage circuit in the dental x-ray machine requires voltage in the range of 65,000 to 100,000 volts. This increase in voltage is achieved by the use of a step-up transformer. An autotransformer also is used in the circuit as a line compensator to control fluctuations in line voltage. The relationship of the input circuit to a variable number of coils is changed in the autotransformer, by the kVp dial on the control panel, to change the quality of the x-rays emitted.

Control panel

The control panel of the dental x-ray machine (Figure 1-15) contains an on-off switch and indicator light, an exposure button and indicator light, timer dial, and kVp and mA selectors. The exposure button is on a 6-foot retractable cord or linked to a remote station. Some machines have preset fixed milliamperage choices, usually 7, 10, or 15 mA or adjustable. The kVp values may be fixed or have a range from 65 to 100.

Timer. As previously discussed, the dental x-ray tube does not emit a continuous stream of radiation but rather a series of impulses of radiation. The number of impulses depends on the number of cycles per second in the electric current being used. In 60-cycle alternating current, there are 60 pulses of x-ray per second (Figure 1-16). Each impulse lasts only ¹⁄₁₂₀ second, since no x-rays are emitted in the negative half of the cycle when the polarity of the tube is reversed. The newer model dental x-ray machine exposure dials are not calibrated in fractions of seconds, but more realistically in impulses. On the timer dial, "24" means 24 impulses per second, which is equivalent to ⅖ or ²⁴⁄₆₀ second of exposure. With the advent of more sensitive or faster films calling for decreasing exposure times, all machines should have electronically controlled timers so that these short exposure times can be achieved accurately and repeatedly. The old mechanical timers with increments of ¼ second, which were usually at least ⅛ to ¼ second inaccurate, are unacceptable for the shorter exposure times in use and are in many instances violations of the radiation code.

The x-ray machine should be turned off after use. Warm-up time is almost instantaneous for the x-ray tube, so there is no need to keep the machine on during the working day. Most offices have a definite setting for mA and kVp that is used for all patients. As will be seen in the next chapter, the kVp is determined by the density

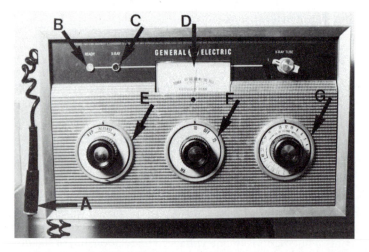

FIGURE 1-15 Control panel of dental x-ray machine. **A,** Exposure control on a 6-foot retractable cord; **B,** "on" indicator; **C,** exposure indicator; **D,** kVp meter; **E,** kVp control; **F,** mA control; **G,** timer control.

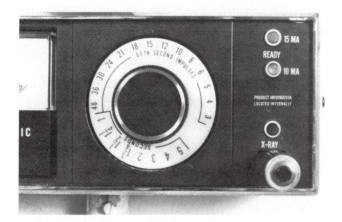

FIGURE 1-16   Timer dial. Note the increments in impulses (⅟₆₀ seconds).

of the object and the type of contrast desired, while the mA is determined by the speed of the film and the exposure time and distance.

The control panel should be checked each day to be sure that the mA and kVp settings have not been changed inadvertently. Some control panels have preset values for different types of patients, and the selectors are labeled with such terms as "large patient," where the kVp is increased, and "child," where the kVp is decreased. If one understands the principles of radiology, this type of panel is unnecessary and very limiting.

X-ray tube

The dental x-ray tube, housed in a large machine, is about 6 inches long and 1½ inches in diameter.

The three basic elements of an x-ray tube needed to produce x-rays are (1) high voltage to accelerate electrons across the tube, (2) a source of electrons within the tube, and (3) a target to stop the electrons.

High voltage. As shown in Figure 1-17, the x-ray tube has a positive side (pole), called the anode, and a negative side, called the cathode. Electric current flows from a negative pole to a positive pole. This voltage can be varied by adjusting the kilovoltage dial that controls the autotransformer, which then affects the step-up transformer and thus the kilovoltage across the tube. The greater the kilovoltage or potential across the tube, the faster the electrons will travel and the greater the energy that will be released when the electrons strike the target at the anode.

Source of electrons. The main source of electrons in the x-ray tube is the tungsten filament found at the cathode. This is a variable source of electrons, unlike Roentgen's tube in which electrons were produced from the ionization of a fixed volume of gas. The tungsten filament is connected to the step-down transformer circuit. The hotter the resistant filament becomes, the more electrons that are produced at the cathode. This production, or boiling off, of electrons from the heated tungsten filament is called the *thermionic emission effect.* The milliamperage dial controls the amount of current in the filament circuit and hence the number of electrons that boil off. The tungsten filament is surrounded by a focusing cup, which directs electrons toward the anode that contains the target.

Target. The target in the x-ray tube also can be called the *focal spot* or area. It is at the anode part of the tube, and when the circuit is complete, it has a positive (+) charge. It is made of tungsten and measures about 0.8 × 1.8 mm. This is the actual target. The effective target or focal area is smaller because of the tilting of the target that geometrically makes the target smaller when viewed from the opening in the tube. All modern dental x-ray machines have approximately the same size target. Tungsten is used as the target material because it has a high melting point and a low vapor pressure at high temperatures and thus is not affected by the heat produced. The element tungsten also is desirable as a target material because of its high atomic number and thus its density, and because when it is bombarded by electrons, x-ray production is more efficient. However, tungsten does not have a high degree of thermal conductivity and must be imbedded in a copper stem. The heat is dissipated into the head of the x-ray machine by the copper stem attached to the anode and cooled by air or oil immersion.

Heat production. The dental x-ray machine is an extremely inefficient machine. That is, of the total energy produced at the anode by the collision of the electrons with the target, less than 1% is x-ray energy; the remaining 99% is in the form of heat. This is why the highly conductive copper sleeve and oil immersion tube surround the target. Care must be taken not to overheat the tube.

Heat production is the limiting factor of the mA setting of a dental x-ray machine. With an mA of more than 15, too many electrons hit the target and too much heat is

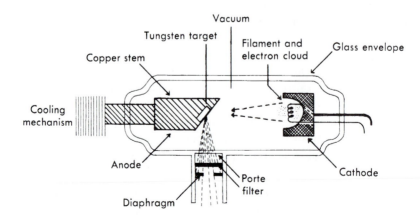

FIGURE 1-17   Components of a dental x-ray tube.

produced. This overheating soon will destroy the target. Some panoramic and extraoral units have rotating anodes to dissipate the heat and thus can use higher mA settings. The standard dental x-ray machine has a fixed anode and a limit to the amount of milliamperage.

Under ordinary use, overheating of a dental x-ray machine is not very likely. Each machine has a duty rating and a duty cycle. The *duty rating* refers to the number of consecutive seconds a machine can be operated before overheating, and the *duty cycle* refers to the portion of every minute that the dental machine can be used without overheating.

X-RAY BEAM

The x-ray photons produced at the target in the dental x-ray tube emanate from and leave the tube as a divergent beam. The x- ray at the center of the beam is referred to as the central ray. The x-rays closest to the central ray are more parallel and those farthest away more divergent. The more parallel rays produce less magnification of the image; thus they are most useful (Figure 1-18).

The x-ray beam is positioned or aimed at the film in the patient's mouth by an open-ended device, either a rectangle or a cylinder, called a *position indicating device (PID)*. These PIDs should be lead lined to prevent the escape of scatter radiation and are usually 8, 12, or 16 inches long (Figure 1-19). Originally, all dental machines had short, 8-inch, plastic, pointed cones as position indicating devices. To this day, people incorrectly refer to open-ended cylinders as cones, although the proper term is position indicating device.

The pointed cone was designed as an easy aiming device, the tip of the cone indicating the position of the central ray. The technique called for aiming the tip of the cone at the center of the film packet placed in the patient's mouth or the extraoral anatomic landmark being used. One of the unfortunate outcomes of this type of instrumentation was that some practitioners came to believe that the x-ray beam was coming out only from the tip of the cone and that the size of the beam was that limited.

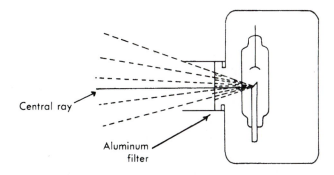

FIGURE 1-18 The divergent x-ray beam. The aluminum filter removes longer wavelength x-rays from the beam.

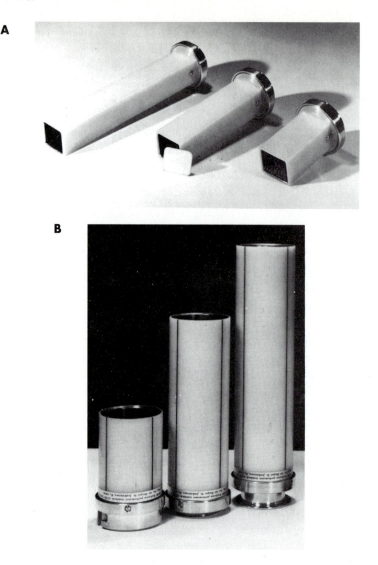

FIGURE 1-19   Position indicating devices, open-ended, lead-lined 8-inch, 12-inch, 16-inch **A,** rectangles; **B,** cylinders. *Courtesy Margraf Dental Mfg., Jenkintown, PA.*

The problem with the pointed plastic cone is the secondary radiation that is produced by the interaction of the primary beam of x-ray photons with the plastic cone (Figure 1-20). These secondary x-rays increase the long wavelength radiation to the patient's face and degrade the diagnostic image on the film. X-rays interact with plastic, even though one might not consider it to be very dense material. X-rays interact and cause secondary radiation with any form of matter from a piece of tissue paper to a bar of steel. The density of the material and the quality of the x-ray beam determine the type and extent of interaction. When the open-ended PID is used, there is no material at the end of the PID with which to interact. Some practitioners

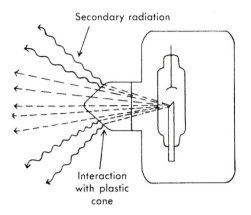

Secondary radiation

Interaction
with plastic
cone

FIGURE 1-20 Production of secondary radiation resulting from interaction of the primary beam with the closed-end plastic cone.

have complained about open-ended PIDs, claiming that they are difficult to aim properly and that "cone cutting" results. In reality, the rectangle or the cylinder is not difficult to use, but the change from using the pointed cone is difficult. Novice students starting instruction in radiology have no more difficulty using open-ended PIDs than their predecessors had with the pointed models.

Radiation protection codes in many states have required the use of open-ended PIDs. It is strongly recommended that even in jurisdictions that allow the use of pointed cones, their use be terminated in favor of using open-ended, lead-lined rectangles or cylinders instead. The state of the art in radiation risk prevention calls for open-ended, lead-lined PIDs.

Quality and quantity of x-rays: milliamperage and kilovoltage

The three parameters of the dental x-ray beam that are adjusted from the control panel by either the dental auxiliary or the dentist are (1) the energy, or penetrating power (quality), of the x-ray beam, (2) the number of x-rays produced (quantity), and (3) the length of time that these x-rays will be produced.

Quality. The quality, or penetrating power, of the x-ray beam is controlled by the kilovoltage. The suitable range for dental radiography is 65 to 100 kVp. Some units can deliver this complete range, whereas others have more limited ranges or even a fixed kVp value. As a rule, the kilovoltage in a dental office remains fixed at one setting for all intraoral radiography. The dentist determines what kilovoltage will produce the most diagnostic radiographs for the particular use of that office. There are some techniques that call for a variable kilovoltage and time with a fixed mA—that is, increased kVp in denser areas and reduced kVp in less dense areas. For every increase of 15 kVp, exposure time is reduced by 50% to maintain the density of the film.

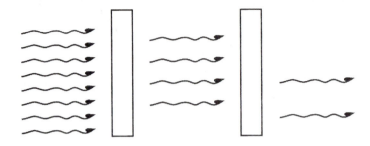

FIGURE 1-21   Schematic representation of half value layer of an x-ray beam.

Dental diagnostic radiology is confined to the 65 to 100 kVp range because the density of the structures dentistry deals with (teeth, bone, etc.) determines the useful penetration range. Kilovoltage settings below 45 would not give proper penetration of the object. Kilovoltage from 45 to 65 would penetrate but not without undue production of secondary x-radiation, and kilovoltage above 100 causes overpenetration. The overall objective of diagnostic radiology is to record differences in densities on the film of the objects being radiographed. A kilovoltage range is chosen that will indicate the difference of penetration and absorption so that the differences in structural densities can be recorded. The choice of kVp setting within the acceptable range will be discussed in the section on density and contrast. Thus we see that a kilovoltage is selected that allows for complete absorption of some x-rays, partial absorption of others, and passage of other x-rays through the object to reach the film.

Differential absorption of the x-ray beam by the object being radiographed produces the radiograph. That is why less dense structures, such as the dental pulp, will appear radiolucent (black) on the dental film, and highly calcified denser structures, such as the enamel, will appear radiopaque (white or gray). The less dense areas in the object allow greater passage of x-rays than do denser areas, and more x-rays strike the film in these areas to darken it.

X-ray machines with a low kilovoltage rating in the 45 to 65 kVp range are no longer considered acceptable, because the radiation produced contains many long, nonpenetrating wavelengths that unnecessarily increase the facial exposure to the patient (see Figure 4-2).

Half value layer. The term *half value layer (HVL)* is more appropriate than kilovoltage to describe beam quality and penetration. Kilovoltage is a description of the electric energy put into an x-ray tube. HVL measures the quality of the x-rays emitted from the tube. Two similar x-ray machines operating at the same kilovoltage may not produce x-rays of the same penetration. The HVL is defined as the thickness of aluminum (measured in millimeters) that will reduce the intensity of the x-ray beam by 50%. For example, a dental x-ray beam could be described as having an HVL of 2 mm. This means the energy of this particular beam is such that a thickness of 2 mm of aluminum would be necessary to decrease its intensity by half (Figure 1-21). Another beam with an HVL of 1 mm would not be as energized because only 1 mm of aluminum is necessary to decrease its energy by half.

Quantity. The milliampere dial determines the number of x-rays produced in a given exposure period by controlling the heating of the tungsten filament at the cathode of the tube. As the kilovoltage determines the quality (penetrating power) of the x-rays produced, the milliamperage determines the quantity of x-rays produced.

It is better to consider the concept of milliampere seconds (mAs) than milliamperage alone. An exposure, at a given kVp, of 1 second using 10 mA is 10 mAs. A 2-second exposure, at the same kVp, using 5 mA would produce an identical film, since the mAs are again 10 ($10 \times 1 = 10$, $5 \times 2 = 10$).

The sensitivity of the film and the focal-film distance used determines the mAs required at a given kilovoltage. The more sensitive the film to radiation, the fewer milliampere seconds required. The advantage of higher milliamperage is that a shorter exposure time can be used. This does not represent a decrease in the patient's x-ray exposure, only a decrease in the time necessary to expose the film. This reduces the chance of blurring caused by patient motion.

Ideally the shortest exposure time and a high milliamperage is the best way to achieve the desired mAs. The range of milliamperage on dental x-ray machines is usually from 5 to 15 mA. As previously mentioned, the limiting factor is the heat produced at the desired small target. Milliamperage higher than 15 would produce too many electrons bombarding the target and thus too much heat. Some x-ray machines in dentistry are made specifically for extraoral radiography and have rotating anodes. A rotating anode is a spinning disk composed of many tungsten targets instead of one stationary target, as found in the standard intraoral x-ray unit. Because the targets are rotating, they are struck by the electrons through only part of their 360-degree rotation. During the rest of the rotation, the targets can cool. Since the heat is dissipated in this manner, an mA of 50 or 100 is used.

Filtration. As we have seen, the x-ray beam that originates at the anode is not homogeneous. It consists of a spectrum of long and short wavelengths. In fact, very few of the x-ray photons produced have energy or penetration power corresponding to the desired kilovoltage called for on the control panel. In other words, if one sets the kVp dial for any desired kilovoltage, only a few of the x-ray photons produced will correspond to this setting. Almost all the x-ray photons produced will have wavelengths longer than those corresponding to the desired setting and thus will be less penetrating. This is partially the result of the electrons in the tube bombarding multiple atomic layers of the tungsten target with the resulting bremsstrahlung and characteristic x-ray production and the effect of alternating current with its sine wave voltage buildup. As shown in Figure 1-22, the x-ray beam is not homogeneous but rather heterogeneous, having a full range of wavelengths. The longer, lower kVp wavelengths will not penetrate tooth and bone and will be absorbed by the skin or produce secondary radiation.

The function of the filter is to remove from the primary beam the long, nonpenetrating wavelength x-rays (see Figure 1-18). After the primary beam has been filtered and collimated, it is referred to as the *useful beam.*

Federal regulations require that for dental x-ray machines operating at kilovoltages up to 70 kVp, 1.5 mm of aluminum filtration is required.[1] For those machines operating from 70 kVp and higher, 2.5 mm of aluminum filtration is required. All new machines must meet these requirements.

Collimation

The size and shape of the x-ray beam as it leaves the tube head are restricted by a collimating device (Figure 1-23). In intraoral radiography, the size of the beam should be just large enough to cover the film packet. Circular collimation allows for a margin of error in positioning (Figure 1-24). A beam size any larger than this would expose the patient's face to unnecessary primary radiation. Historically, the diameter of the x-ray beam measured at the patient's face used in dentistry has been decreasing. From no limitation at all in the early days of dental radiology, the beam diameter has gone to 3½ inches, 3 inches, and presently to 2¾ inches (7 cm).

The collimating device most often used is a lead diaphragm with a circular aperture (Figure 1-25). The size of this aperture, at a selected focal-film distance, determines the beam size. PIDs, be they open-ended cylinders or rectangles, lead lined or made of

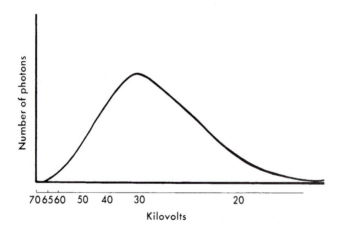

FIGURE 1-22   Graph of spectrum of x-ray beam from dental x-ray machine operating at 65 kVp. Note number of low-energy photons produced.

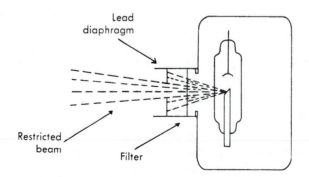

FIGURE 1-23   Collimation and filtration of x-ray beam.

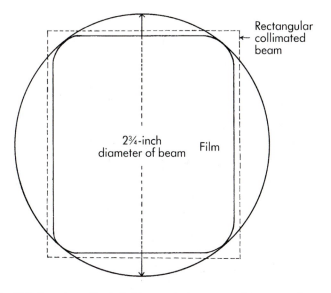

FIGURE 1-24 Relative size of adult film packet compared to x-ray beam 2¾ inches in diameter and rectangularly collimated beam.

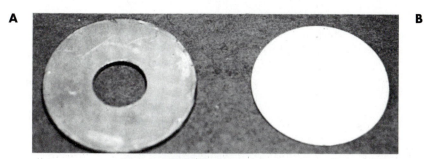

FIGURE 1-25 **A,** Lead diaphragm; **B,** An aluminum filter.

metal, also can serve as collimating devices. Federal regulations presently require that the x-ray beam should not exceed 2¾ inches (7 cm) in diameter when measured at the patient's skin.[1]

Rectangular collimation. The shape of the dental x-ray beam always has been circular. The question can be asked, "Why is a circular beam used when the film packet is rectangular in shape?" The circular beam covers a greater facial area, and it exposes the patient to more primary radiation than a tightly collimated rectangular beam does. The movement in the dental profession is now toward rectangular collimation. It is taught as the primary technique in most dental schools and is recommended by the American Dental Association[2] and the American Academy of Oral and Maxillofacial Radiology. This change to rectangular collimation can be accomplished without an increase in collimator cut-off "cone cutting" with the use of

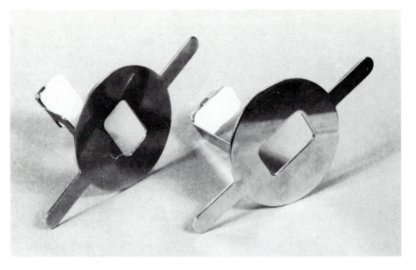

FIGURE 1-26 Rectangular collimating device. *(Courtesy Precision Instruments, Isaac Masel Co., Inc., Philadelphia.)*

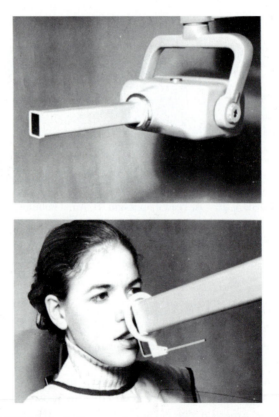

FIGURE 1-27 **A,** Rectangular PID collimator; **B,** With "XCP."

proper equipment. Collimator cut-off occurs when the beam is not centered on the film and thus part of the image is cut off. X-ray beams can be aligned to film easily using the Precision Device (Isaac Masel Co.) (Figure 1-26), the XCP (Rinn Corp.), a metal rectangular PID (Figure 1-27), or many other devices now available. The use of these devices in rectangular collimation is illustrated and described in Chapter 7.

REFERENCES

1. Performance standards for electronic products: diagnostic x-ray systems and their major components, *Fed Register* 37:16461, 1972.
2. American Dental Association, Council on Dental Materials, Instruments, and Equipment: Recommendations in radiographic practices: an update, *J Am Dent Assoc* 118:115-117, 1989.

Chapter

two

Image Formation, Image Receptors

FACTORS INFLUENCING IMAGE FORMATION

No matter what imaging system we use to make radiographs of dental structures, our goal is to produce an image with the proper degree of density and contrast, detail sharpness, and a minimum amount of enlargement and distortion. These factors enable us to gain the most diagnostic information for the amount of radiation expended.

Density and contrast

Density is the degree of blackness on a film, and contrast is the difference in the degrees of blackness between adjacent areas. When comparing a black (dense) area on a film to a white area, we see a great deal of difference, or high contrast. When comparing gray to white or gray to black areas or shades of gray, we see less, or low, contrast. The density of a film is determined by the relative transmissions of the x-rays through parts of the object and by the absorption of the x-rays in the emulsion of the film. These two factors, the object being radiographed (object contrast) and the properties of the film (film contrast) determine the overall density and contrast of the finished radiograph.

Object contrast. The object contrast is determined by (1) the thickness of the object, (2) the density of the object, (3) the chemical composition of the object, (4) the quality of the x-ray beam, and (5) scatter radiation. We cannot control the thickness, density, or atomic number of the structures being radiographed (teeth, bone, etc.), and these parameters determine the range of kVp that is used in dentistry. Therefore we use a kVp range that produces a differential absorption pattern to portray differences in object density on the film. Using a kVp setting greater than 100 in dentistry results in overpenetration, and using a kVp of below 45 conversely results in underpenetration. In both cases the selective penetration desired is not achieved.

The only variables of object contrast are the quality or penetration of the x-rays within the dental penetration range of 65 to 100 kVp and the amount of scatter radiation produced.

The image difference between films produced at the different kVp settings in the dental range is the resulting contrast. By varying the kilovoltage and the quality of the radiation, either high- or low-contrast films can be produced.

Short scale. High-contrast films appear mainly black and white with very few gray tones. They also are referred to as short-scale contrast films and are produced by kilovoltage in the 65 kVp range. These films are said to be "crisper" and more pleasing to the eye, but they may not reveal early pathologic changes. The short-scale film is a "yes" or "no" situation: either the x-ray beam penetrates the object or it does not. Areas appear black or white, radiolucent or radiopaque, with few gray tones in the middle range (Figures 2-1, 2-2, and 2-3). The lower kVp ratings (below 65) are undesirable because they result in increased facial absorption and scatter as a result of their less-penetrating wavelengths.

Long scale. The low-contrast films, also referred to as long-scale contrast, are produced by the high kilovoltage range of 90 to 100 kVp. In these films, there are many tones of gray in addition to the blacks and whites. The long-scale film is not as visually pleasing as the short-scale film, but early changes in object density such as early bone loss or incipient decay may be seen in the gradation of the gray tones because of more selective penetration (Figure 2-1), which is not present in the high-contrast films. Many in the field believe that the human eye can detect changes better in the 70 to 75 kVp range.

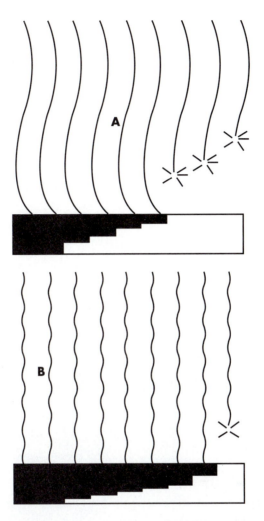

FIGURE 2-1   Diagram of the relative penetrations of an aluminum step wedge and resulting density and contrast of **A,** 65 kVp and **B,** 100 kVp x-ray beam.

In addition to its effect on other parts of the patient's body, scattered radiation produces a uniform exposure or darkening over the film and in doing so reduces the contrast. Scatter radiation is one of the causes of "film fog," and it degrades the diagnostic image. Most scatter radiation originates in the object itself; thus the larger the field, the more that object scatter becomes a factor. As we will see in Chapter 9, grids are sometimes used to eliminate object scatter in extraoral radiography. In intraoral radiography, scatter radiation is reduced by using as small a beam as possible, open-ended PIDs, lead backing in the film package, and kVp settings of 65 and above.

Film contrast. Film contrast is determined by (1) the amount of radiation transmitted (object contrast), (2) the properties of the film, (3) intensifying screens,

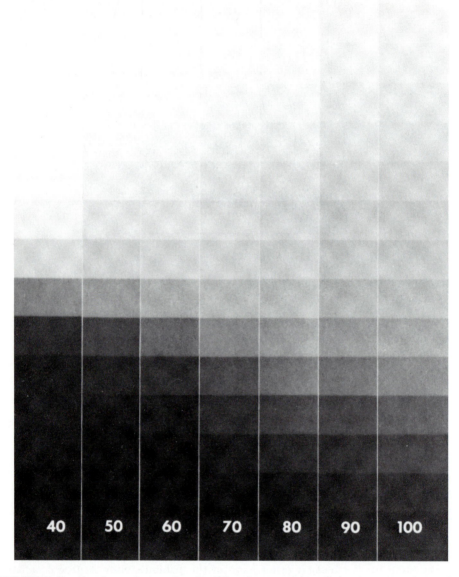

FIGURE 2-2   Aluminum step wedge densities. A step wedge of aluminum is radiographed using increasing kVp (penetration). The thinner portion of the step wedge shows complete penetration at all kVps. At the thicker portion of the wedge, the lower kVp does not penetrate while the higher kVp penetrates as shown by the gray tones. *Courtesy Eastman Kodak Co.*

if used, (4) film processing, and (5) viewing conditions. Each of these factors is discussed in their respective sections. The important fact is that any secondary radiation or light that affects the film decreases the desired contrast, or "fogs" the film and degrades the image.

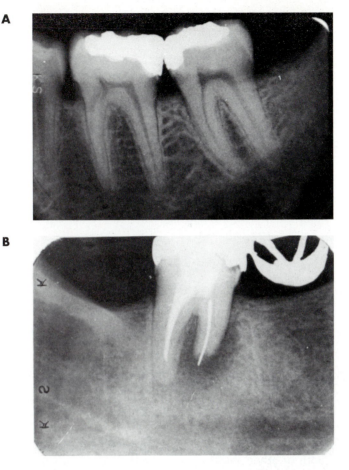

FIGURE 2-3 **A,** High-contrast radiograph taken at 65 kVp. Note predominance of black and white tones. **B,** Low-contrast radiograph taken at 90 kVp. Note predominance of gray tones.

Image detail and definition

Image detail is the visual quality of a radiograph that depends on definition or sharpness. The factors that influence detail are (1) size of the tube focal or target area, (2) focal-film distance, (3) object-film distance, (4) movement of either patient film or x-ray machine, (5) type of intensifying screen, if used, and (6) image contrast.

Size of tube focal (target) area. The smaller the focal area (spot) at the anode (see Figure 1-17) of the x-ray, the better the image detail will be. As discussed in Chapter 1, the heat produced limits how small the focal area can be. The focal area in the tube is tilted, usually at an angle of 20 degrees to the cathode (Figure 2-4), and when viewed from below the focal area appears to be smaller than it actually is and functions as the desired smaller focal area. This is called the *effective focal area,* in contrast to the

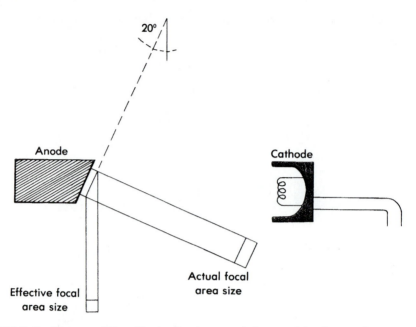

FIGURE 2-4   Diagram of the effective focal area and the actual focal area of an x-ray tube.

actual focal area. The effective area is always smaller than the actual focal area. Most dental x-ray machines are equipped with the smallest fixed focal area possible given the heat production restrictions.

Focal-film distance (FFD) and object-film distance (OFD). The ideal radiograph of a tooth or other object, in terms of definition, image enlargement, and distortion, can be made by meeting the following criteria:

1   Establish a maximum *focal-film distance.* FFD is the distance between the focal spot (target) at the anode and the film in the patient's mouth. The maximum distance enables the more parallel rays from the middle of the x-ray beam to strike the object and the film, and not the more divergent x-rays from the periphery of the beam, which would cause image enlargement on the film (Figure 2-5).

2   Determine a minimum *object-film distance.* The tooth and the film should be as close together as possible. The closer they are, the less enlarged the image is on the film (Figure 2-5).

3   Position the object and the film parallel to each other in their long axes and the central ray perpendicular to both (paralleling versus bisecting).

These are the optimum requirements. Because of anatomic restraints in intraoral radiography, it is impossible to meet all of these requirements at the same time.

Focal-film distance. The most common focal-film distances used in dentistry are 8, 12, and 16 inches. An FFD of less than 8 inches may cause magnification of the image that is larger than the film (Figure 2-6). As the FFD is increased to 12 or 16 inches, the magnification of the image decreases because the image is formed by the more

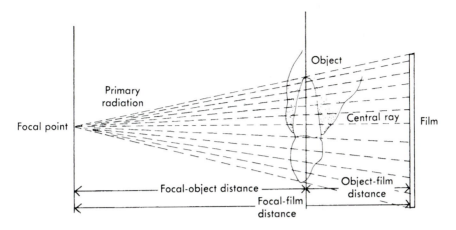

FIGURE 2-5   Relationship between focal point, object, and film.

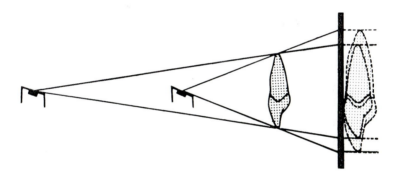

FIGURE 2-6   Comparison of 8- and 16-inch focal-film distance. *Courtesy Rinn Corp., Elgin, Ill.*

parallel x-rays from the center of the beam. However, this decrease in magnification is not a linear relationship beyond 16 inches. Figure 2-7 shows that as the FFD increases beyond 16 inches, the percentage of magnification does not decrease significantly. Therefore using a 24-inch FFD does not give a significantly better image clinically than a 16-inch FFD, and there is no advantage in using this long FFD. The 16-inch FFD is the distance of choice. The extended or 16-inch focal-film distance also results in exposure of less tissue volume (see Chapter 4). The 16-inch FFD produces a better image with less radiation to the patient. For these reasons its use is strongly recommended.[1]

Tube position. The x-ray tube is positioned in the anterior part of the head of the machine close to the PID or "cone" (Figure 2-8). The rest of the head of the x-ray machine contains electric circuitry and cooling devices. The open-ended rectangle or cylinder, placed on the head of the machine, serves as the aiming device for the x-ray beam, and the length of this PID determines the focal distance to be used.

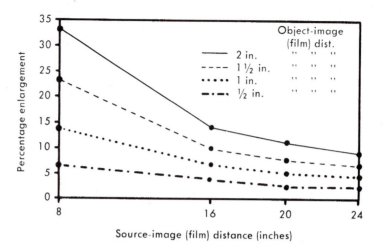

FIGURE 2-7 Relationship of image magnification to object-film distance and focal-film distance. *Courtesy Rinn Corp., Elgin, Ill.*

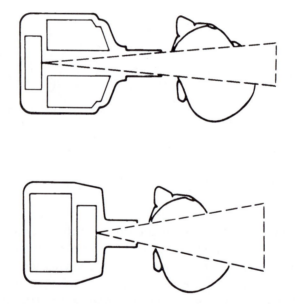

FIGURE 2-8 Long beam tube head *(top)* and conventional tube head *(bottom)*. Note different position of x-ray tube that allows for increased focal-film distance.

Some practitioners objected that the longer PIDs (cones) were bulky, cumbersome, and difficult to operate in small operatories. Others said the long "cone" tended to unbalance the head of the x-ray machine. With the increasing popularity of the paralleling technique and the need for an extended focal-film distance, a new design for the tube head was introduced. Figure 2-8 illustrates the operation of the new design. The x-ray tube is placed in the rear part of the machine's head, and the rest of the components are placed on both sides of the beam. The advantage of the design

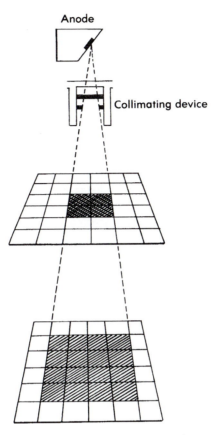

Anode

Collimating device

FIGURE 2-9   Inverse square law. The effect of distance on the intensity of the radiation.

is in the extended focal distance and the elimination of the longer PID. The terms *short "cone"* and *long "cone"* are no longer appropriate. Cones are now outdated because of radiation hygiene, having been replaced by open-ended, lead-lined cylinders and rectangles. In addition, the machine with the short "cone" really may have a long focal-film distance, depending on the placement of the x-ray tube in the head of the machine.

Inverse square law (Figure 2-9). One factor that must be considered when choosing or changing an FFD is the inverse square law: the intensity of radiation varies inversely with the square of the distance. More simply stated, if the FFD doubles, the exposure time quadruples. This assumes that the mA and kVp remain the same. The inverse square law will be discussed again in Chapter 4 in its relationship to radiation protection for the operator.

As seen in Figure 2-9, the intensity of the radiation at 16 inches is much less than at 8 inches, since it is spread out over 16 boxes. To achieve the same intensity of radiation, the exposure time must be increased by a factor of 4. In Figure 2-9 the field size at 16 inches would be kept to 4 boxes by decreasing the aperture of the collimating device.

Before the advent of more sensitive films, the inverse square law presented more of a limiting factor than it does today. For instance, if one were using an 8-inch FFD at 1-second exposure and then changed to a 16-inch FFD, a 4-second exposure time would be necessary to produce a comparable film at the same mA and kVp. This 4-second exposure time would be inordinately long, and there could be patient movement. With the use of faster x-ray film and exposure times in the range of ²⁄₁₀-second at an 8-inch FFD, a 16-inch FFD would need only ⁸⁄₁₀-second exposure time. Clinically, ⁸⁄₁₀-second exposure time, when compared with ²⁄₁₀-second exposure time, presents no more or less problem with the patient movement. The same amount of radiation reaches the film in the 8- and 16-inch techniques; it just takes greater time to achieve required x-ray intensity with the increased distance.

Another clinical application of the inverse square law is in the correction of an error that can cause underexposed light (thin) films. The correct position of the PID is almost touching the patient's face when taking intraoral radiographs. This gives the desired FFD, depending on the length of the PID. If the operator is careless in placement and does not approximate the skin, the result is an increased FFD and decreased intensity of the x-ray beam by a factor of the square of the distance from the patient's face. A small distance, when squared, can produce underexposed film. Most dental offices select an FFD and keep this technique constant.

Object-film distance. The closer the object (tooth, bone, etc.) is to the film, the better the detail and the enlargement (Figure 2-10). The object-film distance depends on the anatomy of the area of the mouth being radiographed and whether the paralleling or bisecting technique is used.

Image distortion and enlargement

Because of the mouth's anatomy it is impossible to satisfy ideal criteria 2 and 3 (Chapter 7 p. 146), which refer to object-film distance and parallelism between the

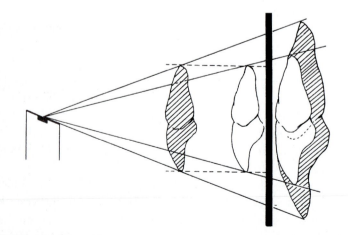

FIGURE 2-10   Comparison of object-film distances and the effect on image magnification.

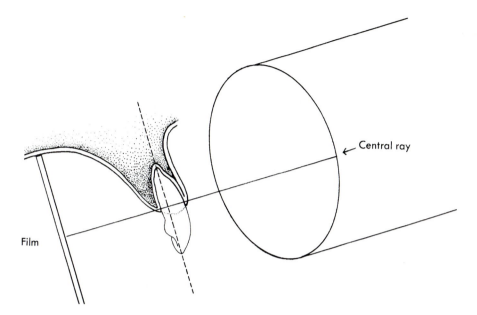

FIGURE 2-11   Relationship of central ray, tooth, and film packet in paralleling technique.

object and the film. If the film is held close to the teeth, then the parallelism is lost; if the teeth and film are to be parallel, there must be increased OFD.

This is the basis for the two techniques used in film placement for intraoral radiography: the paralleling technique and the bisecting-angle technique. The details of performing both these techniques, as well as their advantages and disadvantages, will be described in Chapters 7 and 8.

In the paralleling technique the film is held parallel to the long axis of the tooth. This results in an increased OFD in most areas of the mouth; that is, for the film to remain parallel to the tooth, it must be positioned away from the tooth (Figure 2-11). The compensation for enlargement caused by the increased OFD is using an increased FFD (12 or 16 inches). The use of the increased FFD is the reason for the misnomer "long cone technique." It is not the long cone that is of primary importance but the parallelism between the tooth and the film.

In the bisecting-angle technique the film is held as close to the tooth as possible. At this point the long axis of the tooth and the plane of the film cannot be parallel. A geometric trick is then used to project the proper image of the tooth onto the film. An imaginary line is drawn that bisects the angle formed by the long axis of the tooth and the plane of the dental film (Figure 2-12). The central ray of the x-ray beam then is directed perpendicularly at this bisecting line. This projects the proper linear dimensions of the tooth onto the film without elongation or foreshortening.

Movement. Three types of movement affect image detail: patient movement, film movement, and x-ray source movement. Patient and film movement is controlled by

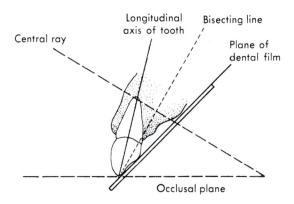

FIGURE 2-12 Relationship of central ray, tooth, and film packet in bisecting-angle technique.

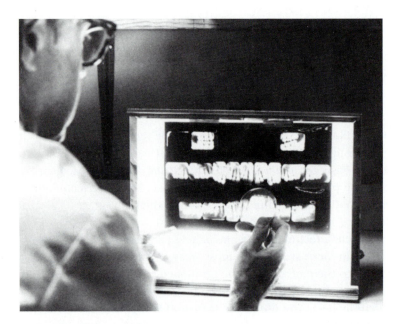

FIGURE 2-13 Dentist viewing radiographs on an illuminating box.

good chairside technique and is discussed in later sections of this book. Source movement, or tube and arm movement, is caused by improper upkeep of x-ray equipment. If the arm or head moves or vibrates, image quality is compromised. There is no excuse for this type of error, and an effective quality control program should detect this malfunction. In many jurisdictions tube or arm movement is a violation of the Radiation Health Code.[2]

Intensifying screens (film screen combinations). The use of intensifying screens and their effects, on image definition are discussed in Chapter 9.

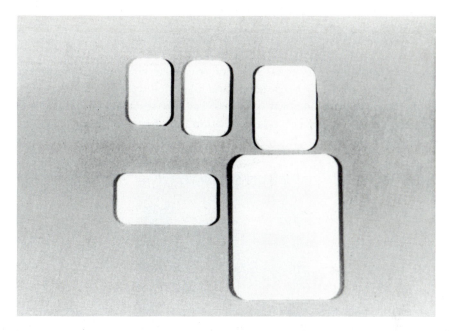

FIGURE 2-14 Intraoral film packet sizes, child (#0) narrow anterior (#1) adult size (#2) preformed bite-wing (#3) and occlusal (#4).

Viewing conditions (Figure 2-13). Radiographs should always be viewed on an illuminator (view box). A magnifying glass can be used to examine fine changes. A dark room is the ideal setting for viewing radiographs. Holding radiographs up to the light on the unit or from the window is no substitute for an illuminator. Valuable information can be lost or never seen if the proper viewing conditions are not used and maintained.

IMAGE RECEPTORS

The image receptors used in dentistry today are film, film screen combinations, and radiation detectors used in intraoral digital imaging and computed tomography. All of these use x-rays to generate an image on a receptor. Some medical imaging systems, such as fluoroscopy, use x-rays, and other systems, such as ultrasound and magnetic resonance imaging (MRI), do not.

Film

Film remains by far the most commonly used image receptor in dentistry. Intraoral packets come in three basic sizes (Figure 2-14): child size, #0; adult size, #2; and narrow anterior film, #1. Occlusal film packets, #4, and preformed long bite-wing films, #3, also are available.

All the film packets must be lighttight and resistant to saliva seepage. These packets must have some degree of flexibility and should be easy to open in the darkroom.

The dental x-ray film packet has an outer, plasticlike wrapper. Inside the wrapper is the x-ray film, covered by black paper, and a lead-foil backing. The lead backing is placed on the side of the film away from the x-ray tube to absorb any unused radiation and prevent back-scattering secondary radiation from fogging the film (Figure 2-15).

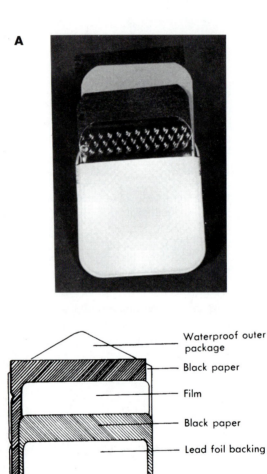

Waterproof outer package

Black paper

Film

Black paper

Lead foil backing

Waterproof outer covering

FIGURE 2-15   A, Back of an opened dental film packet. B, Diagram of A.

A film packet may contain one or two pieces of film. The so-called double film packet requires slightly more exposure time than the single film packet. Some dental offices prefer the double packets to duplicating films.

X-ray film is composed of a clear cellulose acetate film base coated with an emulsion of silver halide (usually silver bromide) grains suspended in a layer of gelatin (Figure 2-16). The emulsion is sensitive to x-rays, visible light, and static electricity. The film base is coated on both sides and thus is called a double emulsion. Less radiation is used than with single-sided emulsion film. Clinically, this means that a radiograph can be viewed correctly from either side. Previously with single-emulsion film, the film had to be viewed from the side with the emulsion on it. The film also has a button or dot on it. This is a small convex-concave area that helps to orient the developed film in mounting (see Chapter 12).

Film sensitivity. The size of the silver halide crystals, the thickness of the emulsion, and the presence of special radiosensitive dyes determine the film speed, or film sensitivity. Film sensitivity determines how much radiation for what period of time (mAs) is necessary to produce an image on the film.

More sensitive films require less mAs and are said to have greater film speed; these are the fast films. Films that require more mAs are less sensitive to radiation and are called slower films. The size of the silver bromide crystals is the main factor in determining the film speed: the larger the crystals, the faster the film.

Film sensitivity is compared or expressed by means of a characteristic or H & D (Hurter and Driffield) curve (Figure 2-17). The curve gives the relationship between radiation exposure to the film and the resulting film density. A fast film requires less exposure to produce a desired density than a slower film.

Different film manufacturers give different brand names to their various film speed types. No slow-speed film is made today. At 65 kVp and 10 mA, slow film would need an average exposure time of about 3 seconds per film. Under the same conditions the intermediate-speed film needs about 1½ seconds and the fast film about ³⁄₁₀-second exposure per film. One manufacturer's "ultraspeed" (Eastman Kodak Co.) may equal

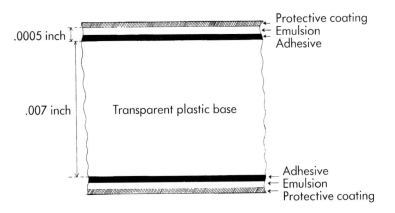

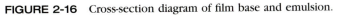

FIGURE 2-16   Cross-section diagram of film base and emulsion.

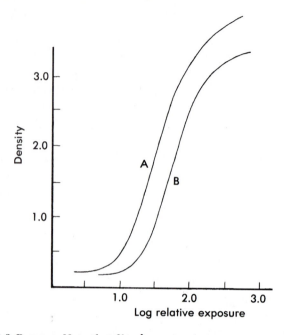

FIGURE 2-17   H & D curve. Note that film **A** requires less exposure to achieve a given film density than film **B**.

another's "lightning" or "very fast" film speed. It is obvious that some standards and nomenclature are necessary. Film speed is designated into groups by the American National Standards Institute (ANSI) using the letters A through F, A for the slowest film and F for the fastest. At the present time E speed is the fastest film available. To get comparable film sensitivities when changing from one manufacturer to another, one should consult the ANSI speed group ratings found on the package and not be misled by descriptive names.

Presently, there are only two film speed groups that should be used, E and D. The American Dental Association (ADA) and the American Academy of Oral and Maxillo-facial Radiology currently recommend that E-speed film should be used.[1] The ADA further recommends that films in a speed group slower than group D should not be used.[1] Certain health codes forbid the use of film slower than group D.[2] Group E film is twice as fast as group D film, and thus the patient receives half the radiation exposure for a comparable diagnostic film.[3]

Film definition and detail.   The definition or detail on a film also depends on the size of the silver bromide crystals. The larger crystals, theoretically, although they allow for reduced exposure time, give poorer definition when compared with the smaller, slower crystals.

The dilemma is whether to reduce the amount of radiation the patient receives by using fast films with large crystals, thereby sacrificing definition, or to increase exposure time by using small crystals to give better definition, thereby increasing radiation exposure. The human eye, which must view the finished radiograph, cannot easily distinguish between the definition on E-speed films and that on D-speed films. The debate today is on the image quality of D versus E film. The literature strongly suggests that it is difficult to tell the difference between films and that the decrease in radiation far outweighs the slight possible loss of definition.[4] Eastman Kodak, the major supplier of E film, recently has improved and changed its group E emulsion; now the film is called "Ektaspeed Plus." The new film has better contrast and is not as sensitive to variations in processing conditions as the original Ektaspeed emulsion.[56] Both these factors were cited as reasons by dentists for not using the E-speed emulsion.

Film fog. An x-ray film is fogged when all or part of the radiograph is darkened by sources other than the primary beam radiation to which the film was exposed. Fogging degrades the diagnostic image, and a good office quality assurance program should be able to minimize its deleterious effects. Here are several sources of fogging:

1   Chemical fog results from an imbalance or exhaustion of processing solutions (see Chapter 6).
2   Light fog results from unintentional exposure to light to which the film emulsion is sensitive, either before or during processing (see Chapter 6).
3   Scatter radiation fog results from radiation striking the film from sources other than the intentional exposure of the primary beam. Examples are scatter from the patient or unprotected storage of films before or after exposure.

REFERENCES

1. American Dental Association, Council on Dental Materials, Instruments, and Equipment: Recommendations in radiographic practices: an update, 1988, *J Am Dent Assoc* 118:115–117, 1989.
2. New York City Health Code, Article 175, February 1981.
3. Silha RE: Methods for reducing patient exposure combined with Kodak Ektaspeed dental x-ray film, *Dent Radiogr Photogr* 54:4, 1981.
4. Kantor ML, Reiskin AB, and Lurie AG: A clinical comparison of x-ray films for detection of proximal surface caries, *J Am Dent Assoc* 111:967–969, 1985.
5. Ludlow J, and Platin E: Densometric comparisons of Ultra-speed, Ektaspeed, and Ektaspeed Plus intraoral films for two processing conditions, *Oral Surg Oral Med Oral Path Oral Radiol Endo* 79:105–113, 1995.
6. Thunty K, and Weinberg R: Sensitometric comparison of Kodak Ektaspeed and Ultra-speed dental films, *Oral Surg Oral Med Oral Path Oral Radiol Endo* 79:114–16, 1995.

Chapter

three

Biologic Effects of Radiation

Much attention has been given, not only in scientific journals but also in the media, about the effects of ionizing radiation, both man-made and naturally occurring, on human beings and the environment. This growing concern about the biologic effects of ionizing radiation is not limited to the scientific community but is evident in the public sector and at all levels of government. On television our patients view demonstrations against nuclear power plants and nuclear weapons; they read about radon gas in homes and hear discussions of arms treaties with destruction of nuclear arsenals. Events such as the near-fatal nuclear accident at Three Mile Island, Pennsylvania, and the catastrophe at Chernobyl in the former Soviet Union have heightened public awareness to the dangers of low-level radiation. The recent and ongoing revelations about human exposure in nuclear testing during the cold war have kept radiation exposure in the headlines. Fear and uncertainty aroused by these events may lead some patients to refuse necessary diagnostic radiographic examinations or avoid dental visits completely. Health professionals need to be informed about risks and benefits of dental radiation and the magnitude of its relationship with these events so that they may anticipate and allay unfounded fears.

Information about ionizing radiation that reaches the public from the media can be misleading and confusing. The latest data indicate that radiation from medicine and dentistry, including nuclear medicine, accounts for about 17% of the average annual dose equivalent to the U.S. population.[1] This is the largest source of man-made radiation to which the population is exposed. At the same time as one talks about the risk of exposure, one should consider the diagnostic benefits and health-preserving or lifesaving consequences of radiation.

Patient reaction can vary from questioning the need for dental radiographs to outright refusal. The dental auxiliary must face this patient reaction and, with the support of the dentist, be able to explain to the patient the biologic effects of dental x-ray exposure and the diagnostic benefits that are derived. Proper dentistry cannot and should not be done without adequate diagnostic radiographs. This is an accepted standard of dental practice. A patient may refuse to have radiographs, but the dentist also can and should refuse to treat that patient.

Ionizing radiation does produce biologic changes in living tissue, and patients should not be misled into believing that dental x-rays have no effect on human cells. The old reply to patient queries regarding radiation safety that claimed "dental x-rays are safe because the dosage is so small it doesn't matter" no longer satisfy informed health care consumers.

The question is no longer whether x-rays pose a risk, but how much of a risk exists. In determining whether radiographs should be used, the dentist must weigh the potential harm of dental x-rays against the benefit the diagnostic information will yield. In dental radiography performed under optimum conditions and when indicated, diagnostic benefits far outweigh potential risks.

Our objective for the patient is to use the least possible amount of radiation to obtain the greatest diagnostic yield. For the dental auxiliary and the dentist, the objective is to achieve occupational radiation exposure as close to zero as possible. To achieve these objectives, the dental auxiliary must fully understand the subjects of radiation biology and protection. Explanations to patients then will be meaningful, and the assistant or hygienist will feel at ease working in an environment where diagnostic radiation is used.

INTERACTION OF X-RAYS WITH MATTER

X-rays interact with all forms of matter. This interaction can result in absorption of energy and thus attenuation of the x-ray beam (a reduction of the intensity of the x-ray beam) and the production of secondary radiation.

Primary radiation is the result of the x-rays produced at the target of the anode in the x-ray tube. Secondary radiation is the result of the interaction of primary radiation with matter (see Figure 4-1).

When x-rays are absorbed by matter, positive and negative ions and secondary radiation are formed from previously neutral atoms. The amount and type of absorption that takes place depend on the energy of the x-ray beam (the wavelength) and the composition of the absorbing matter. The thicker the material that an x-ray beam has to penetrate, the more x-rays that will be absorbed. However, more than thickness determines x-ray absorption. The atomic configuration—the number of orbiting electrons, protons, and neutrons in the nucleus of the atom—also determines x-ray absorption. Heavy elements, those with greater mass, are better absorbers than lighter elements. The more electrons available in an absorbing material, the more x-ray photons that are absorbed. Heavy metals with high atomic numbers (the atomic number indicates the number of protons in the nucleus of the atom), such as lead and gold, absorb x-rays readily.

An important point to be made is that when x-rays are absorbed by any material, that material does not become radioactive, because x-rays have no effect on the nucleus of the absorbing atom. This means that the equipment or walls in a dental operatory do not become radioactive after continuous exposure to radiation. At the atomic level, four possibilities can occur when an x-ray photon interacts with matter. These possibilities are:

1 No interaction (pass through). The x-ray photon can pass through the atom unchanged and leave the atom unchanged (Figure 3-1, A). This happens about 9% of the time in a bitewing examination.[2]

2 Thompson scatter (unmodified or coherent scatter). In effect, the x-ray photon has its path altered by the atom. There is no change to the absorbing atom, but a photon of scattered radiation is produced (Figure 3-1, A). This accounts for about 8% of the interactions that take place in dental radiography.[2]

3 Photoelectric effect. The x-ray photon can collide with an orbiting electron, giving up all its energy to dislodge the electron from its orbit. The photoelectron that is produced has a negative charge, while the remaining atom has a positive charge. This, you will remember, is ionization (Figure 3-1, C). This interaction takes place about 30% of the time with dental x-rays.[2]

4 Compton effect. The x-ray photon can collide with a loosely bound electron in an outer shell of the atom and only give up part of its energy in ejecting the electron from its orbit. This results in a negatively charged, ejected Compton electron, a photon of scattered radiation, and a remaining atom that is now positively charged. This again is ionization (Figure 3-1, B). This interaction takes place about 62% of the time in dental x-rays.[2]

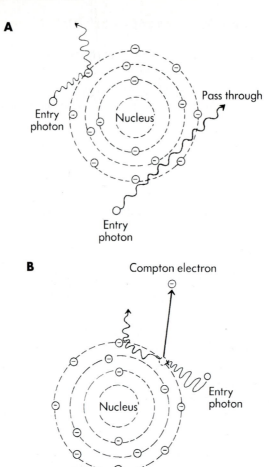

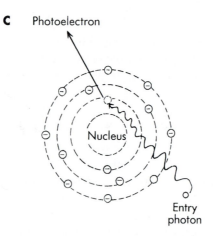

FIGURE 3-1   Interaction of x-rays with matter. **A,** Pass through and Thompson scatter; **B,** Compton effect; **C,** Photoelectric effect.

EFFECTS OF IONIZING RADIATION

Radiobiology is the study of the effects of ionizing radiation on biologic tissue. When a dental radiograph is taken, not all the x-rays reach the film and some even penetrate beyond it. Some of the x-ray energy of the primary beam is absorbed by the skin, bones, teeth, and other body tissues that lie in its path. Tissues that do not lie in the path of the primary beam absorb the energy of the secondary radiation that comes from the patient as a result of the interaction of the primary beam. It is the differential absorption (density) of the x-ray photons by the hard tissues, teeth, and bones that enables us to distinguish various structures on a diagnostic radiograph.

What is the effect of this x-ray energy absorption on the various tissues, and how is it manifested? The human body, like all living organisms, functions through the existence of ions in its organs, tissues, and cells. These ions are electrically charged particles that originate in the water, salts, proteins, carbohydrates, and fats that are the principal components of our bodies. The ions affect the many complex functions that maintain the health of the body and return it to health after illness. Ions are ever present in a finely balanced state, or equilibrium, so that precise control over the reactions concerned with body function can be maintained. If an overabundance of ions occurs, the surplus must be removed immediately if health is to be maintained; illness also occurs if an insufficient number of necessary ions is available for essential functioning. Special ions maintain the proper body environment for such functions as respiration, muscular activity, speech, and digestion. X-ray exposure, depending on the amount, can upset this delicately balanced state because of the x-rays' ability to cause ionization. Let us use the simple example of the ionization of water in human tissue. Water (H_2O) can be ionized to form the ions H (+) and OH (−). The free radicals may affect DNA molecules and cause tissue damage, recombine to form water again and have little effect, or form peroxide (H_2O_2). Peroxide also causes biologic damage.

The mechanism of this ionization or the ability to produce ions has been described previously. In the case of interaction with or penetration of the human body, extra ions become available. These extra ions can upset the fine ionic balance that exists. If the amount of radiation exposure is large, a great ionic upset results, and the body reacts by showing signs of injury or illness. It is important to understand that x-rays are ionizing radiation and, as such, have the potential to affect the health of the human body.

UNITS OF RADIATION MEASUREMENT

Before we can talk logically about the potential effects of dental radiation, we must have some means of measuring the radiation quantitatively. The settings on the control panel of the dental x-ray machine are not measurements of the x-ray energy (ionizing radiation) produced; the kilovoltage and milliamperage are indications of the quality and quantity of the electric energy put into the x-ray machine, and the timer provides a reading of how long the ionizing radiation is produced. The HVL, although a measurement of the x-ray beam, describes the penetration and the quality of the beam. The units of measure that commonly have been employed, each with its own application, have been the roentgen, the *rad* (for radiation absorbed dose), and the *rem* (roentgen equivalent man). To standardize units to the metric system, these conventional units have been replaced by those of the System International (SI). The new units are the coulomb per kilogram (c/kg), the gray (Gy), and the sievert (Sv). This text uses the conventional units with the SI units in parentheses.

Exposure

The unit most commonly used to measure the amount of energy, or ionizing radiation, produced by the x-ray machine is called the *roentgen* and is abbreviated as R. The milliroentgen is $\frac{1}{1000}$ of a roentgen; because exposures in dental radiology are small, they are often expressed in milliroentgens, or mR (1000 mR = 1 R). The SI unit for exposure would be coulomb/kilogram (c/kg), 1 c/kg = 3.88×10^{-3}R.

The roentgen is a measurement of ionization in air. It is defined as the quantity of radiation that produces one electrostatic charge in 1 cc of air. The roentgen is our measuring standard for radiation. Just as we have to know what an inch is before we can compare lengths, we have a standard—the roentgen—to measure radiation. Just as there are rulers and scales, there are ionization chambers calibrated in roentgens. An ionization chamber placed in front of a dental x-ray machine PID can indicate how many roentgens are produced per second (Figure 3-2). This is called the exposure rate or output of the machine. Since it is a measurement of ionization in air, it is measured in roentgens per second. A well-calibrated dental x-ray machine will have an output in the range of 0.7 to 1 R per second. If a patient had a radiograph taken with such a machine and the exposure time was 1 second, the facial exposure of the patient would be 0.7 R (0.7 R/sec × 1 sec = 0.7 R).

Dose

The critical factor in discussing the effects of radiation is not the amount of radiation at a point in air, but rather the amount of energy absorbed by tissue at a specific point.

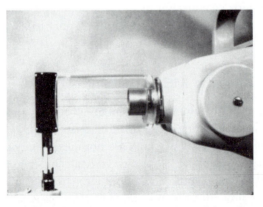

FIGURE 3-2   Ionization chamber measuring output of dental x-ray machine.

To express the amount of energy absorbed by a tissue, we use the rad or the gray. The rad is a unit of absorbed dose (radiation absorbed dose) and is defined as 100 ergs of energy per gram of absorber (tissue). The millirad is $\frac{1}{1000}$ of a rad. The unit for the absorbed dose in SI units is the gray (1 rad = 0.01 Gy or 1 Gy = 100 rads).

Dose equivalent

Different types of radiation on a rad-for-rad basis have different effects on living tissue. Neutrons, for example, will have a greater effect on tissue than will x or gamma radiation. The term *dose equivalent* is defined as the dose multiplied by the quality factor Q and is expressed in units of rem. The millirem is $\frac{1}{1000}$ of a rem. The unit for the dose equivalent in SI units is the sievert (1 rem = 0.01 Sv or 1 Sv = 100 rems). The quality factor by definition for x-radiation and gamma radiation is one *1* so that the dose equivalent in rems (sieverts) is equal to the dose in rads (grays).

In terms of the effects of dental radiation, the rad (gray) and the rem (sievert) are identical and the roentgen is approximately equal to both (roentgen = rad = rem).

RADIATION UNITS

Conventional Unit	Definition	SI Unit	Definition	Conversion
roentgen (R)	1 esu/cc of air	coulomb/kg		1 c/kg = 3876 R
rad	100 erg/g	gray (Gy)	1 j/kg	1 G = 100 rad
rem	rad × Q	sievert (Sv)	Gy × Q	1 Sv = 100 rem

BASIC CONCEPTS
Exposure and dose

Although the terms are often interchanged, there is a very definite distinction between radiation *exposure* and *dose*. Exposure is the measure of ionization in the air produced by x-ray or gamma radiation; it is the quantity of radiation in an area to which the patient is exposed. The radiation dose is the amount of energy absorbed per unit mass of tissue at a particular site. In dentistry, the patient is exposed to a certain amount of radiation, some of which is absorbed by tissue in different parts of the body; this is the dose to the area. Exposure should be expressed in roentgens (coulombs/kg), and dose should be expressed in rads (grays) or rems (sieverts).

Localized radiation and total body exposure (Figure 3-3)

It is important to differentiate between localized radiation and the total body exposure. When a dental radiograph is taken, the patient's face is exposed to an x-ray beam that is 2¾ inches in diameter (with circular collimation). This is a localized exposure and is less than 1% of the total area of the body. A rad of radiation to the localized area means that each gram of body tissue in that area absorbs 1 rad of

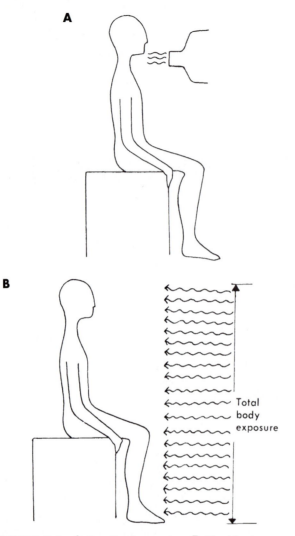

FIGURE 3-3   A, Localized exposure. **B,** Total body exposure.

radiation. A rad of total body radiation means that each gram of tissue in the entire body absorbs 1 rad of radiation. In dentistry, the x-ray machine delivers a localized exposure that results in a total body exposure much less than the facial exposure. In fact, the total body exposure from a dental radiograph is approximately 1/10,000 of the facial exposure.

When discussions of dental x-ray dosages appear in magazine articles, or if patients quote such articles, it is important to determine whether localized exposure or total body exposure is being discussed. For instance, what is the facial exposure of radiation to the patient from a full-mouth survey of radiographs? An average full-mouth survey at 70 kVp, 10 mA, using ANSI group E film, produces a skin exposure to the patient's face of approximately 2 to 3 R (150 mR per film × 20 films). This is not the total body exposure but a localized exposure. If it were a total body dose, it would far exceed the patient's allowable maximum permissible yearly dose. The total body dose could be approximated by dividing the localized dose, 3 R, by 10,000.

The most common misuse of such data occurs when referring to the recommendation of the National Bureau of Standards that the total body dose for the general public for ionizing radiation should not exceed 500 mR in any 1 year. The misstatement is, "You are allowed 500 mR per year, and when your dentist x-rays your entire mouth, you are exposed to 3 R of radiation." The mistakes here are equating the total body dose to the localized dose and using a nonoccupational exposure for a patient exposure. The truer figure to compare the dental facial dose with the 500 mR standard would be 0.0003 R (0.3 mR).

Dose response curve

The dose response curve is an important concept because it illustrates the possible biologic responses to a harmful agent such as ionizing radiation. The responses can be linear or nonlinear, and they can be threshold or nonthreshold. In a linear dose response relationship the response is directly proportional to the dose. In a nonlinear relationship the response is not proportional to the dose. Figure 3-4, *A,* is a threshold curve with both linear and nonlinear responses, indicating that below a certain level (the threshold) there is no response to the agent. Applying this concept to dental radiation would yield a level below which radiographs would be "perfectly safe," since there would be no biologic response below that level. This is not thought to be the case for ionizing radiation (Figure 3-4, *B*). This curve indicates that any dose of radiation, regardless of how small and linear or nonlinear, will produce some degree of biologic response. Therefore dental x-rays do produce biologic changes in the tissues of patients who receive them although no signs or symptoms may be detected and no permanent damage is done to the tissue. It is important to realize that most of the data that produce such a dose response curve for humans come from studying the effects of large doses of radiation on such populations as atomic bomb survivors. In the low-dose range for humans, where dental x-rays fall, little has been documented. The line is therefore an extrapolation based on animal and cellular experiments. The prevailing consensus is that low-dose, ionizing radiation is a linear, nonthreshold relationship.[3]

Somatic and genetic effects

All the cells in the body, with the exception of the reproductive cells (sperm and ova), are included in the grouping of somatic tissue. Changes in these cells are not passed on to succeeding generations of the species. For example, a cancerous skin condition will not be passed on to an offspring. Somatic tissue can be affected by

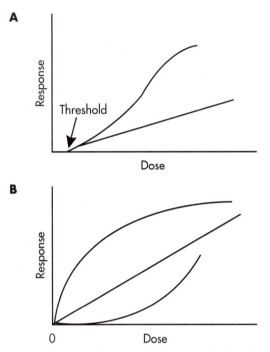

FIGURE 3-4 Linear and nonlinear dose response curves. **A,** Threshold curve; **B,** Nonthreshold type.

radiation, and some cells may die, be altered, or even recover, but none of these effects will be seen in the somatic tissue of the progeny.

Changes in genetic cells cannot be detected in the exposed patient but are passed on to succeeding generations and are referred to as genetic mutations. There are many agents other than ionizing radiation that have been found to be mutagenic, including a variety of chemicals, certain drugs, and even elevated body temperatures. Background radiation also accounts for a portion of naturally occurring mutations. Some of the mutations that have been manifested have been positive and have added to the so-called evolution of the species. A mutation may be recessive and carried in the progeny for many generations before becoming clinically evident.

With the increase in low-level, man-made radiation in recent years, concern focused originally on the possible genetic effects on succeeding generations. Recently the concern has turned to somatic tissue and cancer induction in the blood-forming organs in particular. Leukemia is now believed to be the major risk of chronic low-level radiation.

Acute and chronic effects

The short-term (acute) effects of radiation result from high doses of whole body radiation, usually more than 100 rad. The clinical effect of the exposure, which may vary from mild and transient illness to death, may occur minutes, hours, or weeks after the acute exposure. The median lethal dose for humans is estimated to be 450 rad. It is obvious that in dentistry, we are not concerned with acute radiation doses.

Long-term (chronic) effects of radiation may be seen years after the original exposures. Acute and/or chronic exposures may produce cumulative effects on the somatic cells over the patient's lifetime, as well as genetic effects on future generations.

Direct and indirect effects

The effects of ionizing radiation on tissue may be direct, as when the ionizing radiation alters or destroys cells (DNA molecules) that lie in the direct path of the radiation beam. The effects also may be indirect, as when the impaired function of the radiated tissue adversely influences other tissues in the body. An example of an indirect effect would be the production of a chemically changed hormone that could not properly regulate tissue elsewhere in the body.

Latent period and cell recovery

The latent period is the time that elapses between the exposure to ionizing radiation and the appearance of clinical symptoms. This time may vary from hours to years, depending on the magnitude of the exposure and the tissues involved. Not all radiation-induced changes in tissue cells are permanent. Depending on the time interval, dose, and sensitivity of the affected cells to radiation, the cells' repair processes may be sufficient to effect recovery from the radiation.

Dose rate

The *dose rate,* the rate at which exposure to ionizing radiation occurs and absorption takes place, is a critical factor in determining what the effects will be. Since cells do recover from radiation, a specific dose produces less damage if it is fractionated over a period of time. In dentistry, the time interval between exposures, excluding retakes and working films, is usually months or years, further minimizing the effects.

Long-term effects

The long-term effects of radiation manifest themselves years after the exposure. The latent period is very long. These delayed effects may be from an acute exposure or a series of low-level exposures. A low-level exposure is considered to be under 5 rem (0.05 sieverts).

It is important to remember that no specific disease is associated solely with the long-term effects of radiation. Cancer can be caused by radiation, but it is also caused by smoking, chronic irritants, and exposure to certain chemicals.

Since there is no specific radiation disease, the long-term effects of radiation express themselves in human populations as a statistical increase in the incidence of certain diseases. One can study the incidence of diseases in irradiated populations and compare to nonirradiated groups. The atomic bomb survivors and the incidence of leukemias among them is a good example of this type of evaluation of long-term effects. Evaluating the long-term effects of dental x-rays, where the dose is low, would require large populations over a long period, since the latent period for radiation-induced cancer—even from large doses—ranges from years to decades.[4]

Risk estimates

Since there is no effective way of analyzing the cause of a radiation-induced cancer on a case-by-case basis, we must look to dosages in irradiated populations and the number of cancers in these populations. This number is then compared to nonirradiated populations and the difference is expressed as the risk factor.

Risk factors are expressed as the number of cases or deaths from a specific disease per million persons of population. Estimates have been made of the number of cases of cancer for all body organs induced per 1 million dental examinations. For a full-mouth survey taken with round collimation the estimate is 2.5 to 17 cases per million examinations. If rectangular collimation and E-speed film are used, the risk will be further reduced.[5]

These numbers may seem quite threatening, but they should be compared with risks that our patients take in everyday life. Activities with a fatality risk of 1:1 million in everyday life include traveling 10 miles on a bicycle, 300 miles in an automobile, 1000 miles on an airline, or smoking 1.4 cigarettes a day.[6] It is obvious that we readily accept one-in-a-million risks in everyday living, even though in many cases there is no health benefit.

TISSUE SENSITIVITY

Tissues vary widely in their sensitivity to ionizing radiation and thus the amount of radiation required to produce damage. The same dose of radiation has a different degree of effect on different types of cells in the same organism. Young, rapidly dividing, nondifferentiated cells, such as those found in the abdomen of a pregnant dental patient, are more radiosensitive than older cells. In addition to the age of the cell and its rate of differentiation, tissues vary in their sensitivity to radiation. Grouping tissues and organs in descending order of sensitivity to radiation, we have the following:

High sensitivity:	Lymphoid organs
	Bone marrow
	Testes
	Intestines
Intermediate:	Fine vasculature

Low:
                    Growing cartilage
                    Growing bone
                    Salivary glands
                    Lungs
                    Kidneys
                    Liver
                    Optic lens
                    Muscle

Critical organs

Certain organs and tissues have been designated as "critical" because they are exposed to more radiation than others when dental radiographs are taken. The tissues and organs designated as critical, with their potential risks, are: the skin, carcinoma; thyroid, carcinoma; eye lens, cataract; hematopoietic, leukemia; and genetic tissue, congenital defects or mutations.

Background radiation

Background radiation is a form of ionizing radiation, both naturally occurring and manmade, present in the environment. Naturally occurring radiation always has been present on earth, but the manmade component has been increasing as a result of fallout from nuclear testing and radioactive wastes from industry. It would be helpful to know the level of background radiation and its sources, so that dental radiation exposure can be put in its proper perspective.

An estimate of the average personal exposure, weighted from different sources to approximate a "total body exposure," has been tabulated and is shown in Table 3-1. This report shows an estimated average annual dose of 300 mrem (3 mSv) due to natural background sources. With the addition of the average contributions of medical and dental procedures the total annual average population exposure is about 360 mrem (3.6 mSv). Of the total exposure 55% is from exposure to radon.

These data help to compare dental exposure with background exposure. From the data and from known outputs of dental x-ray machines we can estimate that total body radiation from a four-film, bite-wing examination using rectangular collimation and E-speed film is equivalent to about 12 hours of background. Using a round beam and D-speed film increases exposure to an equivalent of 82 hours of background.

Patient dosage

Ample evidence in the literature substantiates the adverse effects of radiation in high doses. The problem is that, while no direct evidence exists of such effects from dental diagnostic doses, there is also no evidence that proves the absence of adverse effects. To treat a patient without current and diagnostic radiographs is doing a disservice to the patient and leaves the dentist unprotected against possible legal action.

Table 3-1

Average annual exposure to U.S. population

Source	Dose (millirems)
Natural Sources	
Radon	200
Cosmic radiation	27
Soil and building materials	28
Internal radioactivity	39
Occupational	0.9
Nuclear fuel cycle	0.5
Consumer products	9.0
Miscellaneous	0.06
Medical and dental	53

*From National Council on Radiation Protection and Measurements: Ionizing radiation exposure of the population of the United States, Report No 93, 1987, Washington, DC. The Council.

Radiographs are an integral part of modern dental practice. Our goal in dental radiography is to use the least amount of radiation to satisfy the patient's diagnostic needs—that is, minimize the exposure while maximizing the diagnostic yield. In our efforts to minimize the amount of radiation, we also must be guided by the *ALARA principle,* which means "as low as reasonably achievable." The radiation exposure to our patients should be reduced as much as possible within the dental office without excessive cost or inconvenience to the patient.

How do we evaluate these effects of ionizing radiation and the weight of the dental component? No specific disease can be attributed solely to the long-term effects of ionizing radiation. As previously mentioned, leukemia is not caused by x-ray exposure alone but is probably the result of the interaction of several factors. Animal experimentation has been conducted, but direct extrapolation of the results of human populations is not always reliable. Data gained from acute exposures of humans, such as the victims of Hiroshima or industrial accidents, that are then extrapolated downward to low doses also have limitations. Furthermore the incidence of the diseases we are concerned with is low; to relate an increased incidence with population exposure to ionizing radiations, it is necessary to study large populations.

Dental auxiliaries and dentists, because of their involvement with low-level ionizing radiation, should be aware of the consequences of chronic exposure for their patients. In this manner they are better equipped to make the essential risk-versus-benefit decision before making x-ray exposures.

The following examples of specific tissue exposures from dental x-ray exposure and the critical levels of these tissues support the conclusion that the benefits derived from dental x-ray exposure, when used judiciously under proper conditions, far outweigh any possible risk.

Skin. Erythema (reddening of the skin) is the usual effect of radiation and is not a major risk in dental radiography. Its importance lies in that the skin dose is the most commonly reported value for dental x-ray examinations. The skin dose has limitations in that (1) it is easily penetrated and does not reflect a dose to deeper tissues, (2) it varies greatly with the kVp used, and (3) it is less sensitive than many other tissues exposed during dental radiography.

The threshold erythema dose (TED), the amount of radiation needed to produce an erythema or reddening of the most sensitive individual, is 250 R (250 mSv) in a 14-day period. A full-mouth x-ray series using 70 kVp, D-speed film, and round collimation produces a skin dose of 840 mrem (8.4 mSv).[5] With E-speed film the dose would be approximately one half of that. Using ANSI group E film, more than 60 full surveys in a 14-day period would be necessary to produce an erythema in the most sensitive patient. Clinically, this is an absurd possibility, and it is not surprising then that no cases of erythema have been reported as a result of exposure to dental radiographs. Risk for the earliest type of skin cancer is not evident below dose levels of 25,000 mrem (250 mSv).[7]

Eyes. Exposure to ionizing radiation in high doses to the lens of the eye can induce cataract formation. The required dose to produce this change has been reported in the range of 200,000 to 500,000 mrem (2,000 to 5,000 mSv),[7] while the mean corneal surface dose for a full-mouth series is about 60 mrem (0.6 mSv). The lens of the eye is exposed to radiation during intraoral radiography, but the risk of cataract formation is extremely low.

Thyroid. The thyroid gland, which is particularly radiosensitive, may lie in the beam of primary radiation in some dental views. Malignant changes have been reported in the thyroid glands in a group of patients who received x-ray therapy for tinea capitis (ringworm of the scalp).[8] The dose to the thyroid in these patients was estimated to be 6 rad. Presently, the thyroid exposure for a full-mouth series is about 94 mR (0.94 mSv).[5] The dose to this radiosensitive tissue should be kept to an absolute minimum, especially in children. This can be accomplished by the use of a lead thyroid collar and the paralleling technique.

Bone marrow. It is now thought that the greatest somatic hazard to patients from dental x-rays is leukemia induction.[9] The red bone marrow is one of the blood-forming organs of the body. The significant hematopoietic bone marrow exposed to dental x-rays is located in the mandible, the calvarium of the skull, and the cervical spine. The calvarium and cervical spine are exposed to primary radiation in extraoral and panoramic radiography. The bone marrow of the mandible and maxilla are the major dental concern and, when exposed to radiation in a full-mouth survey, still only represent 5% of the total body bone marrow.

White and Rose[10] published a report that will help the auxiliary and dentist discuss the risk of leukemia with patients. They compared the higher background radiation in

Denver due to high elevation and thus increased cosmic ray exposure to bone marrow exposure from dental examinations. The report states, "If a person in an average location in the United States were to receive a full-mouth intraoral periapical and panoramic examination every 4 months for the rest of his life, he would incur only the same risk, in terms of bone marrow exposure, as a person living in Denver who was not exposed to dental radiography."

The leukemia risk, then, is very low but still exists. However, with judicious use of radiation and proper technique, the diagnostic benefit derived outweighs the slight risk.

Numerous demonstrations have produced no changes in the complete blood count (CBC) after dental x-ray examination.[11] This refutes an outdated report, still often cited in the lay press, that claimed significant blood changes after dental x-rays.[12]

Gonads. The reproductive cells (sperm and ova) are very radiosensitive. Sterilization from an acute exposure from the dental x-ray beam is an impossibility; 400 R is needed in the male and 625 R in the female to cause sterility. The dose to the gonads from dental radiographic procedures is in the form of secondary radiation. For a full-mouth series without using a lead apron the gonadal dose is 0.5 mrem (0.005 mSv).[13] With the use of a lead apron this dose can be reduced by about 95%. The gonadal exposure for a full-mouth series with a lead apron is about ½ the average daily gonadal exposure of the U.S. population from background radiation.[13] This background dose, of course, nearly doubles at higher elevations such as Denver.

Pregnancy. As previously mentioned, the nondifferentiated, rapidly dividing fetal cells are extremely radiosensitive; hence the concern for pregnant patients.

A panel of dental radiologists recently considered the appropriateness of dental radiographs for pregnant patients.[13] They concluded that the guidelines for taking radiographs for patients (discussed in Chapter 4) need not be altered for the pregnant patient. They pointed out that the concept of avoiding radiography during pregnancy generally applies to procedures in which the fetus or embryo would be in or near the primary x-ray beam. In dentistry the primary beam is limited to the head and neck region, and the only radiation the fetus would be exposed to would be secondary radiation. Uterine doses for a full-mouth series without using a lead apron have been shown to be less than 1 mrem.[14] As we have seen, the uterine dose from naturally occurring background during the 9 months of pregnancy can be expected to be about 225 mrem (2.25 mSv) based on the background doses of 300 mrem (3 mSv) per year. With these factors there seems to be no scientific reason to preclude an indicated dental x-ray examination during pregnancy. Radiographs in some cases may have to be deferred during pregnancy for purely psychological reasons.

As we will see in Chapter 4, no occupational hazard for the pregnant dentist or auxiliary exists. When appropriate precautionary procedures are followed, the occupational dose is zero.

REFERENCES

1. National Council on Radiation Protection and Measurements: Ionizing radiation exposure of the population of the United States, Report No 93, 1987, Washington, DC, The Council.
2. Goaz PW and White SC: Oral radiology, St. Louis, 1994, Mosby Year Book Inc.
3. National Academy of Sciences, National Research Council: The effects on populations of exposure to low levels of ionizing radiation (BEIR V), Washington, DC, 1990, National Academy Press.
4. Bebbe GW, Kato H, and Land CE: Studies of the mortality of A-bomb survivors 1950–1974, *Radiat Res* 73:138–201, July 1978.
5. White SC: 1992 Assessment of radiation risk from dental radiography, *Dentomax Radiol* 21:118–126, 1992.
6. Wilson R: Risks caused by low levels of pollution, *Yale J Biol Med* 51:37–51, 1978.
7. Langland OE, Sippy FH, and Langlais RP: *Textbook of dental radiology,* ed 2, Springfield, Ill. 1984, Charles C. Thomas.
8. Pentel L: Current perspectives on radiation, *NYJ Dent* 45:3, March 1975.
9. White SC and Frey NW: An estimation of somatic hazards to the U.S. population from dental radiography, *Oral Surg* 43:1, January 1977.
10. White SC and Rose TC: Absorbed bone marrow dose in certain dental radiographic techniques, *J Am Dent Assoc* 98:553–558, 1979.
11. Budowsky J et al: Lack of effect of exposure to radiation during intraoral roentgenographic examinations as post examination blood studies, *J Am Dent Assoc* 55:199, August 1957.
12. Nolan WE: Radiation hazards to the patient from oral roentgenography, *J Am Dent Assoc* 47:681, December 1953.
13. U.S. Department of Health and Human Services, Public Health Service, FDA: The selection of patients for x-ray examinations: dental radiographic examinations, HSS/PHS/FDA 88-8273:10–21, 1987.
14. Gibbs SJ et al: Radiation doses to sensitive organs from intraoral dental radiography, *Dentomax Radiol* 17:15–23, 1987.

Chapter

Radiation Protection

Now that we have discussed the mechanism and the effects of ionizing radiation on human tissue, we can apply these principles to the clinical environment. The issue of radiation protection can be discussed from the perspective of two major concerns:

the patient and the operator. Of the two we will see that concern for the operator is the easier to deal with, because we can can quantify and easily adhere to exact limits.

PATIENT PROTECTION

In patient protection the objective is to use the least amount of radiation to achieve the maximum diagnostic results. The patient must be protected from excessive or unnecessary primary radiation and the resulting secondary radiation. This goal can be met through the use of safe, well-calibrated x-ray machines, rectangular collimation, film-holding devices, E-speed film, lead aprons, rare earth intensifying screens and thyroid collars, proper shielding, good chairside and darkroom techniques, and sound professional judgment in selection criteria.

Primary radiation is the energy contained by the x-rays that comes from the target of the x-ray tube. The primary radiation is collimated by the lead diaphragm and filtered of its softer, less penetrating wavelengths by aluminum filters. Thus it is known as the *useful beam.* All other radiation can be considered secondary radiation. *Secondary radiation* is defined as radiation that comes from any matter struck by primary radiation. The scattered radiation that results from the interaction of the useful beam and the patient's face is a form of secondary radiation (Figure 4-1). Secondary radiation, besides being harmful to both patient and operator, degrades the diagnostic image of the film, because the scattered rays produce film fog on the radiograph.

EQUIPMENT

All dental x-ray machines manufactured after 1974 must meet federal diagnostic equipment performance standards.[1] No federal standards existed for x-ray machines manufactured or installed before 1974. It is important to remember that the federal standards do not regulate diagnostic equipment users such as dentists, dental hygienists, and dental assistants but only the equipment itself. However, most state or local governments also regulate equipment and have radiation health codes that pertain to the use of radiation. The federal government regulates the manufacture and installation of x-ray machines, while state and local governments may regulate equipment as well as how the x-ray units are used. Depending on the local radiation code, dental offices, clinics, and dental schools may be inspected every 1 to 3 years to monitor equipment performance and the barriers and procedures used when taking radiographs. Usually a fee is charged for this inspection, and many jurisdictions also require a fee for licensure to use x-ray machines.

Tube head and arm

Head leakage.   The term *head leakage* refers to radiation that escapes through the protective shielding of the x-ray tube head. The only radiation that should leave the tube head is the primary beam. Radiation leakage exposes the patient unnecessarily and should not occur in a properly functioning x-ray unit. Leakage is a violation of the

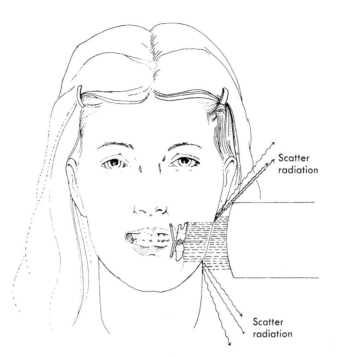

Scatter
radiation

Scatter
radiation

FIGURE 4-1 Production of scatter radiation of primary beam by interaction with patient's face.

federal performance standards and local radiation codes.[1] This is not a common problem, because x-ray units are well built; if the unit is not abused in use or moving, head leakage is unlikely to occur.

Drift. The tube head of the dental x-ray machine should not move, or drift, in any direction after positioning for an exposure (see Figure 1-1). The movement can cause a blurred image or position the central ray off the film, resulting in a cone cut. If the tube head drifts, the arm should be repaired immediately. The patient or the auxiliary should never hold the tube head in place during an exposure. Checking for tube head drift in all directions is an important step in an office quality assurance program.

Kilovoltage and milliamperage seconds. These technique factors control proper penetration and film density and contrast. As explained in Chapter 2, film speed and FFD determine the mAs' contribution to the patient's radiation exposure. The choice of kVp, however, affects the contrast of the film and radiation dose. The patient's skin exposure decreases as the kVp increases, but the dose to deeper tissues and the amount of scatter radiation increases. At present, some debate focuses on the best kVp within the 65 to 90 range that should be used in dentistry.[2] A kilovoltage that is best suited for the diagnostic needs should be used. There is no question that kVp below 65 should not be used, because the exposure to the patient per film is nearly doubled when using a kVp below the acceptable range (Figure 4-2).

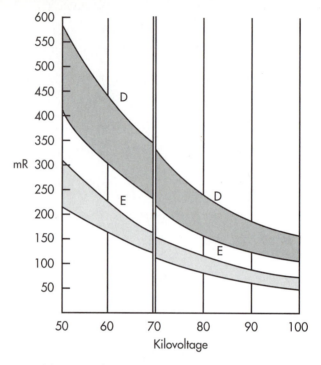

FIGURE 4-2   Acceptable x-ray exposure ranges for group D and E films. Note the increased exposure in the low kVp range and that the exposure with group E is about half that of group D. *Courtesy Department of Health and Human Services.*

Filtration. Because of the enactment of the federal performance standards and the enforcement of local health codes, filtration is no longer a major concern in patient protection—compliance is almost 100%. The purpose of filtration is to remove the long (soft), nonpenetrating x-ray photons from the x-ray beam (see Chapter 1). These photons either would be absorbed by the overlying tissues or give rise to secondary radiation to the patient and degrade the diagnostic image.

Collimation. The collimation of the x-ray beam limits the size of the area exposed by the primary beam and the amount of scatter produced. The beam size was discussed in Chapter 1 and at present a 2¾-inch (7.0 cm) circular beam measured at the skin is required. If the size and shape of the x-ray beam were changed to a rectangle that is slightly larger than the film, the volume of tissue exposed could be reduced by more than half (Figure 4-3). The American Dental Association and the American Academy of Maxillofacial Radiology strongly recommend the use of rectangular collimation (Figure 4-4).[3] Rectangular collimation is the single most effective factor in reducing radiation to the patient.

Timing device. The use of more sensitive x-ray film with extremely short exposure times makes the use of electronic timers imperative. All new x-ray machines come equipped with these devices.

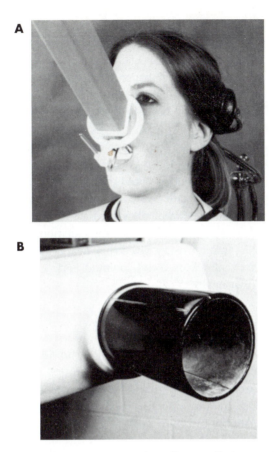

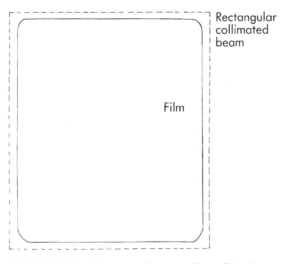

FIGURE 4-3   **A,** Open-ended metal rectangular collimator. **B,** Open-ended lead-lined cylinder.

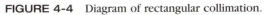

FIGURE 4-4   Diagram of rectangular collimation.

The mechanical timers existing on older machines are inaccurate at short exposures, are usually calibrated down to ¼ second, and can have a ¼ second margin of error. It is impossible to use a mechanical timer with group D and E films and make accurate exposures. Unfortunately, those using mechanical timers often compensate for the unavoidable overexposure by underdeveloping and in this way produce a diagnostic radiograph. The electronic type timer should be used.

Position-indicating devices (PIDs). Open-ended, lead-lined (shielded) rectangles (Figure 4-3, *A*) or cylinders (Figure 4-3, *B*) are the only type of PIDs that should be used.[3] The use of closed-end, pointed cones is contraindicated (see Chapter 1). These cones increase scatter radiation to the patient because of the interaction of the primary beam with the closed end of the cone (see Figure 1-18). It is somewhat disconcerting to note that in an era of concern for radiation, as recently as 1984 a radiation survey of practicing dentists reported that 18% of those surveyed still used the pointed cone.[4] Any existing closed-end, pointed cone can be replaced by the recommended types of PIDs.

Receptor (film) holders

Film holders that align the x-ray beam with the film in the patient's mouth should be used.[3] These devices reduce the possibility of cone cutting. Some of these devices also produce rectangular collimation (Figure 4-5). A film holder should never be held in place for the patient by the operator. Some of the more commonly used film-holding devices are shown in Figure 7-8.

Film

Decreasing the exposure time by the use of a more sensitive receptor (film, film-screen combinations, digital detectors) is one of the most important factors in reducing radiation exposure to the patient. As discussed in Chapter 2, film slower than group D should never be used.[3] Group E film, when compared with group D film, reduces the radiation exposure by 50% (Figure 4-2). At present the American Dental Association recommends the use of E-speed film. The E film is a major step forward in patient protection. Its use requires an electronic timer and strict adherence to time-temperature processing, because the film has very little leeway for error. The new film has not been accepted universally by practitioners because of claims of lost diagnostic ability. Many recent reports of clinical tests of D versus E film show that no significant clinical difference exists between the films.[5,6] The Eastman Kodak Company recently changed the shape of the silver halide grains of its E-speed film to increase the sharpness and give higher contrast images with less dependence on processing conditions. This improvement was designed to overcome the profession's reluctance to universally accept the use of E-speed film.

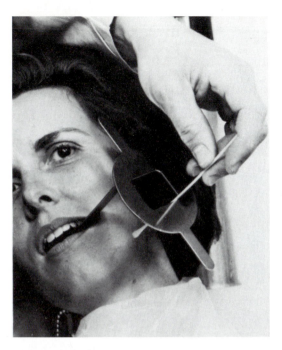

FIGURE 4-5   Precision device. *Courtesy Isaac Masel Co., Inc., Philadelphia.*

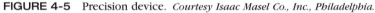

Lead aprons and collars

All patients should be draped with a lead apron for all exposures, and a thyroid collar should be used (Figure 4-6) for intraoral exposures. This rule holds regardless of the patient's age or the number of films exposed. The use of lead aprons and thyroid collars can reduce radiation to the thyroid and gonads up to 94%. The apron should cover the patient from the thyroid to the gonadal area. Lead aprons with attached cervical (thyroid) shields are available. Separate thyroid collars can be purchased to use with existing lead aprons. The aprons available are usually the equivalent of 0.25 mm lead, relatively light and flexible, and not uncomfortable for the patient. The dose to the gonads is very small during dental exposures but can be reduced even further with the lead apron. The thyroid gland, except with rectangular collimation and more specifically with the bisecting-angle technique, may lie in the path of the primary beam. The dose may be small but can be decreased significantly with the use of the thyroid collar. There is no valid reason not to use the lead apron and collar for every intraoral exposure. Many states have enacted legislation that makes this procedure mandatory.

Lead aprons should not be folded but rather hung up when not in use. Folding eventually cracks the lead and allows leakage. The positioning of lead aprons in taking panoramic films must be modified as discussed in Chapter 10.

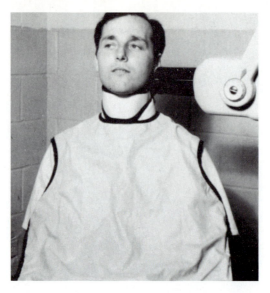

FIGURE 4-6   Lead apron with thyroid collar.

TECHNIQUE

Retakes

One of the major sources of unnecessary exposure to radiation in the dental office is retaking films as a result of poor technique in either taking or processing films. Every retake represents an unnecessary doubling of radiation exposure to the patient for that film. Both the dental auxiliary and dentist are obligated to perfect their intraoral technique so that retakes are unnecessary.

Exposure

Films should be exposed properly. A technique that employs overexposure with under-development subjects the patient to unnecessary radiation. If exposed films come out too dark with time-temperature processing, the exposure time or the kVp, not the developing time, should be reduced. An overexposure and a shortened processing time used to expedite patient treatment is unconscionable in relation to good patient radiation hygiene. Figure 4-7 shows an acceptable range of x-ray exposure. The exposures are expressed in milliroentgens and not impulses or seconds. If one knows the output of the dental x-ray machine (mR/sec), then the exposure can be expressed as mR instead of impulses to see whether the exposure falls within the acceptable range. Film packets also come with recommended exposure times, so there is no excuse for overexposure.

Paralleling technique

In addition to a more accurate diagnostic image, the paralleling technique results in lower dose levels to the thyroid gland and the lens of the eye (Figure 4-8).

"D" Speed Film ★			**"E" Speed Film ★ ★**		
kVp	Lower Limit	Upper Limit	kVp	Lower Limit	Upper Limit
50	425	575	50	220	320
55	350	500	55	190	270
60	310	440	60	165	230
65	270	400	65	140	200
70	240	350	70	120	170
. . . .			. . . .		
75	170	260	75	100	140
80	150	230	80	90	120
85	130	200	85	80	105
90	120	180	90	70	90
95	110	160	95	60	80
100	100	140	100	50	70

*Exposure Conditions

10mA
 8" S.S.D.
50- 70 kVp - 1.5 mm Al
71-100 kVp - 2.5 mm Al

**Exposure Conditions

10 mA, 12" S.S.D.
50- 70 kVp - 1.5 mm Al
71-100 kVp - 2.5 mm Al

FIGURE 4-7 Acceptable range of x-ray exposure. *From Department of Health and Human Services: Dental exposure normalization technique (DENT) instruction manual.*

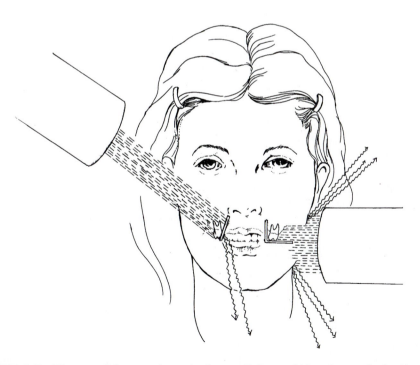

FIGURE 4-8 Diagram of the x-ray beam in the paralleling and bisecting method and scatter radiation to the thyroid gland.

Focal-film distance

Increased FFDs, up to 16 inches, are recommended with the paralleling technique to compensate for the magnification of the image caused by the increased object-film distance (see Chapter 2). Another important advantage of an increased FFD is that less total tissue volume is in the path of the primary beam at 16 inches than at 8 inches. As the distance increases from 8 to 16 inches (Figure 4-9), the x-ray beam becomes less divergent, and less total body area is irradiated by the primary beam after it penetrates the skin. The shorter FFD, with a more divergent beam, irradiates a far greater volume of tissue. The diameter of the primary beam is still 2¾ inches at the skin in both cases. The difference is in the beam divergence after the skin entry and film exposure.

Darkroom

Every effort should be made to establish darkroom procedures that produce films with the maximum diagnostic yield. As previously mentioned, underdevelopment should not compensate for overexposure. There is no excuse for darkroom errors that cause film retakes. This subject is discussed thoroughly in Chapter 6.

Viewing finished radiographs

To get maximum diagnostic yield for the radiation expended, the manner in which radiographs are viewed for interpretation is extremely important. The only proper way to view a radiograph is in front of an illuminator (viewbox), preferably with a variable light source. Using sunlight in front of a window or the lamp on the dental

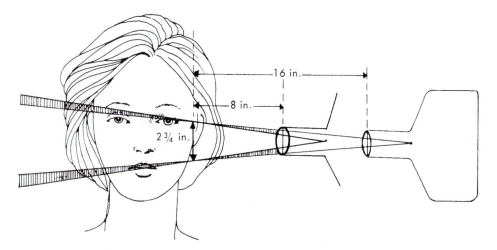

FIGURE 4-9   Focal-film distance and tissue volume exposed. Shaded areas represent tissue exposed at 8-inch FFD but not in the beam at 16-inch FFD because of the more parallel and less divergent x-rays.

unit is unsatisfactory. The film mount used for the full-mouth survey should cover the entire illuminator, and empty windows in the mount should be covered with an opaque material. This prevents light that escapes around the periphery or through the mount from distracting the viewer. Ideally radiographs should be viewed in a darkened room to avoid excessive reflection.

CLINICAL JUDGMENT
Radiation history

Specific questions regarding the patient's prior radiation exposures should be part of every history. This should include medical, dental, and therapeutic radiation. Questions of this type may help determine whether dental radiographs have been taken recently that might be available and still diagnostically valid. These radiographs also help to give historical data, show previous dental disease, and the result of treatment. A history of radiation therapy is important not so much because of the added dental dose but of interest in the areas radiated. Radiation to the head and neck region may leave the patient susceptible to radiation caries and osteoradionecrosis. Radiation history is valuable and pertinent information in treatment planning. Patients may not volunteer such information, because they may not recognize its importance.

Selection criteria

Selection criteria are descriptions of clinical conditions (signs and symptoms) and historical data that identify patients who are most likely to benefit from a particular radiographic examination. They help the dentist select which patients need radiographs and determine which radiographs are needed. The final decision rests with the individual dentist and is determined by professional judgment.

An expert panel of dentists sponsored by the Public Health Service has developed guidelines for the prescription of dental radiographs.[7] Using these guidelines the dentist can decide when, what type, and how many radiographs should be taken. The practice of taking dental radiographs based on a time interval rather than on patient needs, as determined by clinical examination and dental history, is not considered an appropriate way to practice dental radiology.[3] The dentist should decide whether to take radiographs after examining the patient. There are no routine dental radiographs. Radiograph needs are not determined by the calendar but rather by evaluating the overall health needs of a patient after a clinical examination and history. This is true for new patients, for emergencies, and for recall visits.

These guidelines, the asymptomatic ones are shown in chart form in Figure 4-10, cover three general categories of patients: those with positive historical findings, patients who are symptomatic, and those who are asymptomatic. Asymptomatic patients are divided into three main categories: (1) children with primary and transitional dentitions, (2) adolescents with permanent dentition, and (3) adults,

Patient category	Child	
	Primary dentition *(prior to eruption of first permanent tooth)*	Transitional dentition *(following eruption of first permanent tooth)*
New patient All new patients to assess dental diseases and growth and development	Posterior bitewing examination if proximal surfaces of primary teeth cannot be visualized or probed	Individualized radiographic examination consisting of periapical/occlusal views and posterior bitewings *or* panoramic examination and posterior bitewings
Recall patient Clinical caries or high-risk factors for caries	Posterior bitewing examination at 6-month intervals *or* until no carious lesions are evident	
No clinical caries and no high-risk factors for caries	Posterior bitewing examination at 12- to 24-month intervals if proximal surfaces of primary teeth cannot be visualized or probed	Posterior bitewing examination at 12- to 24-month intervals
Periodontal disease or a history of periodontal treatment	Individualized radiographic examination consisting of selected periapical and/or bitewing radiographs for areas where periodontal disease (other than nonspecific gingivitis) can be demonstrated clinically	
Growth and development assessment	Usually not indicated	Individualized radiographic examination consisting of a periapical/occlusal *or* panoramic examination

FIGURE 4-10   Selection criteria chart. *Courtesy Department of Health and Human Services.*

Continued

Adolescent	**Adult**	
Permanent dentition *(prior to eruption of third molars)*	Dentulous	Edentulous
Individualized radiographic examination consisting of posterior bitewings and selected periapicals. A full-mouth intraoral radiographic examination is appropriate when the patient presents with clinical evidence of generalized dental disease or a history of extensive dental treatment.		Full-mouth intraoral radiographic examination *or* panoramic examination
Posterior bitewing examination at 6- to 12-month intervals *or* until no carious lesions are evident	Posterior bitewing examination at 12- to 18-month intervals	Not applicable
Posterior bitewing examination at 18- to 36-month intervals	Posterior bitewing examination at 24- to 36-month intervals	Not applicable
Individualized radiographic examination consisting of selected periapical and/or bitewing radiographs for areas where periodontal disease (other than nonspecific gingivitis) can be demonstrated clinically		Not applicable
Periapical *or* panoramic examination to assess developing third molars	Usually not indicated	Usually not indicated

FIGURE 4-10   *Cont'd.*

including dentulous and edentulous patients. Each patient category is further divided into new patient and recall patient categories. In addition, the recall patient category is subdivided into clinical caries or high-risk factors for caries, no clinical caries or high-risk factors, periodontal disease, and growth and development assessment.

Using these guidelines we can see that all new patients should have a recent full-mouth survey of some type on file before treatment is instituted. The radiographs may be taken by the current dentist or may be duplicates of those taken by a previous dentist. The full-mouth survey is essential for case planning, baseline data for future reference, and medicolegal reasons.

Recall radiographs should not be taken on all patients as a matter of routine. As we can see in Figure 4-10, very few patients need radiographs at 6-month intervals. Caries susceptibility, for example, is a major factor when determining the time frame for recall radiographs. The diagnostic radiographic needs of a decay-prone teenager are quite different from those of a middle-aged periodontal recall patient whose last filling was placed 20 years earlier.

Administrative radiographs

Administrative radiographs are those required for reasons not related to the patient's immediate health needs. Included in this category are teaching films, those required by state examination and licensing authorities, and radiographs taken to verify treatment for compensation by insurance companies or other third-party carriers. Radiographs should *never* be taken for administrative reasons. If it produces no diagnostic benefit to the patient, the radiograph should not be taken. This is not to say that radiographs should not be submitted to insurance carriers; films taken for diagnostic purposes, or their duplicates, can be submitted because no unnecessary radiation is used. Many states have laws that prohibit the use of administrative radiographs, and the FDA recommends that insurance carriers and others refrain from requiring administrative radiographs.[8]

Postoperative radiographs are indicated only when they have diagnostic value—for example, confirming the retrieval of a root tip in surgery or the placement of filling materials in endodontic procedures. The use of radiographs to check the fit, contact, contour, and seating of restorations is discouraged. These checks are best done with a mirror, explorer, and floss, thus saving the patient the radiation exposure.

Working films in endodontics, surgery, and restorative post and pin preparations may be necessary for proper treatment, but every effort should be made to keep the number of exposures to a minimum.

OPERATOR DOSAGE AND PROTECTION

As we noted earlier about the concerns of protecting operator and patient from radiation, it is much easier to deal with the protection of the operator. The sources of potential exposure to the dental auxiliary are the primary beam, head leakage from the tube, and secondary radiation originating from the patient, x-ray machine, or objects in the operatory. Through the use of careful technique in a well-designed, well-equipped, and well-monitored office, the occupational exposure to dental auxiliaries and dentists can be kept to a minimum, well below the recommended maximum. Exposure should be zero.

Maximum permissible dose

At present the maximum permissible dose (MPD) of whole-body radiation for persons occupationally concerned with ionizing radiation, such as dental auxiliaries and dentists, is 5000 mrem (50 mSv) per year, or 100 mrem per week. This is in contrast to the recommended MPD of 500 mrem (5 mSv) for the general public. In addition, the operator should not receive more than 3000 mrem (30 mSv) in any 13-week period. Dental personnel also should not exceed an accumulated lifetime dose of (N −18) × 5000 mrem. In this formula, N is the operator's age.

The current stated MPD is 5000 mrem, but historically the MPD has been higher. Thus we may see this figure revised downward. The International Commission on Radiation Protection (ICRP) has recommended that the yearly MPD be reduced to 2000 mrem (20 mSv). Dental auxiliaries and dentists should strive for an occupational dose of zero. If one's occupational dose is zero, any downward change would produce no cause for concern since "zero is zero." Zero exposure is not difficult to achieve in an office with an awareness of radiation hygiene. Dental auxiliaries should not fear working with x-rays, but they should be knowledgeable about their use and abuse.

Exposure technique

The dental auxiliary or dentist should never be in the path of the primary beam. Film packets should never be held in the patient's mouth, nor should a drifting tube head be held by the person making the exposure. There are *no exceptions* to this rule. The operator should not make the mistake of saying, "I'll just hold the film for the patient this one time." Ideally the operator should be a minimum of 6 feet away from the tube head and behind a suitable barrier when the exposure is made. At 6 feet the minimum occupational exposure does not exceed the MPD. At 6 feet and behind the barrier, the occupational exposure is zero.

Federal and state regulations require that every x-ray machine be equipped with either a 6-foot retractable exposure cord or a remote switch that permits such operator positioning. The remote switch is preferable because it prevents lapses in operator technique. Though not as crucial as distance and shielding, knowing where areas of minimum scatter are is important to the operator. These areas are at right angles to the x-ray beam and toward the back of the patient (Figure 4-11). The areas of highest scatter are in back of the tube head and behind the patient. Correct positioning of the operator still necessitates the minimum 6-foot distance or adequate barrier protection.

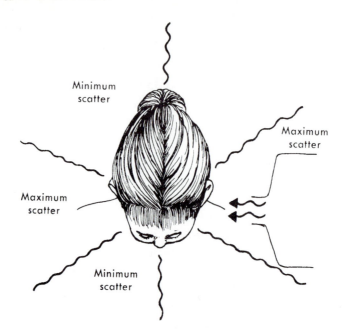

Minimum
scatter

Maximum
scatter

Maximum
scatter

Minimum
scatter

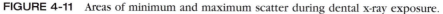

FIGURE 4-11   Areas of minimum and maximum scatter during dental x-ray exposure.

Radiation monitoring

How can dental auxiliaries and dentists know the amount of occupational exposure of radiation they receive? Concerned personnel can use two methods to measure the levels of radiation and potential exposure. First, a health physicist can perform a radiation survey, using ionization chambers to determine radiation levels during exposures at all locations in the office. This type of survey checks the reliability of the x-ray machine and protective barriers. It does not monitor the day-by-day activity of the concerned personnel.

The second method is to have personnel wear pocket dosimeters or film badges. Of the two methods, film badges are less expensive and more widely used. Film badge service is readily available from many radiation survey companies at a nominal monthly cost. The badge (Figure 4-12) is usually worn for a 3- or 4-week period and contains a film packet, similar to dental film, embossed with the wearer's name and identification number. At the end of the prescribed reporting period, the film packet is returned to the survey company where it is processed; the density on the film is compared with standards and the exposure determined. The report returned to the dental office contains not only the exposure for the reporting period but also the accumulated quarterly, yearly, and lifetime exposure of the individual (Figure 4-13). Using the 100-millirem weekly MPD limit, the dental auxiliary's radiation exposure can be evaluated easily. The film badge should be worn in the office at all times to provide an accurate reading of occupational exposure. If clipped to a pocket, it should not be covered with a pen or piece of jewelry that might shield the film. Auxiliaries should not wear the badge outside the office, especially in bright sunlight, and they

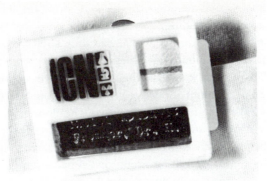

FIGURE 4-12   Film badge attached to pocket on operator's uniform. *Courtesy ICN Pharma-ceuticals, Inc., Cleveland.*

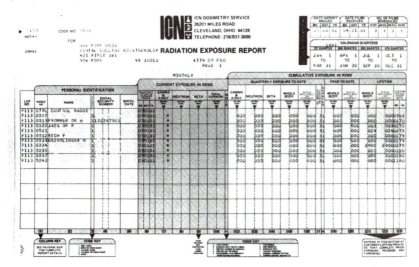

FIGURE 4-13   Film badge report. This monthly report gives current and cumulative exposure for the listed personnel.

should remove it if they are having medical or dental x-rays, because it is intended to measure only occupational exposure.

Protective barriers

The walls, floor, and ceiling of the x-ray operatory must be of such construction that the surrounding areas are shielded from both primary and secondary radiation. This does not mean they must be lead lined. Many materials used in construction today in the proper thickness provide protective shielding.

Because of the relatively low workload and the low x-ray energies used (65 to 90 kVp), dental offices with concrete or cinder block walls have enough inherent shielding in wall construction materials. Drywall construction, if of proper thickness, is also sufficient for dental shielding.[9]

The shielding or barrier requirements are based on such factors as workload, use and occupancy factors, maximum kilovoltage, and distance from the tube head. The formula W × U × T is used to calculate the guide number. In this formula, W is the workload (in milliampere minutes per week) and U is the use factor. The walls in dental radiography have a higher use factor than the floors or ceiling, because the central ray is never directed straight up or down. T is the occupancy factor, which accounts for whether a person is behind the barrier (1) all the time, as one seated at a desk; (2) sometimes, as in a waiting room; or (3) occasionally, as in a passageway. The guide number is correlated to the proper kVp and distance in reference tables found in Report 35 of the National Council on Radiation Protection.[10] These tables give the specifications of materials necessary for adequate shielding for the given conditions.

Pregnancy

The pregnant dental auxiliary, in relation to occupational exposure, should not be compared with the pregnant patient discussed in Chapter 3. In a well-designed and well-monitored dental office, the occupational exposure is zero. If a pregnant auxiliary follows proper procedure in such an office, there is no risk to the fetus. If a pregnant auxiliary is apprehensive, she should wear a film badge to document occupational exposure and allay any fears.

QUALITY ASSURANCE

It is important to establish quality assurance programs in dental offices to check and monitor x-ray machines, darkroom equipment and procedures, and chairside technique to make sure that ionizing radiation is used properly and that the maximum diagnostic yield is achieved for the energy expended. This is an important part of a radiation protection program. A quality assurance program is easy to establish and maintain. It reduces exposure to patients and dental personnel and helps provide better dental care.

The American Academy of Dental and Maxillofacial Radiology has published an outline of preventive maintenance procedures for radiographic systems.[11] Of the six categories listed in this report, the dental auxiliary, in most offices, is the person most likely to perform and be responsible for these procedures. The monitoring, calibrating, and inspection of the x-ray generator would be handled by a government agency, repair service, or health physicist. The auxiliary is involved in these categories:

1 Properly storing and handling all films, cassettes, screens, grids, and chemicals
2 Posting current technique charts, including time-temperature for processing, x-ray exposure factors, and x-ray equipment measurements
3 Maintaining proper conditions of processing tanks and automatic processors

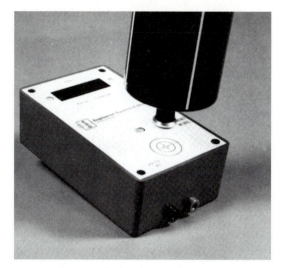

FIGURE 4-14   X-ray pulse counter. This instrument is used to check timer accuracy.

4   Maintaining optimal darkroom conditions by periodic checks for light tightness and adequacy of safelighting, cleanliness, and temperature control of the water supply

5   Maintaining the condition of protective devices such as lead aprons, thyroid shields, barriers, and film-holding devices

The quality assurance steps regarding film processing and the darkroom are discussed in detail in Chapter 6.

Periodic testing of the x-ray machine's performance is essential to a quality assurance program. Some state and local regulatory agencies provide such equipment inspection as part of their registration and licensing programs for x-ray machines. The x-ray machine should be checked for timer accuracy, beam quality, collimation, beam alignment, electrical calibration, barrier adequacy, and tube head stability (Figures 4-14 to 4-16).

Another part of a quality control program is the maintenance of high levels of chairside competence. Using programs of self-evaluation, intraoffice peer review, and continuing education, superior levels of chairside technique can be maintained and retakes kept to a minimum.

PATIENT CONCERN AND EDUCATION

The auxiliary and dentist should understand and be sensitive to the patient's concern and possible fear of dental radiographs. Recent years have been marked by a rise of consumerism and an increasing mistrust of health care providers. The media have been replete with stories warning of the danger of medical and dental radiographs.

The dental auxiliary, through knowledge and understanding, must be able to allay fears and explain the necessity of radiographs for proper dental treatment. Patients

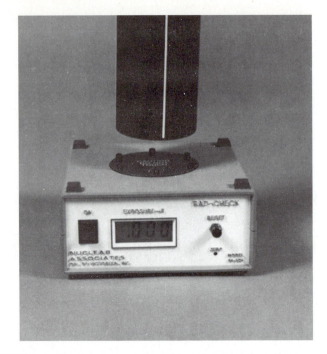

FIGURE 4-15 Exposure meter with a digital readout in roentgens.

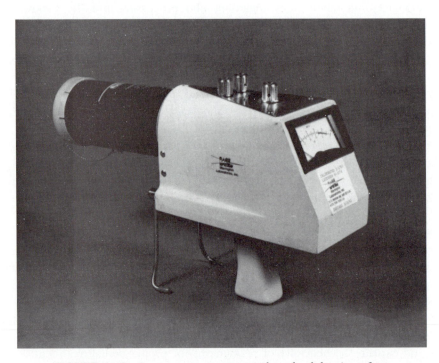

FIGURE 4-16 Survey scatter meter used to check barrier safety.

are likely to question the auxiliary rather than the dentist about the danger of radiographs. It may be helpful to explain to the patient how essential radiographs are in detecting diseases and planning treatment. Patients also can be informed of federal and local laws enacted for their protection. Patient educational material, such as the American Dental Association's pamphlet *Dental X-rays: Your Dentist's Advice* or the Food and Drug Administration's *X-rays Get the Picture on Protection,* can be placed in the waiting room or given to interested patients.

REFERENCES

1. Performance standards for electronic products: diagnostic x-ray systems and their major components, *Fed Register* 37:16461, 1972.

2. Brooks SL and Joseph LP: Basic concepts in the selection of patients for dental x-ray examinations, U.S. Department of Health and Human Services (FDA) 85:8249, September 1985.

3. American Dental Association, Council on Dental Materials, Instruments, and Equipment: Recommendations in radiographic practices: an update, 1988, *J Am Dent Assoc* 118:115-117, January 1989.

4. Kangers GE, Broga DW, and Collett WK: Dental radiologic survey of Virginia and Florida, *Oral Surg* 60(2):225-229, 1984.

5. Kantor ML, Reiskin AB, and Lurie AG: A clinical comparison of x-ray films for detection of proximal surface caries, *J Am Dent Assoc* III:967-969, December 1985.

6. Kanter ML et al: Efficacy of dental radiographic practices: options for image receptors, examination selection, and patient selection, *J Am Dent Assoc* 119:259-268, August 1989.

7. U.S. Department of Health and Human Services Public Health Service, FDA: The selection of patients for x-ray examinations: dental radiographic examinations, *HSS/PHS/FDA* 88-8273:10-21, 1987.

8. Recommendations on administratively required dental x-ray examinations, *Fed Register* 45:40976-40979, 1980.

9. Macdonald JCF, Reid JA, and Berthoty D: Dry wall construction as a dental radiation barrier, *Oral Surg* 55:319-326, 1983.

10. National Council on Radiation Protection and Measurements: Dental x-ray protection, Report 35, Washington, DC, 1970, *NCRP Publication.*

11. American Academy of Dental Radiology, Quality Assurance Committee: Recommendations for quality assurance in dental radiography, *Oral Surg* 55:421-426, 1983.

Chapter

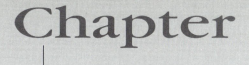

Infection Control

Infection control has become a major concern of patients, regulatory agencies, and health care workers in the practice of dentistry. The dental profession has been or should have been practicing infection control at all times as dental personnel have always been at risk for infection from cuts, breaks in the skin, and contact with body secretions and inhalants. The emergence and identification of acquired immunodeficiency syndrome (AIDS) in 1981, the highly infectious hepatitis B virus (HBV), and the resurgence of tuberculosis have brought the issue to the forefront.[1] Diseases such as tuberculosis, hepatitis, and herpes always have been a risk for dental workers, but it took the fatal consequences of AIDS to heighten the interest and awareness of the public, the government, and the profession to the importance of infection control in the dental office. Dentistry came into the spotlight of public and media attention with the report of an incident in Florida of possible HIV infection during an invasive dental procedure. A female patient, whose lifestyle did not put her in a high-risk category, was reported infected with a strain of HIV closely related to that of her HIV-infected dentist. The resulting inquiry revealed that seven other patients in the practice had HIV, and five of them carried a strain similar to that of the infected dentist. The exact nature of the transmission, if it occurred at all, is still unknown, but the public has become alarmed and federal and state agencies at all levels are imposing requirements for office procedures and required courses in infection control.

INFECTION CONTROL IN DENTAL PRACTICE

Any comprehensive infection control policy in dentistry must include protocols for radiology, including both chairside technique and darkroom procedures. Radiology is not exempt from infection control even though radiographic procedures do not involve the aerosol spray produced by the dental handpiece, needles, or the cutting of tissue and the spatter of blood. Infectious disease can be transmitted by the cross contamination of equipment, supplies, and film packets and cassettes used to take or process radiographs. In addition, dental radiographic procedures are in almost all cases performed in the same dental units that are used for more invasive procedures. The American Dental Association, the Center for Disease Control (CDC), and Occupational and Safety Health Agency (OSHA) all state that gloves must be worn when contact with saliva or items or surfaces contaminated with saliva is anticipated. Masks, eyewear, and protective clothing are required only when spatter is anticipated, and the use should be left to the judgment of the dentist. We believe that masks, eyewear, and gowns should be used at all times as these precautions fall under the rule of ALARA: "as low a risk as reasonably achievable." Gowns, masks, and gloves are easily achievable.

If we understand and practice infection control, we can protect our patients, our fellow workers, and ourselves from harm. Our objective is to be educated so that we can work in a concerned manner—not in a fear-induced, hysterical atmosphere. We are educated professionals, and we should act in a manner befitting our profession.

Immunization

All dental personnel should have the appropriate immunizations, including that for the hepatitis B virus (HBV). OSHA's new standard covering blood-borne pathogens requires health-care employers to offer a three injection HBV vaccination series free to all employees exposed to blood or other potentially infectious fluids or materials. The OSHA standard also states that should routine booster doses of hepatitis vaccine be recommended at some future date, the employer also should make these boosters available to employees at no cost.

Presently there is no immunization for the AIDS virus. However, hepatitis B remains a greater risk for dental workers, even though it does not have the certainty of fatal consequences that the AIDS virus does.[2] There has been great concern among dental personnel and in some cases refusal to receive the hepatitis B vaccination; they fear contracting AIDS because the original vaccine was derived from the serum of people who might have been at high risk for or who had AIDS. These fears have been shown to be unfounded, and the new vaccine for hepatitis B (Recombvax HB) now is produced artificially by a recombinant DNA technology and is in no way related to the serum of human donors. All dental personnel should receive the hepatitis B vaccine.

Patient history

Every patient should have a current medical history. The dentist and/or the dental auxiliary should obtain this history at the initial or recall visit, using a questionnaire and/or direct questioning of the patient. Information gained by the history will alert the dental team to the presence or history of infectious disease or to those who are in high-risk categories. Unfortunately, many potentially infectious patients cannot be identified by history or examination. Thus a rational infection control policy should not distinguish between patients who are known to be infected and those who are not. Every patient should be treated in the same manner and all infection control procedures carried out at all times. There are no exceptions. If there are no exceptions, there can be no surprises.

SOURCES OF INFECTION

Through contact with saliva, blood, and nasal and respiratory secretions, many instruments and pieces of equipment can become the means of transmission of pathogens. A pathogen is a microorganism that can cause disease. Everything we touch after glove contamination by oral cavity fluids during radiographic procedures is a possible transmitter of pathogens. Our concern then must be with film-holding devices, instruments, the x-ray machine PID (cone), the tube head, the control panel and exposure switch, clothing, countertops, dental chair, lead apron, the light handle, walls, doorknobs, processors, and patient records. In short, any object that the operator touches after placing the packet in the patient's mouth can be considered contaminated and a source of transmission to the operator or other patients. On the other hand, any object the operator touches before working in the mouth is a potential source of transmission to the patient. Thus barriers to the transmission of infective microorganisms must be used. Barriers include gloves, masks, protective eyewear, gowns, and surface coverings. If contamination does occur, as it will in the dental office, steps must be taken to remove or destroy the pathogen to prevent further transmission.

BARRIERS

Dental personnel always should wear gloves, masks, and protective eyewear when working on patients (Figure 5-1). Just as there is no excuse for not standing 6 feet away from the x-ray machine, there is no excuse for not protecting oneself from infection. Blood is the most common and easily recognized transmission route of the human immunodeficiency virus (HIV) and the hepatitis B virus (HBV). HIV has been

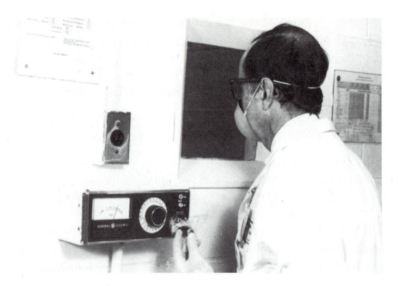

FIGURE 5-1   Operator making exposure wearing gloves, eyeglasses, and mask.

isolated in the saliva of some patients. It is true that no cases of HIV transmission have been documented via the salivary route by casual contact, but this should not serve as an excuse for not wearing gloves, masks, and eyewear. Saliva can be contaminated by blood and therefore poses a potential for transmission.[3]

Any object that the operator touches after placing the film in the patient's mouth must be covered with some removable barrier or disinfected after the patient leaves. A good maxim to remember is "the less you touch, the less you have to worry about." Household plastic wrap, plastic bags, or aluminum foil are good barriers. The material should be placed over the chair headrest, the countertop, the arm and PID (cone) of the x-ray machine, control panel, and exposure button (Figures 5-2 through 5-5). If barriers are not used, these objects must be disinfected after the radiographic procedure is completed. Disinfecting solutions such as Iodophor have the drawback that they may not reach irregular surfaces and have the potential to affect electrical connections (Figure 5-6).

Sterilization and disinfection

Sterilization produces the absence of all microorganisms, including spores. The most common methods of sterilization in the dental office are steam autoclaving or the use of the dry heat oven.

Disinfection is the process that results in the absence of pathogenic organisms but not spores. Disinfecting agents are usually employed on surfaces but not on human tissue. Iodophors, chlorines, and synthetic phenolics are examples of disinfectants commonly used in the dental office.

"Cold sterilization" of instruments with quaternary ammonium compounds or glutaraldehyde, so often used in the dental office, is really a type of disinfection and

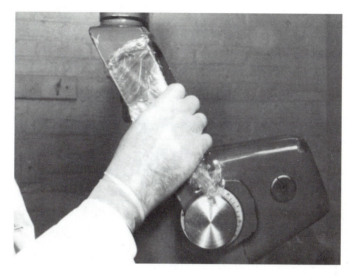

FIGURE 5-2   Plastic wrap covering yoke of the x-ray machine.

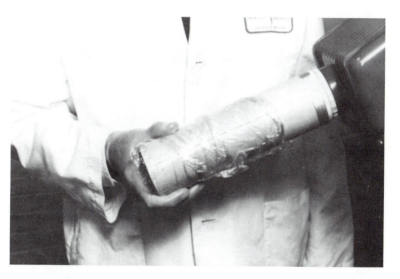

FIGURE 5-3   Plastic wrap covering PID (cylinder).

not sterilization. Those methods do not meet today's standards and are not acceptable. Some instruments such as plastic film holders, bite blocks, or localizing rings may be damaged by heat sterilization and thus are usually cold sterilized. Dental offices either should quit using these instruments or place them in protective plastic wrap covers. Most radiographic devices manufactured today are autoclavable and are clearly marked so.

Antiseptics are agents used on human tissue that are either bacteriostatic or bacteriocidal. In dentistry they are used mainly for hand washing.

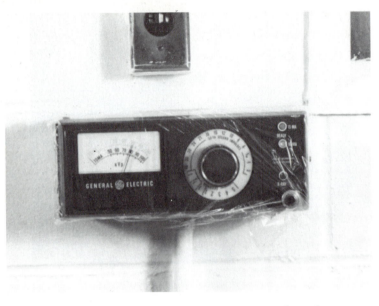

FIGURE 5-4   Plastic wrap covering control panel.

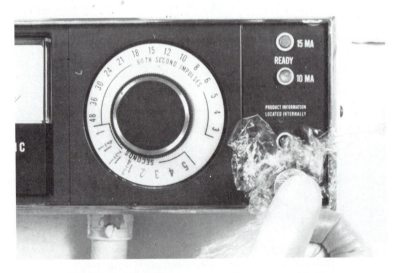

FIGURE 5-5   Plastic wrap covering exposure button.

In dental radiography, sterilization, disinfection, and antiseptic agents are employed.

Film packets

Other than the operator's hands the film packet is the main vector of cross contamination. The packet remains in the patient's mouth, and when removed it is coated with saliva or possibly with blood. The film packet is handled in the operatory

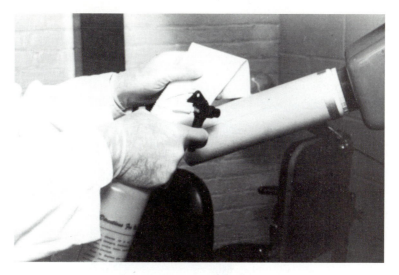

FIGURE 5-6 Disinfecting the x-ray machine.

and then transported to the darkroom. Three methods can help prevent transmission of microorganisms by the film packet to other parts of the operatory or the darkroom: (1) sterilization or disinfection of the exposed packet, (2) use of barrier protection for the packet, and (3) handling technique.

1 Sterilization and disinfection of the film packet is impractical and time consuming, and may degrade or ruin the radiographic image; therefore, these methods are not recommended.[4] Autoclaving or sterilizing by dry heat destroys the image. Immersing the packet in a disinfecting solution for the required time results in penetration of the solution to the film emulsion. Thus neither sterilization nor disinfection is recommended.

2 The Eastman Kodak Company now markets a barrier envelope for film packets. Its D- and E-speed film (size #2) may be purchased already inserted into barrier envelopes, or the barrier envelopes may be purchased separately and individual film packets (size #0 through #2) may be inserted in them before exposure.

   The film packet is placed and sealed in the barrier envelope before beginning the radiographic procedure. All film packets to be used are prepared in this manner. The film packet in the barrier envelope is then exposed, dried of saliva, and brought to the darkroom in some type of a receptacle. The operator wears gloves to open the barrier envelope, taking care not to touch the film packet, and the packet is allowed to drop onto a clean surface. The gloves and the barrier envelope are then discarded. With clean hands or new gloves the operator opens the film packet and processes the film (Figure 5-7).

3 If the barrier film packet is not used or contaminated, by saliva or blood, film packets should be placed in a receptacle that is outside the operatory and carried to the darkroom when all the exposures have been made. Operators should always remember that the gloves they wear are contaminated, so they should touch nothing on the way to the darkroom. They can change gloves after the

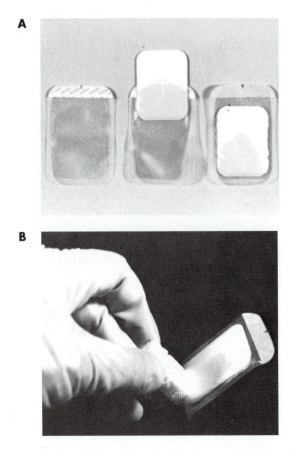

FIGURE 5-7 Barrier pack. **A,** with film packet. **B,** in film holder.

exposures have been made if touching surfaces and objects such as a doorknob is unavoidable. Once operators are in the darkroom under safelight conditions, they can open film packets, taking care not to touch the films as they are allowed to drop onto a clean surface. The contaminated gloves are then discarded and the films processed either manually or by automatic processing (Figure 5-8). If there are two people in the darkroom (admittedly this is not common in most offices), one gloved person can open the contaminated packet, and the other can remove the film from within the packet without touching the outside. This process will avoid contamination of the film.

Automatic processing

Operators should load film into an automatic processor with the same concern and method for cross contamination as with manual processing film hangers. The problem is with the automatic processors used with daylight loaders. Using daylight loaders is discouraged, because it is almost impossible to avoid contamination because of the

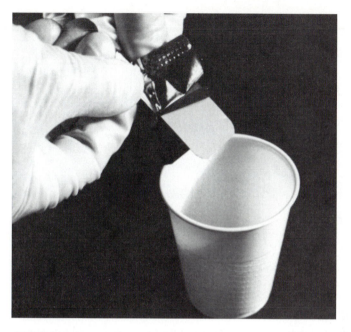

FIGURE 5-8   Opening contaminated film packet in darkroom.

tight-fitting hand baffles, which then serve as a source of cross contamination.[5] It is also very difficult to remove the film from the film packet and to put on one's gloves within the confined space of the daylight loader and then take off the contaminated gloves and feed the film into the uptake slots. If operators must use a daylight loader, they should follow this protocol:[6]

1   Prepare the interior of the daylight loader by placing a barrier on the bottom surface. Place the cup with the exposed film packets, a pair of gloves, and a second cup on that surface and then close the top of the daylight loader.
2   Place clean hands through the sleeve baffle and put on the gloves.
3   Open packets, allowing the films to drop into the second cup.
4   Remove gloves and place uncontaminated films in the processing slots and then remove ungloved hands through the sleeves.
5   Open top of loader and wrap all trash in the barrier and remove.
6   Wash hands.

Processing solutions

The developing and fixing solutions used in the dental darkroom have not been shown to act as sterilizing agents.[7] This is a common misconception. Any contaminated film that is processed emerges from the processing still contaminated. In automatic processors the rollers and tracks can be contaminated by the film, as can the film hangers in manual processing.

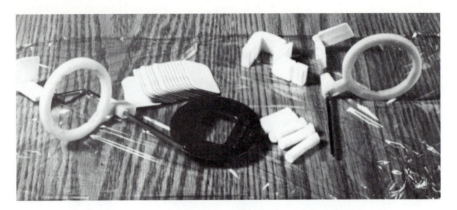

FIGURE 5-9   Plastic wrap covering necessary items on work surface.

Chairside exposure procedures

1 Cover all appropriate surfaces with plastic wrap or aluminum foil. This should include but not be limited to the PID and arm of the x-ray machine, the control panel and exposure button, and the working surfaces where unexposed films are placed (Figure 5-9). Plan in advance. Set out all anticipated supplies (film, film holders, cotton rolls, etc.).

2 Seat the patient and drape in the appropriate manner with the lead apron.

3 Wash hands with antiseptic soap and put on gloves.

4 Make the required exposures, taking care to touch only the covered surfaces. If the procedure is interrupted and you have to leave the room and touch anything (e.g., the telephone), remove the gloves, dispose of them, and put on a new pair before resuming work. Each exposed film packet should be wiped dry of saliva and put in a disposable cup outside the operatory.

5 If no other dental procedures are to be done, dismiss the patient. Dispose of all contaminated barriers and supplies in the operatory and then disinfect the lead apron and other appropriate surfaces.

6 Remove contaminated gloves and carry the film container to the darkroom.

Processing.

7 Put on new gloves.

8 Under safelight conditions with gloved hands, remove the films from the film packet or the film packets from the barrier envelopes by allowing them to drop onto a clean surface. Do not touch the film with gloved hands. The gloves are considered contaminated, since they touched the film packet.

9 Dispose of the film packet wrappers and carrying cup, and remove and dispose of the gloves.

10 Process the uncontaminated film on the clean surface either manually or automatically.

11   Since the film is not contaminated, gloves are not needed for processing or mounting.

Panoramic x-ray units. Because the panoramic radiography is an extraoral procedure, fewer areas are contaminated from the patient's saliva. The patient bite block should be covered by a plastic cover and the chin rest, ear rods, and patient hand grips should be disinfected after use. Processing presents no problems because the cassette does not contact the patient; thus the procedure for preventing film contamination is not necessary. The only possible contaminant in the darkroom would be the operator's gloves. These gloves should be removed before taking the cassette from the panoramic unit.

ANTIBIOTIC PROPHYLAXIS

It is accepted and required procedure to premedicate certain patients with antibiotics prior to invasive dental procedures. Patients with positive medical histories of heart murmur, mitral valve prolapse, shunts, and artificial joint replacement fall into this category. Any procedure including probing that might produce bleeding should be considered invasive. The question then arises whether intraoral radiography is an invasive procedure because in rare instances it may produce bleeding. A recent survey shows no consensus on this subject.[8] It is prudent because of the immense risk to the patient to premedicate if any bleeding is expected. Patients with advanced periodontal disease with positive medical histories are a good example of this type of need.

REFERENCES

1. Facts about AIDS for the dental team, ed 2, Chicago, 1988, *American Dental Association.*
2. Klein RS et al: Low occupational risk of human immunodeficiency virus infections among dental professionals, *N Engl J Med* 318:86-90, 1988.
3. Centers for Disease Control: Update: universal precautions for prevention of transmission of human immunodeficiency virus, hepatitis B virus, and other blood-borne pathogens in health-care settings, MMWR37, 1988.
4. Infection control in modern dental practice, Rochester, NY, 1992, Eastman Kodak Co.
5. American Academy of Oral and Maxillofacial Radiology: Infection control guidelines for dental radiographic procedures, *Oral Surg Oral Med Oral Pathol* 73:248-249, 1992.
6. Glass BJ: Infection control in dental radiology, *NY State Dent* 60:42-45, April 1994.
7. Stanczyk D and Pavnovich E: Microbiologic contamination during dental radiographic film processing, *Oral Surg Oral Med Oral Pathol* 76:112-119, 1993.
8. Jones GA: Radiographic protocol for patients needing antibiotic prophylaxis, *JADA* 125: 602-605,1994.

Chapter

six

Film Processing
the darkroom

The processing of exposed x-ray film either manually or by automatic processing is an important, but often neglected and abused step in the radiographic process. It is at this point in the chain of events that a visible image is produced from which a diagnosis can be made. The x-rays that have penetrated the hard and soft tissue in the patient's mouth have created a latent image on the exposed x-ray film. The processing of this film converts the latent image into a visible image.

The darkroom is one of the areas in a dental office for which the dental auxiliary has complete responsibility. In addition to processing film, the auxiliary must keep the darkroom clean, change solutions regularly, keep accurate records of radiographs processed, and maintain a quality assurance program. Only through meticulous attention to detail can proper darkroom technique be maintained. It is important to realize that the processing of films is vital in the production of the diagnostic radiograph. Errors in the darkroom can easily ruin what would otherwise have been good films, making it necessary to retake the films with the resultant loss of time and increased radiation exposure to the patient. Good chairside radiographic technique must be coupled with good darkroom technique.

The lack of attention to detail and of concern for film processing in many dental offices has been reported in the literature. Beiderman et al, in their study of radiographs submitted to an insurance company for reimbursement, reported that a majority of the radiographs were substandard.[1] Of these substandard radiographs, 20% were judged unsatisfactory because of poor density or improper processing. A study done in Nashville, Tenn., reported equally disturbing findings.[2] About 15% of the facilities changed their processing solutions less frequently than recommended, and severe light leaks in the darkroom were found in 10% of the facilities. More than 40% of the darkrooms did not have a thermometer, and more than 20% did not have a timer. The most alarming finding was that offices using the sight development techniques showed a much higher mR exposure per film than offices using the time-temperature technique.

It is much easier to prevent darkroom errors than chairside errors. Yet a great many dental patients receive excess radiation because of poor processing technique. It is important for the dental auxiliary to have a working knowledge of the chemical reactions taking place in film processing. This understanding helps prevent and correct errors. To process films without understanding is a "cookbook" technique that leads to errors and to a lack of appreciation for the importance of the processing task. The importance of eliminating darkroom errors, with the increased radiation dose consequences to the patient, should be uppermost in the minds of dentists and auxiliaries.

DESIGN AND REQUIREMENTS OF THE DARKROOM

The darkroom is that room in the dental office set aside for radiograph processing. It should be used only for that purpose, and it should not be combined with a dental laboratory or used as a lounge where the coffee pot is kept. The essential requirements and components of a darkroom are that it should be light-tight and have safelight and white light illumination, processing tanks, a thermostatically controlled supply of water, thermometer, timer, film hangers, drying racks, and storage space.

Location and size

A properly planned and located darkroom is an important, but often overlooked, feature in a dental office. Darkrooms are placed in unused spaces, closets, and laboratories without proper concern for the function or importance of the procedures to be conducted there.

Dental auxiliaries should have some knowledge of planning, although in most instances they work in previously established facilities. However, office renovation or relocation of a practice occurs frequently, and the knowledgeable auxiliary can have valuable input in the planning and design of a new office.

The darkroom should be a space unto itself, located near the rooms where the x-ray units are placed. This eliminates the necessity of personnel walking the length of the office with wet readings, thereby saving time, eliminating dripping of processing solutions, and reducing office traffic.

The darkroom should be a minimum of 16 square feet (4 × 4), allowing enough room for one person to work comfortably. The factors that should be considered in determining the space needed are (1) the volume of radiographs to be processed, (2) the number of auxiliaries handling the processing, (3) the type of processing to be done (manual, automatic, or both), and (4) space required for duplicating, drying, and storage.

The walls of the darkroom should be a light color that reflects the safelighting; darkroom walls do not have to be black. The surface of the walls and floor should be of materials that resistant can be cleaned of the processing solutions that inevitably spill or splash on them.

The darkroom must be completely lighttight so that, when the safelight is on, it is the only illumination in the darkroom. Because x-ray film is sensitive to white light, any light leaks fog the film. A fogged film is less diagnostic and in some cases may be useless. The easiest way to check for light leaks is to stand in the darkroom in complete darkness; any leaks around the door are apparent and can be corrected with either black masking tape or weather stripping. The darkroom door should have an inside lock so that the door cannot be opened inadvertently while films are being loaded.

The darkroom should be well ventilated to exhaust the moisture from the drying films and, if a dryer is used, the heat, and to maintain comfortable working conditions. Keeping the darkroom at a reasonable temperature makes it easier to maintain desired processing solution temperatures. Another consideration is film quality: if unexposed film is stored in the darkroom, high temperatures (above 90° F) will cause film fog.

Lighting

A well-designed darkroom has five different light sources: (1) an illuminating safelight, (2) an overhead white light, (3) a viewing safelight, (4) an x-ray viewbox, and (5) an outside warning light.

Illuminating safelight. When film packets are opened, when film is attached to hangers, or when film is processed, safelight conditions must be maintained. As previously mentioned, white light fogs x-ray film. *Safelight* is any illumination that does not affect the x-ray film (Figure 6-1). It is a low-intensity light composed of long wavelengths from the orange/red range of the spectrum. X-ray films are more sensitive to the blue/green region of the light spectrum where the wavelengths are relatively short. Red lighting was used previously as safelighting but has been replaced by yellow, because one can see better with yellow lighting. Not all yellow and red lights are safe. The determining factors are the sensitivity to the type of light of the x-ray film used, and the position and intensity of the light source. Usually a 7½- to 10-watt bulb with a yellow filter (e.g., Kodak yellow Morlite M-2) placed 3 to 4 feet from the work surface is used when working with intraoral film. If extraoral screen film is used, a Kodak GBX-2 Safelight Filter with a 15-watt bulb is needed because of the film's increased sensitivity to light. This filter also can be used for intraoral film.

A simple and reliable test of a safelight is to place a coin on an unwrapped, unexposed piece of dental film under safelight conditions. After 3 minutes of exposure to the safelight, the film is developed. If the film shows an outline of the coin, the light is not safe; the uncovered part of the film should have been as unaffected as the part covered by the coin (Figure 6-2).

Panoramic and other extraoral films used with intensifying screens are more sensitive to light than periapical films. As previously mentioned, screen film must be used with a different filter (e.g., Kodak GBX-2). Periapical films can be processed with the GBX filter, or, in offices where both screen and nonscreen (periapical) films are used, the darkroom can have two safelights of different intensity.

Overhead white light. The only requirement for overhead white light is that it provide adequate illumination for the size of the room. The switch for this light should be placed in a position inside the darkroom where it cannot be bumped accidentally and turned on, exposing films to white light.

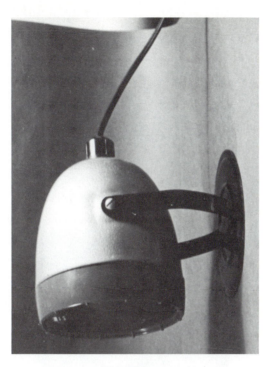

FIGURE 6-1 Safelight mounted on wall of darkroom. This light is placed 3 to 4 feet from working surface and has a 10-watt bulb with a appropriate filter.

Viewing safelight. Most dental offices use wet readings for emergencies and working films. In these cases it is convenient to have a viewing safelight mounted on the wall behind the processing tanks. Then films can be removed from the fixer after 3 minutes and checked by safelight to see if they have cleared enough for washing and reading. If a viewing safelight is not located behind the processing tanks, the operator would have to hold the wet film up to the overhead safelight with the obvious problem of the dripping and staining of the fixer solution. Auxiliaries should never check for clearance or the lack of murkiness on fixed film by holding it to the overhead white light or viewbox; in the uncleared state, the film still can be affected by the white light.

X-ray viewbox. The ability to read wet films in the darkroom is a great convenience. A proper diagnosis can be made only by having an adequate viewing mechanism. The darkroom should have a viewbox to suit these needs. A diagnosis should not be made by holding a wet radiograph up to the overhead light.

Outside warning light. This light should be wired so that when the safelight is on in the darkroom, the warning light is on outside the darkroom. This is a double check on the inside lock on the door and helps to prevent entry into the darkroom when safelight precautions are in effect.

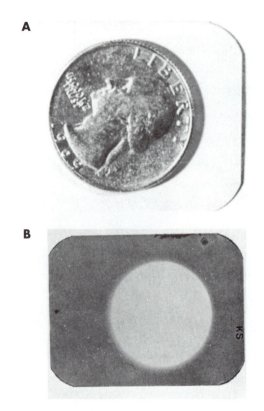

FIGURE 6-2 Coin test for safelighting. **A,** Coin placed on unexposed film under safelight. **B,** Developed film showing outline of coin indicating that safelight intensity is too great and not safe.

Plumbing

The darkroom requires intake lines of hot and cold water with an adequate drainage line. There should be a thermostatically controlled intake valve to maintain constant temperatures of the solutions. The disposal line should be made of materials that resist the action of the processing chemicals. If automatic processors are used, the flow rate of the incoming water should be considered in planning darkroom plumbing, because automatic processors have individual requirements.

A sink with a gooseneck faucet is extremely convenient for tank cleaning and solution changing. This is often overlooked in darkroom planning, but auxiliaries will realize that oversight the first time they carry processing tanks to the nearest sink for cleaning and replenishing. The gooseneck faucet is essential, because a normal-size faucet neck does not allow enough room to place the tanks under the faucet for cleaning.

Contents

Processing tanks. Most dental offices have processing units that contain either 1- or 2-gallon developer and fixer inserts suspended in a tank of running water (Figure 6-3).

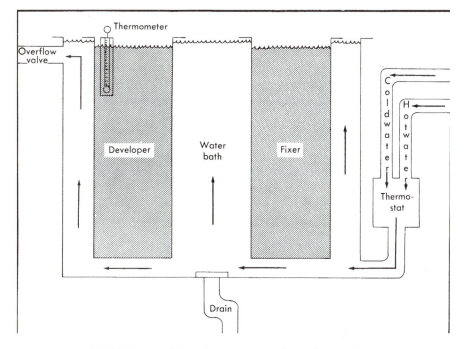

FIGURE 6-3 Typical processing tanks in dental office.

The tanks should be made of stainless steel, and the water bath should have a thermostatically controlled flow valve to keep the solutions at the desired temperature. The tank is equipped with a lid that should be kept on at all times. The cover protects developing films from accidental exposure to white light and prevents oxidation and evaporation of the processing solutions.

Solutions. The developer and fixer solutions are usually supplied as liquid concentrate that must be diluted. Some commercial services deliver prepared solutions in 1-gallon containers. Extra amounts of prepared solutions should be stored either in dark bottles or opaque plastic containers away from heat and light sources.

Under normal working conditions, developer and fixing solutions should be changed at least every 3 to 4 weeks. A normal workload is considered to be 30 intraoral films per day. If many panoramic films are processed, solutions should be changed more often, because more chemical is needed per film area. The chemical solutions lose strength when exposed to air and should be replaced even if normal workload minimums have not been met. This means that the times that an office is closed for vacation still are counted when determining time to change solution. Remember that film development is a chemical reaction: every time the developer and fixer solutions affect a film emulsion, the solutions become weakened. In a busy office the auxiliary may need to change solutions more frequently than every 3 weeks. Weak developer and fixing solutions do not bring out the optimum image on the film and thus do not provide the maximum diagnostic information for the radiation exposure.

Replenishing. Developer and fixer solutions should be replenished daily. Commercially prepared replenishment solutions are available, but it is usually easier to use the standard developer and fixer solutions that fill the tanks. Approximately 8 ounces of replenishment is required each day for the developer and fixer solutions. Commercial replenishers include manufacturer's instructions. The replenisher is added in respective tanks directly to the existing solutions to bring them to the proper fluid level. The level of solutions always should be kept at the top of the tank to ensure that the immersed films are covered with solution. Water should never be added to the solutions to bring them to tank top level; this dilutes the strength of the chemicals.

Table 6.1 lists the main ingredients of developer and fixer and their function.

Timer and thermometer. No darkroom is complete without a timing device and a thermometer. The most modern radiographic equipment cannot produce optimum results without time and temperature control in the darkroom. There is no other correct way to process films. The timer is used to determine the length of time the films stay in the developer solution. This depends on the temperature of the developer—not the temperature of the water in the surrounding tanks or that of the water entering through the flow valve. To determine temperature of the developer, a thermometer must be suspended in the developer tank. Early in the day, developer solutions may be cold or hot, depending on the overnight office temperature. It may take some time for equalization of temperatures between the water tank and the developer tank. That is why the temperature of the developer bath is read, not the

Table 6.1

Chemicals for development process

Ingredient	Function
Developer	
Elon or Metol and hydroquinone (developing agent)	Reduces the energized silver bromide crystals to silver
Sodium sulfite (preservative)	Prevents oxidation of developer
Sodium carbonate (activator)	Provides alkaline medium and softens gelatin to allow developing agents to reach silver bromide crystals
Potassium bromide (restrainer)	Controls activity of developing agents and prevents chemical fog
Fixer	
Sodium thiosulfate (clearing solution)	Removes undeveloped or unexposed silver bromide crystals from the emulsion
Sodium sulfite (preservative)	Prevents the decomposition of the thiosulfate clearing agent
Potassium aluminum sulfate (hardener)	Shrinks and hardens gelatin
Acetic acid (acidifier)	Maintains acid medium

temperature of the water entering the surrounding water tank (Figure 6-4). It is ironic that some dental offices have thousands of dollars invested in radiographic equipment but are missing a timer and thermometer, which together cost $40.

A time-temperature chart, similar to the following, appears on every package of developer-fixer solution. These charts may vary slightly from manufacturer to manufacturer. A chart like this should be posted in every darkroom.

80° F 2½ minutes in the developer
75° F 3 minutes in the developer
70° F 4 minutes in the developer
68° F 4½ minutes in the developer } Optimum
60° F 6 minutes in the developer

Film hangers. Intraoral film hangers come in various sizes and contain clips for 2 to 20 films. In all cases the films should be unwrapped and attached to the clips using the techniques described in Chapter 5 without touching the films with one's fingers (Figure 6-5). This can be accomplished easily by using the wrapping paper in the film packet. The working surface on which the hanger is loaded should be clean and dry to prevent film staining. Film hangers should be numbered or have the patient's name written on the hanger to avoid mix-ups. The implications of a film series with the wrong patient's name are obvious. Hangers with defective clips should be discarded because the defective clip can scratch films on adjacent hangers in the solution. Defective clips also lead to lost film in the solutions. The idea that one would remember which clip is defective and avoid using it is not realistic. If the film hanger is in any way defective, it should be discarded.

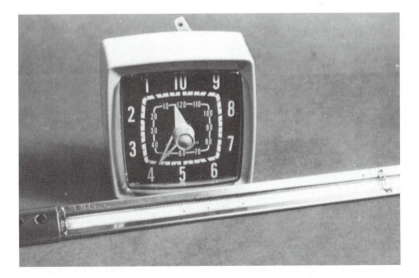

FIGURE 6-4   Darkroom timer and thermometer, essential parts of time-temperature technique.

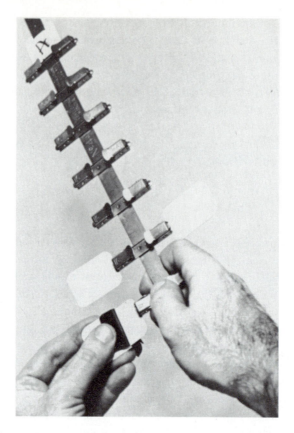

FIGURE 6-5   Placing film on hangers in darkroom under safelight conditions after gloves have been removed. Note that fingers do not touch film. (Barrier Pack Technique)

Dryer. After films have been washed for 20 to 30 minutes they are ready for drying. This can be accomplished with the use of an x-ray dryer or simply by hanging them on towel racks and letting the films air-dry. In either method the films should not touch one another or they will stick together; separating them will rip the emulsion. Drying racks should be out of the way in a clean room. One of the major objections to laboratory-darkroom combinations is that the dust and dirt of the grinding and polishing done in the laboratory contaminates the dental films.

THE DEVELOPMENT PROCESS
Procedure

1   Lock the darkroom door from the inside and record the patients' names whose films are to be processed on film hanger.
2   Stir the solutions to equalize the temperature and the chemical distribution of the processing solutions. Use a different stirring paddle for each solution to prevent cross contamination. Check the level of solutions and replenish if necessary.

3   Check the temperature and set the timer. The temperature of the developer solution should be checked with an accurate thermometer. Refer to the time-temperature chart, which should be posted in the darkroom, and set the time for the desired interval.

4   Turn off the white light and turn on the safelight.

5   Put on gloves and open the film packets, dropping the films onto the working surface. Discard contaminated film packets and/or barrier wraps, remove gloves, and load the film hangers. Work carefully, avoiding finger marks or film scratches. Be sure the film is securely fastened to film hanger clips.

6   Immerse the film hanger in developer and activate the timer. After immersing the film, immediately raise and lower the hanger a few times so that the film surfaces are covered totally by solution. Remaining in the darkroom while the films are in the developer is the preferred procedure, but auxiliaries can leave if the tank lids are securely in place.

7   Remove the film rack from the developer when the timer sounds (under safelight conditions).

8   Rinse thoroughly for 20 seconds in the water bath (under safelight conditions).

9   Place the film rack in the fixer solution. Agitate the rack up and down immediately after the initial placement. Films should remain in the fixer for a minimum of 10 minutes (approximately twice the developer time) for permanent fixation but may be removed after 3 or 4 minutes for use as a wet reading. After fixing, with the tank lids firmly in place, normal lighting can be resumed in the darkroom. Safelighting is not needed after the timer signals that fixation is complete and films are moved from the fixer to the water bath.

10   Place the films in the running water bath for 20 minutes.

11   Dry the films. Remove the films from the water bath and suspend them from rack holders to dry.

Explanation and discussion

Latent image. Radiographs, after having been exposed, are said to contain a latent image. The silver halide on the radiographic emulsion is energized by the x-ray beam. The pattern of this energizing of the silver halide depends on the density of the objects being radiographed. For instance, the silver halide crystals on the film that lie behind a metallic restoration receive almost no radiation because the density of the metal absorbs all the x-ray energy. Silver halide crystals on the film that correspond to an area such as the pulp of the tooth or a cavity receive more radiation energy since these areas are less dense and absorb little x-ray energy (Figure 6-6).

Developing. Exposed dental film packets that contain a latent image should be processed as soon as possible. In the darkroom under safelight conditions the x-ray films are removed from the packets and placed on film racks. The developer is the first solution into which these film racks are placed. The developer has a pH above 7 and thus is basic compared with the acidic fixing solution. The developer chemically

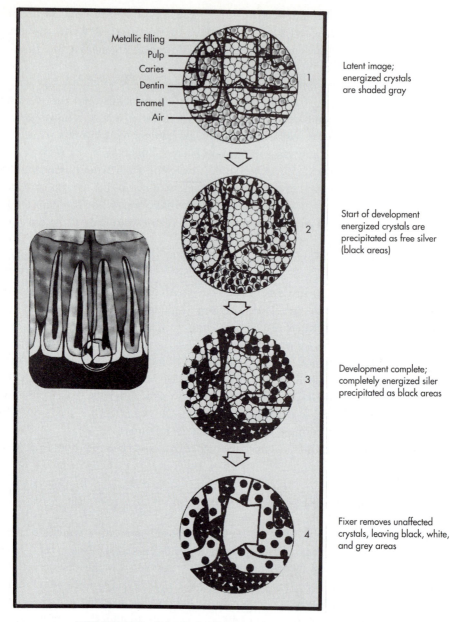

Metallic filling —
Pulp —
Caries —
Dentin —
Enamel —
Air —

1   Latent image;
     energized crystals
     are shaded gray

2   Start of development
     energized crystals are
     precipitated as free silver
     (black areas)

3   Development complete;
     completely energized siler
     precipitated as black areas

4   Fixer removes unaffected
     crystals, leaving black, white,
     and grey areas

FIGURE 6-6   Schematic drawing of x-ray film development.

reduces the energized silver halide crystals by precipitating silver on the film base. This precipitation corresponds to the black (radiolucent) areas on the radiograph. An area of less density, such as the pulp, allows greater penetration of x-rays; therefore more x-rays reach that part of the film. The silver halide crystals are more greatly energized, and more silver precipitates to give a black, or radiolucent, outline to the pulp chamber.

This is a chemical reaction. The optimum amount of precipitation of silver for the amount of x-ray energy delivered to the object takes place in a specified amount of time with the developing solution at a certain temperature. This is the basis and importance of the time-temperature technique.

If films are left in the developing solutions too long, more silver precipitates than was intended and dense and less dense structures lose their distinctions. A completely overdeveloped film results when all the silver is precipitated by the developer and the film is totally black.

Crystals of silver halide that have received small amounts of radiation have correspondingly less silver precipitated and appear gray. The silver halide that was unenergized by radiation, such as the area on the film behind a gold crown, precipitates no silver and appears white or radiopaque on the x-ray film.

Washing (stop-bath). The main purpose of washing is to remove the developer from the film so that the development process stops. This also removes the basic developer so that it does not contaminate the acidic fixer. This is usually accomplished by agitating the film hanger in a water bath for about 20 seconds. Safelight conditions must be maintained when transferring the films from the developer to the wash tank and then to the fixing solution.

Fixing. The acidic fixing solution removes the unexposed and undeveloped silver halide crystals from the film emulsion and rehardens the emulsion, which has softened during the development process. For permanent fixation the film is kept in the fixing solution for a minimum of 10 minutes. However, films may be removed from the fixing solution after 3 minutes for viewing. This procedure is known as the *wet reading* and is useful when films are needed immediately. For example, a wet reading of a film would be used to check that all the root tip has been removed in an extraction before dismissing the patient. As previously mentioned, a film is ready for a wet reading if it is cleared enough for washing and reading. Operators should always check for clearance or the lack of murkiness under safelight conditions.

Since all films should be made part of the patient's permanent record (archival), they should be returned to the fixing solution to complete the required 10 minutes. Films not fixed properly fade and turn brown in a short time.

Washing and drying. The film is washed for about 20 minutes in the water tank to remove the fixing solution from the emulsion. The film is then dried in a clean, dust-free area.

TIME-TEMPERATURE VERSUS SIGHT DEVELOPMENT

The only correct way to process dental x-ray films is by the time-temperature method described in this chapter. This scientific method portrays optimum information on the film. Even so, many dental offices develop x-ray films by sight. The usual technique is to immerse the film hanger in the developer, removing it at frequent intervals to hold it up to the safelight, until fillings or root shapes are visible. At that point the films are washed and placed in the fixer. This is obviously an inexact, unacceptable technique. The usual reason given for the use of the sight development method is, "We have always done it this way, and it works well." This continual acceptance of lower standards of the quality of radiographs leads dentists and dental auxiliaries to believe that this is the way the radiograph should appear. Sight development is unfair to the patient because it does not provide the maximum amount of diagnostic information for the radiation exposure. The time-temperature method, performed either manually or by automatic processors, is the only acceptable way to process dental radiographs.

RAPID PROCESSING

Rapid processing of dental radiographs is done with the use of higher solution temperatures, concentrated solutions, agitation of the film, or a combination of these. It is sometimes called *hot processing,* referring to the temperature of the solutions. Rapid processing does not require an increase in radiation to the patient, but the images produced by this technique are not comparable in density and definition to films processed by standard methods.[3] The clinical indications for the use of rapid processing are when time is more important than exacting detail of the image. For example, it may be used when a patient has just had an extraction, and a radiograph is taken to make sure no debris is left in the socket before suturing. The degree of definition needed to visualize anything in the socket is not as important as suturing as soon as possible.

The use of regular-strength developing solutions at 92° F with agitation of the film can produce acceptable diagnostic images in less than 1 minute (20 seconds developing, 3 seconds washing, and 30 seconds fixing). There also are concentrated processing solutions available that can be used at room temperature. The increased chemical activity of these solutions makes the rapid processing possible. Some of these solutions use a two-bath technique, developer and fixer; others use a single-bath technique, or monobath, that contains the developer and the fixer (Figure 6-7).

Rapid processing can be helpful with endodontic working films and postoperative films in oral surgery where a high degree of definition is not essential. It should not be used for routine processing of films.

EXTRAORAL AND PANORAMIC FILMS

These films are processed in the same manner as intraoral films using the time-temperature technique with the same solutions. As mentioned earlier, the only precaution that must be taken is to check safelight intensity. Those extraoral films that are used in combination with intensifying screens (screen films) are more sensitive to light than nonscreen films. Darkroom illumination that may be safe for intraoral films may adversely affect screen films. The safety of the light can be checked by using the coin test discussed earlier.

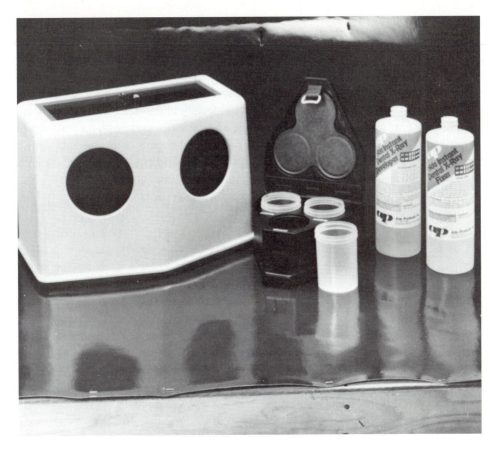

FIGURE 6-7 Rapid processing system *(left to right):* lighttight working area with hand baffle, solution receptacles, and processing chemicals. *Courtesy Ada Products/Block Professional Dental Products Co.*

CARE AND MAINTENANCE OF THE DARKROOM

Although darkroom maintenance may seem like a housekeeping chore, it is really a means of ensuring quality control. Maintenance should be likened to our regard for sterility to avoid contamination and subsequent infection. Contaminants in the darkroom or other errors resulting from sloppy techniques may ruin diagnostic radiographs and require retaking of films, with an unnecessary increase in the patient's radiation burden.

Cleanliness

The working surface, where films are stripped and placed on hangers, always should be clean and dry. Developer, fixer, and water are the most common stains. Drying films should not be placed above the working surface without catch pans. If the working surface is made of formica, it can be cleaned easily with a mild detergent.

Film hangers should be clear and dry when loading films. Hangers used for wet readings are the most likely ones to be insufficiently washed and contain residual fixer that can stain the next film. Hangers should be washed after each use, and clean, dry hangers always should be used.

Processing tanks should be cleaned thoroughly when solutions are changed. This includes not only the insert tanks that hold the developer and fixer but also the water reservoir. The water tank accumulates sludge and algae, especially under the metallic lip and in the overflow tube. Operators can use a bland detergent or preferably one of the tank cleaners made specifically for this purpose. It is in this routine tank cleaning that one appreciates the sink and gooseneck faucet in the darkroom.

Solutions

Solutions should be brought to the optimal temperature at the beginning of the working day and kept at that temperature by the thermostatic control on the mixing valve.

Tanks should be kept full by the use of replenishers, not by adding water, since such an addition dilutes the concentration and weakens the solutions. If the tanks are not kept full, the films or portions of the films on the top clips of the film rack may not be immersed fully in solution and will not be developed.

As mentioned before, both the developer and fixer solutions should be changed at least every 3 to 4 weeks regardless of use. In some practices with heavy film volume, it may be necessary to change solutions as often as once a week.

The lids of the processing tanks always should be closed when the tanks are not in use to prevent oxidation and weakening of the solutions.

Record keeping

Two types of records are important in the darkroom. The first is the supply inventory, including the date of the next scheduled solution change. It is helpful to have the date of the next scheduled solution change posted in a prominent place.

Film identifications are the second important type of records in the darkroom; accurate records are essential when processing radiographs. The patient's name, the number of films, the number or letter of the rack the films were placed on, and the date should be recorded. This eliminates the likelihood of lost films and mixed x-ray series.

ENVIRONMENTAL CONCERNS

Dental professionals must be aware of and comply with the growing number of environmental laws that regulate the management of waste materials. It is our professional responsibility to be aware of these federal and local regulations as they apply to our office and to comply.

Dental radiology generates three types of waste: waste solid, x-ray processing solution effluent, and medical waste. Waste solid is the x-ray film packaging, including the lead foil. The effluent is the liquid waste coming from the x-ray processing chemicals. Medical waste is the intraoral dental packets that have been contaminated by blood or blood components and/or saliva.

The federal statute that regulates discarded material is the Resource Recovery Act of 1976. Professionals who create hazardous wastes are referred to in this statute as *generators.* Most dental offices in the United States would be classified as "conditionally exempt small quantity generators" because the small amount of hazardous waste they generate is exempt from federal regulations.[4] State and local laws vary and exemption from federal regulation does not mean automatic exemption from local laws. Large dental clinics and dental schools because of their volume may be classified as "small quantity generators" and may fall under federal regulation.

There are two sources of silver retrieval in the dental office. In the category of waste solid are the old, no longer needed, or unusable processed radiographs, and second, the exhausted fixer solution, which falls under the effluent category.

Silver can be recovered from the processed radiographs by ashing the film above the melting point of silver. The economic benefit of this endeavor is limited, but it is an environmentally sound practice and is much preferred to ordinary disposal. A pound of radiographs is worth less than $25. In a litigious society dental offices may be better off saving old radiographs, even beyond the statute of limitations, than using the ashing process. Discarded film is generally not a regulated waste.

The discharge of processing solution effluent into a sewer system or a septic tank is not recommended and in many localities is prohibited by law, depending on the concentration of silver in the effluent. The concentration depends on the amount of films processed. Chemical precipitation or electrolysis can retrieve residual silver from the fixer and the wash water. There is no residual silver in developer solution. Electrolysis units that can be inserted into dental processing tanks or connected to automatic processors cost about $100 (Figure 6-8).

Throwing the lead foil inserts of film packets in regular trash is not environmentally sound. Eastman Kodak now offers to their film users, for the cost of the prepaid shipping label, cardboard holding boxes for collecting and shipping the foil to qualified disposal facilities (Figure 6-9).

AUTOMATIC PROCESSING

In recent years automatic dental x-ray film processing units have become available and more popular. They are not an essential component of a darkroom but a substitute for manual time-temperature processing. Their major advantage is the maintenance of standardized procedure; these units provide solutions of proper strength, correct temperature, and regulated processing time. In short, they provide automated time-temperature processing. Other advantages of the units are the time saved and the increased volume of films that can be processed when compared to the manual method. However, these units are costly, and they still require maintenance and a quality control program. Some offices that use automatic processing still maintain a backup system of manual processing tanks.

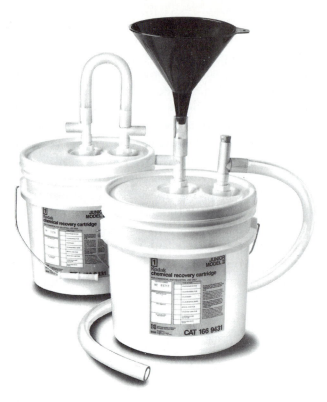

FIGURE 6-8   Silver retrieval unit. *Courtesy Eastman Kodak Co.*

The typical automatic processor has three solutions—developer, fixer, and wash—and a drying chamber (Figure 6-10). A transport system of either rollers or tracks driven by gears, belts, or chains moves the film from solution to solution and then into the drying chamber. Finished film is produced in 4 to 7 minutes, and some units have the capacity to process faster by elevating the temperature of the solutions.

Automatic processors vary in the size film they can accept, their safelight and plumbing requirements, and the option of automatic replenishment. Freestanding units are not connected to water and waste lines and may be kept in the operatory as films are fed into the unit through a daylight loader.

Size of film.   Some units accept only periapical and bite-wing size film (#0, #1, #2, #3) (Figure 6-10), while others can accommodate all sizes including 8 × 10, 5 × 12, or 6 × 12 inch panoramic film (Figure 6-11).

Safelight.   Some processors must be located in the darkroom because safelight procedures are required for stripping and inserting the film. Units with daylight loaders do not have to be in the darkroom as they have lighttight baffles into which the hands are placed while stripping and inserting film into the rollers (Figure 6-12). The problems of infection control with daylight loaders was discussed in Chapter 5.

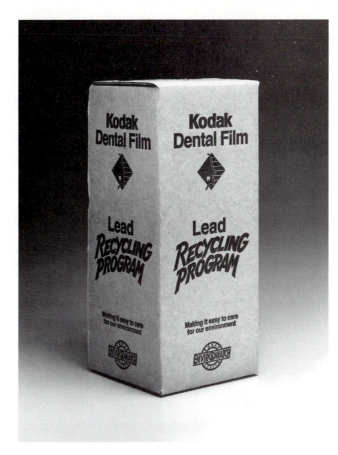

FIGURE 6-9   Mailing package for lead foil disposal. *Courtesy Eastman Kodak Co.*

Plumbing. If there is a constant flow of water in the wash chamber, plumbing is required. This arrangement is more desirable than a freestanding chamber where the water level may drop and constant change is necessary.

Automatic replenishment. More sophisticated processors maintain solution concentration and levels by automatic replenishment. Each time a piece of film is fed into the unit, a few drops of fixer and developer are added automatically to the baths to maintain solution strength.

Care and maintenance

Automatic processors need daily or weekly cleaning, depending on the volume of films processed. The rollers should be cleaned at the beginning of the day by running an extra oral-size film or cleanup film that is designed to clean through the rollers. This removes any residual gelatin or dirt from the rollers. The rollers should be removed weekly from the processor and soaked in a water bath for about 20 minutes.

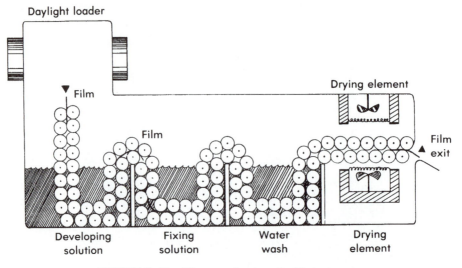

FIGURE 6-10   Diagram of automatic film processor.

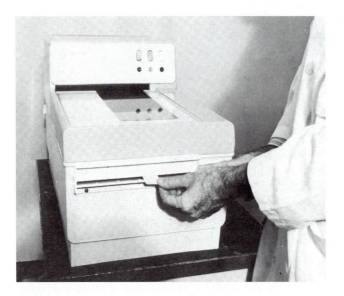

FIGURE 6-11   Automatic processor being used in darkroom under safelight conditions. Note gloves have been removed after taking film from packet.

Solution levels should be checked at the beginning of every day and replenished when necessary. Quality assurance checks are also necessary. The processors are only as good as the care their operators give them.

Technique remains important and cannot be neglected just because the machine runs automatically. Films should not be fed into the rollers too quickly. Operators should maintain at least a 10-second interval between films on the same track. This

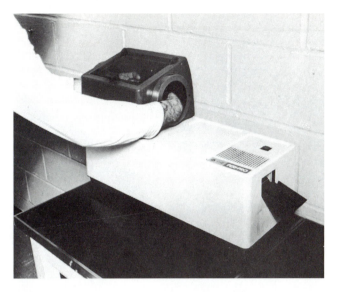

FIGURE 6-12 Automatic processor with daylight loader being used in operatory. Gloves have been removed inside daylight loader.

prevents overlapping of films in processing and the inability of chemicals to reach overlapped portions of the film. In fact, a good practice is to alternate tracks when feeding film into the processor. Carelessness can lead to feeding the film with the black paper or lead foil still attached. Not only does this ruin the film, but the foil and paper also may stick to the rollers, ruining subsequent films.

QUALITY ASSURANCE

An effective quality assurance (QA) policy for the darkroom is the prime responsibility of the dental auxiliary. A quality assurance program in the darkroom is as important as, and much easier to conduct than, the QA monitoring of the x-ray machine. At least monthly the auxiliary should check the safelighting, lighttightness of the darkroom, and the accuracy of the timer and thermometer. The auxiliary should monitor daily the cleanliness of countertops, condition of the film hangers, and the strength and level of processing solutions.[5]

The chemical strength and level of processing solutions in both manual tanks and automatic processor must be monitored on a daily basis. This is the most critical part of a QA program. Processing solutions should be changed at a maximum of every 3 to 4 weeks. There are better ways to determine when solutions should be changed than just using the calendar.

An easy way to check solution strength in an office, although admittedly a rough estimate, is by comparison to a standard (Figure 6-13). A processed periapical film of ideal density should be kept taped to the darkroom viewbox for comparison of densities with films that are processed daily. A lessening of the film density in the

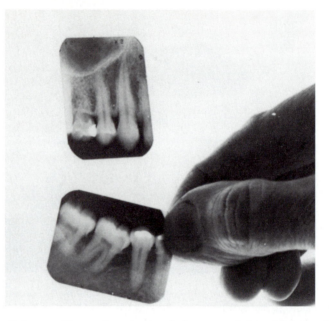

FIGURE 6-13 Reference film used to check solution strength by comparing densities.

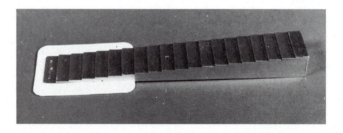

FIGURE 6-14 Step wedge and film prior to exposure.

processed film indicates a weakened solution and signals the need for solution change. Do not wait until the films lose their diagnostic usefulness to change solutions; this type of reasoning offers little comfort to the last patient before the solution change, whose films become useless.

A better and more scientific way to check the strength of solutions is to make a test exposure at the beginning of every working day. This test exposure is done through a step wedge or a predetermined density (Figure 6-14). The film is then processed and compared with standard film densities. In the device shown in Figure 6-15, the processed film is placed in a slot, and the numbered densities are moved until a visual match of densities is achieved. If the test densities are too light, the solutions are either weak or cold. If the densities are too dark, the solutions are either too concentrated or too warm. Either case is a "no go" situation, and processing cannot begin until conditions are optimum.

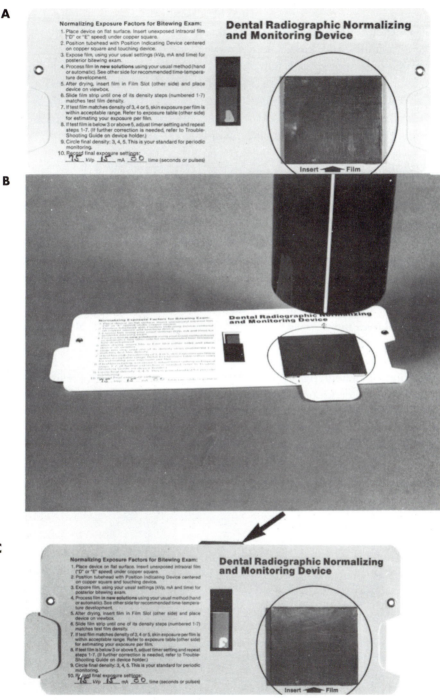

FIGURE 6-15 **A,** Dental radiographic normalizing and monitoring device. **B,** Test film inserted beneath copper plate and exposure made. **C,** Processed test film *(arrow)* inserted in device and compared to numbered densities.

The strength of the fixer can be gauged by noting the length of time needed to clear films. Fresh, full-strength fixer clears films in 2 to 3 minutes. If clearing requires more than 4 minutes, the fixing solution is weakened and should be changed.

Unexposed and unprocessed film should be stored in a cool dry location. High storage temperatures increase film fog. Film should be stored at temperatures between 50° F and 70° F and between 40% and 60% relative humidity.[6] Film should be used before the date of expiration clearly marked on each box, and film boxes should be placed on the shelf so that the oldest film is in the front.

DUPLICATING RADIOGRAPHS

In recent years, with the increase in dental insurance programs and a more mobile patient population, dental offices receive many requests to provide radiographs to insurance carriers or forward films to the patient's new dentist. Coupled with this has been the increase in the number of dental malpractice suits for which the defendant/dentist's records are of utmost importance. Radiographs are an essential part, if not the most important, of these records. The use of radiographic duplicating film can satisfy requests for radiographs and still maintain the integrity of office records. Radiographs should never leave the dental office unless they have been duplicated. There should be no exception to this rule. We live in a litigious society, and we must protect ourselves.

Duplication of radiographs is a relatively easy process that requires only a few additions to normal darkroom equipment, namely duplicating film, appropriate-sized film hangers, a light source (ultraviolet is preferable), and a photographic printing

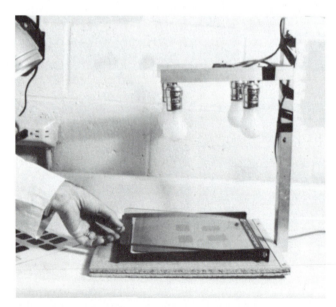

FIGURE 6-16   "Homemade" setup for radiographic duplication.

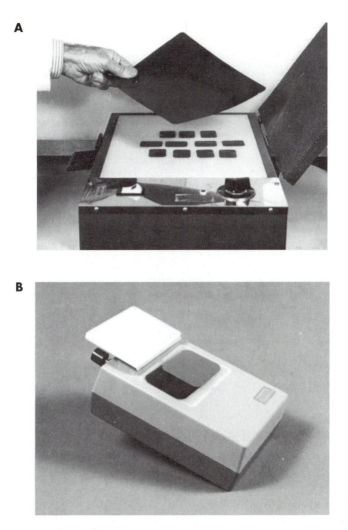

FIGURE 6-17 A and **B,** Radiographic duplicators. **B** *Courtesy Rinn Corp., Elgin, Ill.*

frame (Figure 6-16). Duplicating devices are also commercially available that can duplicate all film sizes or just one film (Figure 6-17, *B*).

Radiographic duplicating film is readily available from dental supply firms and is supplied in 8 × 10 or 5 × 12 inch sheets and individual periapical-sized duplicating film. The photographic emulsion is coated on only one side of the film. Under safelight conditions the emulsion side appears dull when compared with the shiny, nonemulsion side. The duplicating film is a direct positive film; therefore if more film density is required (darker film), the exposure time is shortened. Conversely, if decreased film density is desired (lighter film), the exposure time is increased. This is the opposite of time requirements for exposing dental films to x-rays. The key to remember is to think the opposite of what you do normally. Duplicating films do not have an orientation dot as standard intraoral films do, and so the films must be labeled right and left.

Procedure

Under safelight conditions the radiographs to be duplicated are placed in close contact with the emulsion side of the duplicating film. A photographic printing frame is ideal for this, because it has a rigid frame with a glass front that will hold the original radiograph against the duplicating film. This frame is placed on a tableandexposed to a light source for 4 to 5 seconds with the light source about 2 feet from the film. Since intensities of light sources may vary from office to office, trial exposure should be made to standardize time and light source distance. After the exposure is made, the duplicating film is processed on an 8 × 10 inch film rack in the same manner that x-rays are, using either manual or automatic technique. An original radiograph can be copied without limits. Close positive contact between the radiograph and duplicating film is essential, or image definition will be compromised. The glass top of the printing frame should provide this contact. Films always should be removed from the mounts to achieve tight contact.

When using a manufactured duplicating device the principles are the same. The auxiliary should follow the unit's operating procedures.

COMMON DARKROOM ERRORS

The following are the most common errors made in the darkroom.

Fogged film (Figure 6-18). Fogged film has an overall gray appearance because of diminished contrast. This can be caused by light leaks in the darkroom, improper safelighting, or improper film storage.
Remedy. Safelight conditions can be tested with a coin (see pp. 104-105). All doors should be checked for possible leaks, and old film should be used first.

Underdeveloped film: thin image (Figure 6-19). Underdeveloped film is light in appearance and does not contain all possible diagnostic information. This results when the optimum amount of silver has not been precipitated because of weak or cold developing solutions or insufficient developing time. This type of film is identical to the thin image produced by chairside technique errors.
Remedy. The developer and fixing solutions should be changed every 3 to 4 weeks, and the time-temperature method should be used. That is, the temperature of the developer should be checked before immersing films in the solution, and the timer should be set for the appropriate time as given in the manufacturer's specifications, referring to density comparison standard mounted on the viewbox. Daily QA checks should be performed to determine solution strength.

Overdeveloped film: dense image (Figure 6-20). Overdeveloped film may vary from dark to totally black, depending on the degree of overdevelopment. This type of film is of no diagnostic value. It results when too much silver has been precipitated on the film base; in the case of the totally black film all the silver from

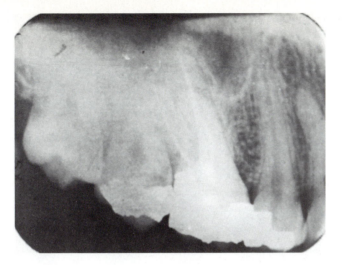

FIGURE 6-18   Maxillary molar radiograph that has been fogged. Note lack of definition and contrast.

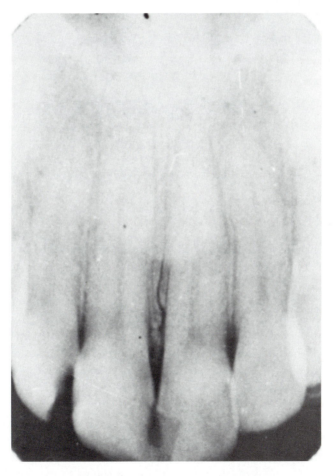

FIGURE 6-19   Underdeveloped film.

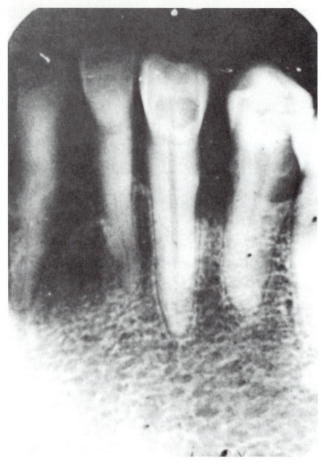

FIGURE 6-20 Overdeveloped film.

the silver bromide has been precipitated. This error can be caused by hot developing solutions or prolonged developing time. Chairside errors also can produce a dense image.

Remedy. The time-temperature method of processing always should be used. The timer should have a bell or buzzer that rings when the developing time has elapsed. This enables the dental auxiliary to leave the darkroom while the films are processed. Without the bell the dental auxiliary may be distracted by other duties and forget to remove the films from the developer at the proper time. Operators should perform daily QA checks on solution strength.

Developer cutoff (Figure 6-21). Cutoff film shows a straight radiopaque border on what was the upper edge of the top film on the processing hanger. This is an undeveloped area of the film. When the solutions are allowed to deplete in the processing tanks, the films on the top positions on the racks may not be covered by

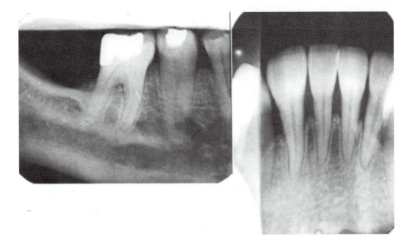

FIGURE 6-21   Radiographs with developer cutoff.

solution when the racks are placed in the tanks. This error should be differentiated from "circular collimation" cone cutting, which may give a curved radiopaque border. In cone cutting the film portion is unexposed; in developer cutoff the film portion is undeveloped.

Remedy. The dental auxiliary always should make sure that processing tanks are full. If the level of solutions has dropped, water should not be added; this will only dilute the solution and result in underdeveloped films. Proper replenisher solutions should be added to maintain the desired level.

Clear films (Figure 6-22). Films are clear because the entire emulsion has been washed off. This occurs when films are overfixed or left in running water baths for 24 to 48 hours. This type of film is identical to an unexposed film that is developed and processed. With unexposed film the fixer removes all the unaffected silver bromide crystals.

Remedy. Films should never be left in water baths overnight. Processing should be complete before one leaves the office. Films should not be left in the fixer overnight or for prolonged periods beyond the recommended 10 minutes; the fixer will lighten and finally remove the image. It is a common misconception that films cannot be overfixed.

Stained films (Figure 6-23). If the working surface in the darkroom is wet and dirty, films can be stained either before or after processing. There is no excuse for this error.

Remedy. Darkroom work surfaces must be kept clean and dry.

Discolored films. Films that have not had adequate fixation (approximately twice the developing time) turn brown after a period of time and are useless as part of the patient's permanent record.

FIGURE 6-22   Clear film. This can result from excessive washing or fixing or an unexposed film.

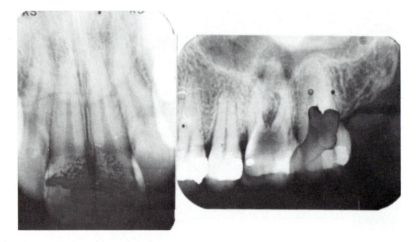

FIGURE 6-23   Stained radiograph.

Remedy. All films must have adequate fixation time (10 minutes). All wet readings should be returned to the fixation tank after the patient has been treated.

Torn emulsion (Figure 6-24). If films that are drying are allowed to touch and overlap, they stick together. In separating the films the emulsions are usually torn off the film base in the overlapped area, rendering the film useless for diagnosis.
Remedy. Film racks should be checked to be sure that drying films from different racks are not touching.

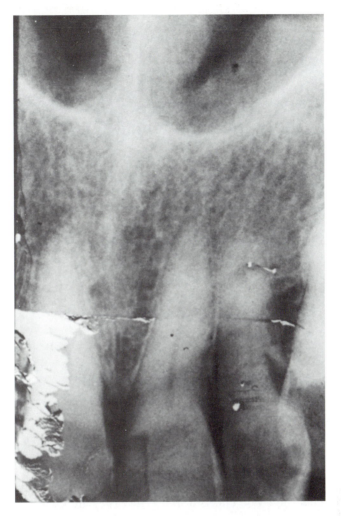

FIGURE 6-24   Radiograph with torn emulsion.

Scratched films (Figure 6-25). A radiopaque line on a film is usually an artifact caused by scratching the emulsion on the film base in film processing. Most often it is caused by putting a second film rack into a tank that already contains a film rack. It also can be caused by fingernails scratching the film while unpacking the film and placing it on a rack.

Remedy. When film racks are put into the processing solution, care should be taken to avoid touching those already immersed. Any film racks should be discarded if they have sharp edges or broken clips that could scratch other films.

Lost film in tanks. If films are not firmly clipped onto the hangers, they may fall off in any of the three processing baths. A lost film necessitates a retake or results in a "wet elbow" in an attempt to retrieve it from the processing solution.

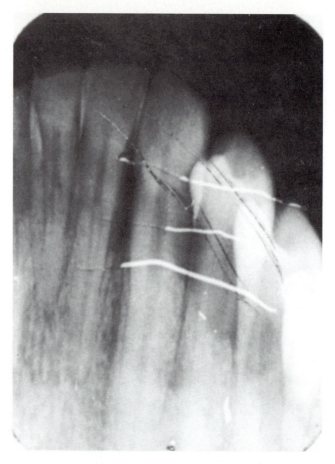

FIGURE 6-25   Scratched radiograph.

Remedy. All films should be checked to see that they are clipped securely to the hangers before processing.

Fluoride artifacts (Figure 6-26). Some fluorides, especially stannous fluoride, produces black marks on radiographs.
Remedy. After working with fluoride, the auxiliary should wash hands thoroughly with soap and a weak acid, such as vinegar or lemon juice, before handling films in the darkroom.

Reticulation (Figure 6-27). If film is developed at an elevated temperature and then placed in a cold water bath, the sudden change in temperature causes the swollen emulsion to shrink rapidly and give the image a wrinkled appearance called *reticulation.*
Remedy. Sharp contrasts in temperatures between processing and the water bath should be avoided.

Air bubbles (Figure 6-28). If air bubbles are trapped on the film as it is placed in the processing solutions, the chemicals cannot affect the emulsion in that area.

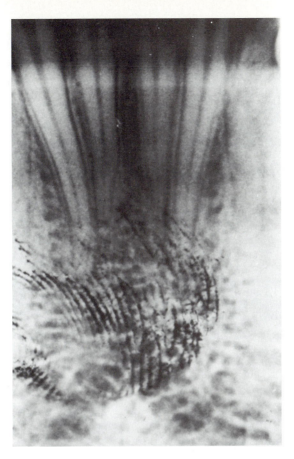

FIGURE 6-26 Fluoride artifact. Operator's fingertip contaminated by fluoride touched film when stripping and placing film on hanger.

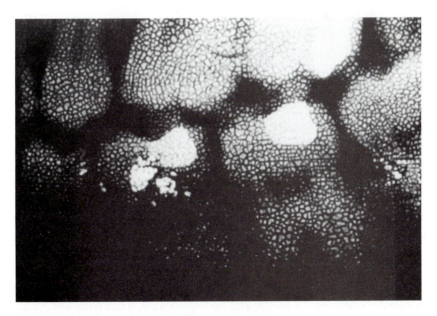

FIGURE 6-27 Reticulation.

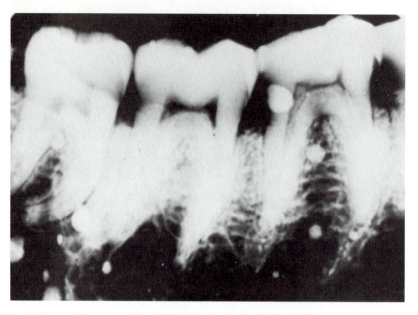

FIGURE 6-28   Artifact caused by air bubbles trapped on the film, preventing processing solution from touching film in the area.

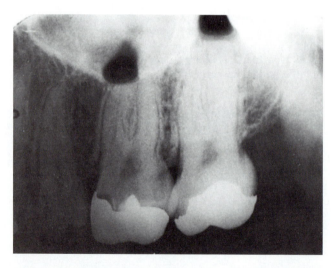

FIGURE 6-29   Periapical radiograph with static marks.

Remedy. The film hangers always should be agitated when they are placed in the processing solutions to dislodge any trapped air bubbles.

Static marks (Figure 6-29). Static electricity can be produced when intraoral film packets are opened forcefully in the darkroom. This is not common for intraoral film in new film packets. The static electricity produces multiple black linear streaks

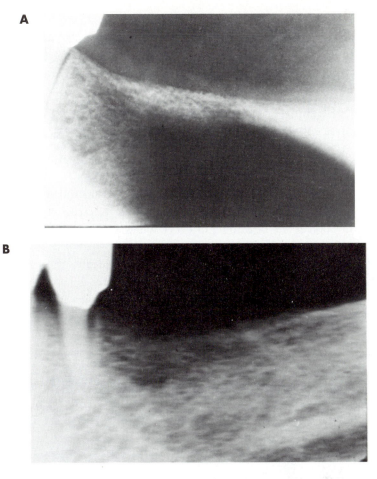

FIGURE 6-30 **A,** Artifact caused by light leak in daylight loader resembling a large pathologic area in bone. **B,** Normal radiograph of same area.

on the radiograph. The same effect occurs much more frequently on extraoral films. With these films static electricity may result when removing the piece of film from a full box; the sliding of the film out of the tightly packed box may produce static electricity. It also may be produced when loading and unloading flexible cassettes in panoramic machines as the film is slid in or out between the intensifying screens. In addition, walking around a carpeted office may produce static electricity. If the auxiliary does not touch a conductive object before unwrapping the film, charge marks may result. Static electricity occurs most often on cold, dry days.

Remedy. Operators should ground themselves by touching any conductive object in the darkroom before handling film and should avoid friction of any kind against the film that will produce static electricity.

Daylight loaders: light leaks (Figure 6-30). Film fog, a ruined film, or unusual artifacts can be caused by removing one's hands from the baffle (see Figure 6-10) before the film has entered the processor.

Remedy. The operator's hands must be kept on the film until it has been completely taken up by the rollers. The material that makes up the baffle should fit tightly around the hands. Rips and tears should be repaired immediately and stretched elastic replaced. It is a good idea to remove wristwatches and bracelets, because they tend to tear the baffle material.

Automatic processing

Dirty rollers (Figure 6-31). If the rollers are not cleaned periodically, radiolucent bands appear on the finished film.
Remedy. Rollers should be cleaned periodically by removing and soaking them in accordance with the manufacturer's recommendations. A piece of extraoral film should be run through at the beginning of every workday.

Overlapped films (Figure 6-32). If the films are fed into the processor too quickly, they overlap and the processing solutions cannot reach the emulsion.
Remedy. The operator should wait 10 seconds before putting a following film into each processing track.

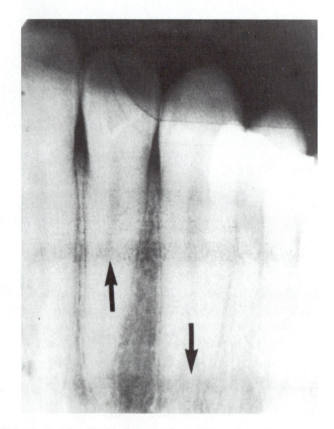

FIGURE 6-31   Bands of stain *(arrows)* from dirty rollers of automatic processor.

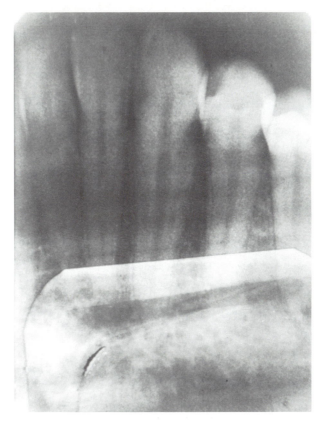

FIGURE 6-32 Overlapped films during automatic processing.

REFERENCES

1. Beiderman RW et al: A study to develop a rating system and evaluate dental radiographs submitted to a third party carrier, *J Am Dent Assoc* 89:1010, November 1976.
2. Bureau of Radiological Health: Nashville dental project: an educational approach for voluntary improvement of radiographic practice, US Department of Health, Education, and Welfare Publication (FDA) 76-8011, Rockville, Md, July 1975.
3. Alcox RW and Jameson WR: Rapid dental x-ray film processing for selected procedures, *J Am Dent Assoc* 78:517, March 1969.
4. *Waste management guidelines,* Rochester, NY, 1994, Health Sciences Division, Eastman Kodak Co.
5. American Acadamy of Dental Radiology, Quality Assurance Committee: Recommendations for quality assurance in dental radiography, *Oral Surg* 55:421-426, 1983.
6. *Quality assurance in dental radio-graphy,* Rochester, NY, 1989, Health Sciences Division, Eastman Kodak Co.

Chapter

seven

Intraoral Radiographic Technique:

the paralleling method

THE FULL-MOUTH SURVEY

The full-mouth intraoral radiographic survey is one of the cornerstones of a complete oral diagnosis. No dental examination or treatment plan can be considered complete without current or valid radiographs, and in almost all cases the full-mouth survey is the radiographic procedure of choice. The full-mouth survey is a difficult procedure to do correctly and requires time and meticulous attention to detail. It bears with it the responsibility of exposing the patient to the least amount of ionizing radiation to obtain the maximum diagnostic yield. Unnecessary radiographs or those of poor quality that have no diagnostic value do not serve the patient's needs and only add to the patient's radiation burden. Whether the dentist or dental auxiliary takes the radiographs is not important, as long as the same standards are maintained.

The full-mouth radiographic survey is usually composed of 14 or more periapical films and, where possible, four posterior bite-wing films. This text will discuss a 15-periapical and four bite-wing film technique, using two films for the maxillary central and lateral incisors. A 14-periapical film series would use one film projection for these four teeth. Some series of more than 15 periapical films include distal maxillary molar projections, vertical bite-wings, anterior bite-wings, and individual radiographs using #1 size film of the six maxillary and four mandibular anterior teeth.

The number of radiographs in a full-mouth survey can be modified to include extra or fewer projections, depending on the size of the patient's mouth or tooth position. In all cases the minimum number of films that satisfy the diagnostic requirements of a full-mouth survey should be used. Film mounts are available in combinations of number and size of film. The radiographic survey should not be determined by the film mount available but by the diagnostic needs of the patient. The recommended film projections (Figure 7-1) are as follows.

Maxillary	Mandibular	Bite-wing
Right and left central and lateral incisors	Central and lateral incisors	Right and left premolars
Right and left canines	Right and left canines	Right and left molars
Right and left premolars	Right and left premolars	
Right and left molars	Right and left molars	

A periapical film shows the entire tooth from occlusal surface or incisal edge to apex and 2 to 3 mm of periapical bone. This film is necessary to diagnose normal or pathologic conditions of tooth crowns and root, bone, and tooth formation and eruption (Figure 7-2).

The bite-wing film can be taken only if there are opposing teeth to hold the film in position with their occluding surfaces. This film projection shows the upper and lower teeth in occlusion. Only the crown of the teeth are seen. It is used for detecting interproximal decay, periodontal bone loss, recurrent decay under restorations, and the fit of metallic restorations (Figure 7-3). Bite-wing films can be taken of the anterior teeth but are usually unnecessary if the paralleling method is used.

The full-mouth survey shows all of the teeth in the mandible and maxilla as well as the surrounding bone. Each tooth is shown at least twice in the survey; that is, the maxillary second premolar can be seen on the premolar periapical film and on the premolar bite-wing film. Some teeth may be seen in three or four views. This gives the diagnostician an opportunity to view the tooth from different radiographic angles and eliminates the possibility that an artifact could be mistaken for caries or other pathologic conditions.

All the teeth-bearing areas of the jaws are covered in a full-mouth survey. However, the survey includes more than teeth: A clinically edentulous area may have residual root tips, unerupted teeth, or other pathologic conditions in the bone. One should not assume that because no teeth are present, everything is all right. The full complement of periapical films should be taken on all patients.

Pedodontic full-mouth series

Depending on the child's age and the size of the child's mouth, the composition of the full-mouth series may vary. A report of the Selection Criteria Panel[1] recommends

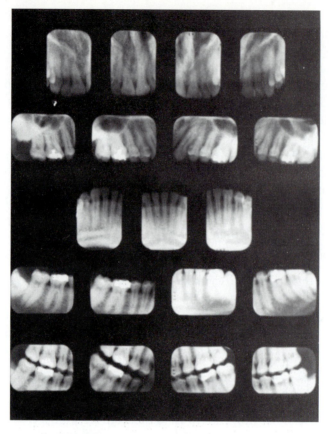

FIGURE 7-1   A 19-film full-mouth survey.

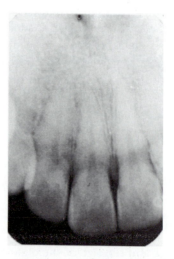

FIGURE 7-2   Periapical radiograph of the maxillary central incisor area. Note that the entire tooth and surrounding periapical bone are shown.

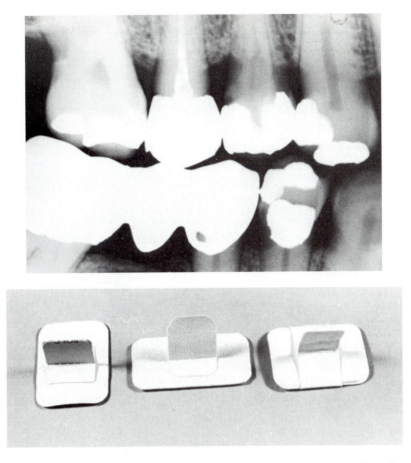

FIGURE 7-3 *Top,* Bite-wing radiograph. Note that only the crowns, alveolar ridge, and a small part of the roots of opposing teeth are seen. *Bottom,* Types of bite-wing films: *left,* vertical; *middle,* long posterior; and *right,* standard.

that for the asymptomatic pediatric patient with closed posterior contacts only two bite-wing films be taken. For asymptomatic pediatric patients with open posterior contacts, no radiographs are necessary.

For patients up to age 5 who need a full-mouth series, the operator should use the pedodontic-size film #0 for anterior, posterior, and bite-wing projections. The full-mouth series at this age entails 12 films: three maxillary anterior films, three mandibular anterior films, four mandibular and maxillary premolar-molar projections, and two bite-wing projections. The size of the child's mouth does not necessitate separate premolar and molar films. For the same reason, only one bite-wing film is taken on each side.

In the 6- to 9-year-old group the pedodontic film or narrow adult film size #1 can be used for anterior projections, since the child's arch shape at this age can still be very narrow. For posterior projections, adult size #2, narrow adult, or pedodontic film is used, depending on the size of the arch. At this age two posterior periapical films

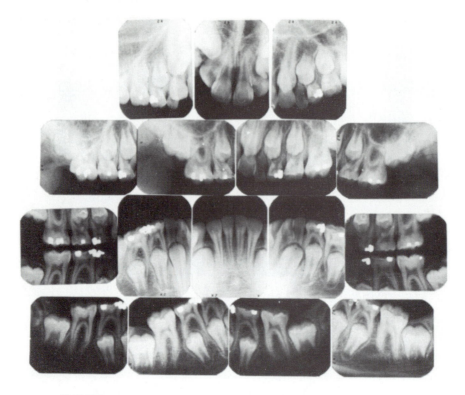

FIGURE 7-4 Full-mouth pedodontic survey of a 9-year-old patient.

in each quadrant are taken, since the 6-year molars have erupted and the dental arch has lengthened. One bite-wing film on each side also is used.

After age 9 the full adult series is taken, using the narrow adult film where necessary. These age guidelines are flexible and depend on the growth and development of the child. As a rule it is best to use the largest film size that the patient can accommodate comfortably (Figure 7-4).

In the pedodontic series the chair position, film placement, point of entry, and vertical and horizontal angulations follow the same rules as in the adult series.

CRITERIA FOR INTRAORAL RADIOGRAPHS

The criteria for judging whether a single radiograph or a full-mouth survey is diagnostically acceptable are:

1 The radiograph should show proper definition and detail, and a degree of density and contrast so that all structures can be delineated easily.
2 The structures should not be distorted either by elongation or by foreshortening.
3 The radiograph should show the teeth from the occlusal or incisal edges to 2 to 3 mm beyond their apices.
4 In a full-mouth survey, the entire alveolar processes of the mandible and maxilla must be seen—as far distal as the tuberosity in the maxilla and the beginning of the ascending ramus in the mandible.

5   All interproximal surfaces of the teeth should be seen without overlapping, providing the teeth are not overlapped in the mouth.

6   The x-ray beam should be centered on the film so there are no unexposed parts of the film ("cone cuts" or "collimator cutoff").

7   The radiograph should not be cracked or bent or have any other artifacts.

8   The radiograph should be processed properly (see Chapter 6).

If a single radiograph does not meet these criteria and provide diagnostic value, it must be retaken. In a full-mouth survey, those areas and structures that do not appear on the primary film may be seen on adjacent films in the series. Although a technically perfect full-mouth survey is the ideal, retakes should not be done unless judged necessary for proper diagnosis.

Quality assurance

These criteria should be used to evaluate radiographs taken by dentists and dental auxiliaries as part of a quality assurance program. This can be accomplished by either self-analysis and criticism of one's work or by peer review. In this manner, technical errors can be corrected and high-quality diagnostic radiographs produced.

PARALLELING TECHNIQUE

The basic principle of the paralleling technique for intraoral periapical films is that the film packet and the long axis of the tooth being radiographed must parallel each other, and the central ray of the x-ray beam must be directed perpendicular to both (see Figure 2-11). To accomplish this parallelism, the object-film distance must be increased. This distance can be sizable in some areas, such as the maxillary molar projection where the film may have to be held at the midline of the palate to achieve this parallelism.

The increased object-film distance results in loss of image sharpness; using a 16-inch FFD compensates for these problems (Figure 7-5).

Unfortunately, the paralleling technique has too often been called the *long cone* technique. This terminology emphasizes the length of the PID rather than the parallel relationship of the object and the film. Better names for this technique are the *extension paralleling* or *right-angle technique,* both of which stress the important components of the technique.

Advantages and disadvantages of the paralleling technique compared with the bisecting technique

When comparing the paralleling and bisecting techniques, the first point is that general consensus backs the paralleling method as the technique of choice.[2] The paralleling technique produces better diagnostic images, less exposure to critical organs such as the thyroid and lens of the eye, a smaller exit dose, and easier standardization and execution than the bisecting technique. This text takes the position that the paralleling technique is the method of choice.

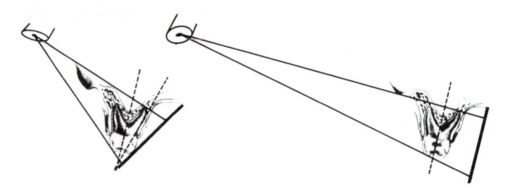

FIGURE 7-5 Bisecting, 8-inch focal-film distance technique and paralleling 16-inch extended-cone technique. Note superimposition of zygomatic arch on apices of maxillary molar in bisecting technique. *Courtesy Rinn Corp., Elgin, Ill.*

Advantages. The major advantage of the paralleling technique is that when performed correctly it forms an image on the film with both linear and dimensional accuracy to support a more valid diagnosis. The key terms are *dimensional accuracy* and *dimensional distortion.*

The bisecting technique correctly represents the teeth linearly but produces dimensional distortion. The bisecting technique can project the images and surrounding structures on the film in a true linear relationship without elongation or foreshortening. When radiographed with the bisecting technique, performed ideally, a tooth 22 mm in length is shown on the radiograph as 22 mm long. The teeth and bone, however, are three-dimensional objects, and although their overall length may be recorded accurately, the relationship of one part of the tooth to another is distorted dimensionally (Figure 7-6). Those parts of the tooth that lie farthest from the film—for example, the buccal plate of bone and buccal roots—are foreshortened although their lingual linear counterparts are not. A classic clinical example is comparing the length of the buccal roots to palatal roots in maxillary first molars. Clinicians who have used the bisecting technique for many years may come to believe that the buccal roots are much shorter than they really are because of dimensional distortions. One may argue that this may not be clinically important, except in an initial endodontic measurement, but when this distortion is applied to periodontal evaluation of alveolar bone levels, the clinical importance becomes apparent (Figure 7-7). In the bisecting technique the image of the buccal bone level is figuratively added to the palatal bone height to give a distorted image. A diagnosis and treatment plan could be made of adequate bone for restorations, fixed splinting, and so forth based on distorted radiograph images.

With the paralleling technique, it is possible to diagnose and evaluate caries and alveolar bone height accurately on all radiographs and not rely on the bite-wing projections, as the users of the bisecting technique do. It is interesting to note that bite-wing projections in both techniques are paralleling films.

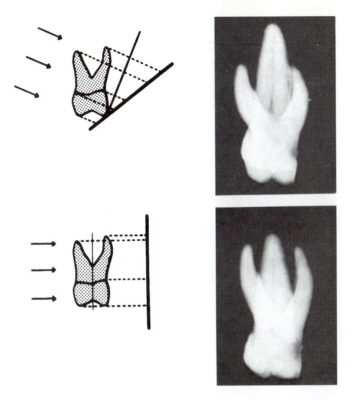

FIGURE 7-6   Radiographs of maxillary molar taken with bisecting technique *(top)* and the paralleling technique *(bottom)*. *Courtesy Rinn Corp., Elgin, Ill.*

In the bisecting technique the radiopaque image of the zygomatic arch is often superimposed on the apices of the maxillary molars, making diagnosis difficult, if not impossible. This superimposition is understandable because the point of entry of the central ray for molar projections is along the zygomatic arch.

The paralleling technique produces no superimposition, since the central ray, which is perpendicular to the long axis of the molars, enters below the level of the zygomatic arch (Figure 7-5). Also, in the paralleling technique the vertical angulation of the primary beam is rarely more than plus or minus 10 degrees, compared to vertical angulation of plus 40 to 50 degrees in the bisecting technique. The lack of extreme vertical angulation reduces the exposure to the thyroid gland and lens of the eye as they no longer lie in the path of the primary beam. The literature reports thyroid exposure of 25 mR for a full-mouth survey using the paralleling technique compared with 60 mR for the bisecting technique.[3] In addition, the 16-inch focal-film distance employed with the paralleling technique reduces the volume of tissue irradiated when compared to the 8-inch focal-film distance used in bisecting (see Figure 4-8).

The paralleling technique is easier to standardize than the bisecting technique, and serial comparison radiographs of the same area have greater validity. This is especially

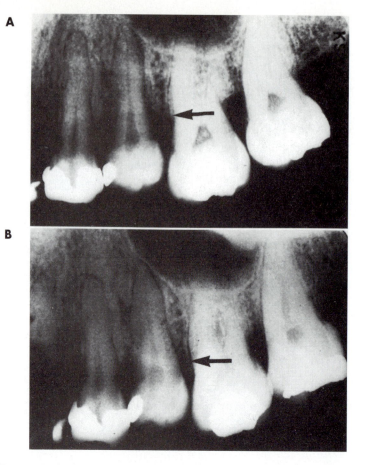

FIGURE 7-7 Radiographs of the same area: **A,** taken with the paralleling technique, and **B,** the bisecting technique. Note the difference in alveolar bone height as indicated by arrows.

important in evaluating alveolar bone levels of periodontal patients at recall examinations.

If a film-holding device with a localizing ring is used, in the paralleling technique the patient does not have to be positioned so that the occlusal plane of the jaw being radiographed is parallel to the floor. This is especially helpful in contour chairs or where patients are treated in the supine position. In both these instances it is difficult to position the patient with the occlusal plane parallel to the floor.

Disadvantages. One of the objections most often raised about the paralleling technique is the difficulty in placing and the degree of discomfort caused by the devices used to hold the film parallel to the long axis of the tooth. For patients with small mouths, for children, and for patients with low palatal vaults, this may present some problems, but the more adept an operator becomes with the technique, the less these problems are a factor.

It is said that paralleling is more difficult to learn and takes clinically longer to do. Experience with novice students has disproven this argument.[4] At the least, the time element is the same, and learning the paralleling technique is as easy or easier than learning the bisecting technique.

Objections also focus on the "long, bulky" 16-inch position-indicating device that is used in the paralleling technique. The claim is that these PIDs are difficult to work with in small operatories. The difference is 8 inches, and in a well-designed office this cannot be a factor. This objection has no validity in the newer x-ray machines with the extended FFD within the tube head (see Figure 2-8).

Another supposed disadvantage of the paralleling technique is that with the 16-inch FFD, longer exposure times are necessary, resulting in a greater chance of patient movement. With the use of faster film this is no longer true. We are comparing exposure times of $\frac{1}{5}$ versus $\frac{4}{5}$ second (inverse square law), and the difference in possible patient movement within these time frames is not significant. Previously, with the use of slower film, the possibility of patient movement with a 4-second exposure, compared with a 1-second exposure, was greater, and the objection was valid.

EXPOSURE ROUTINE

Regardless of which technique is used, certain basic rules must be followed regarding barrier technique, preparation of the patient, and radiation hygiene. Operators should develop a routine to avoid mistakes that necessitate retaking of films. Retaking a radiograph because of operator error adds unnecessarily to the patient's radiation burden.

The patient should be seated comfortably in the chair, with the back well supported and the head positioned so that the jaw can be radiographed correctly. Except when localizing rings are used, the occlusal plane of the jaw being radiographed must be parallel to the floor when it is in the open position.

The patient should remove any nonfixed prosthetic appliances from his mouth, as well as eyeglasses and facial jewelry, such as nose rings. Failure to do this is a common error. Glass and any metallic frame are radiopaque and may be superimposed on the film in the maxillary canine and premolar areas.

The patient should be draped with a lead apron. This is done routinely on all patients, for a single film as well as the full-mouth series. Then the operator turns on the x-ray machine and selects the desired kilovoltage and milliamperage.

The infection control procedures outlined in Chapter 5 should be followed. Most dental offices have a semiautomatic, lead film dispenser in each operatory. This enables the operator to withdraw one film at a time. The operator should take care not to touch the dispenser with the gloved hand after it has been in the patient's mouth. If a dispenser is to be used, it should be activated with the upper part of the arm or elbow. The exposed films are placed in a paper cup within a lead receptacle. If there is no lead dispenser, the desired number of films, as well as additional supplies such as bite-wing tabs and bite blocks, should be brought near the operatory at this time.

If there are no lead film dispensers and no exposed film receptacles, both the exposed and unexposed films must be kept out of the room where the x-ray machine is used. Many diagnostic dental films are fogged by secondary radiation and thus made unacceptable because they are left on the bracket table in the dental operatory when other films are being exposed. Again, poor technique on the part of the operator leads to film retakes and unnecessary exposure for the patient.

One of the more important general principles of intraoral radiographs is to have the positioned film in the patient's mouth for as short a time as possible. This decreases the likelihood of gagging and patient movement. The desired exposure time on the machine always should be set before placing the film in the patient's mouth. Many seconds can be wasted in consulting exposure charts and setting the timing dial while the film is in the patient's mouth.

While the exposure is made from the required 6-foot distance, the operator should watch the patient. If the patient moves, the operator can see the problem and retake the film immediately. A properly designed office permits this observation from behind a suitable barrier.

After the exposure has been made, the operator removes the film from the patient's mouth, dries it of saliva, and places it in the exposed film receptacle.

Some definite order should be followed for a full-mouth series of radiographs. Skipping from area to area without a set pattern often results in an omitted film. A good place to start is with the maxillary central incisor film; it is probably the easiest to position and the easiest for the patient to tolerate. One should never start with the maxillary molar film, because this is the projection most likely to excite the gag reflex; once the reflex is excited, the patient may gag on films that normally could be tolerated. After starting with the maxillary central incisor, the maxillary canine, premolar, and molar are radiographed in that order. The opposite side of the maxilla is then radiographed. It is poor technique to radiograph left canine, right canine, left premolar, and so forth. This necessitates moving the tube head constantly from one side of the patient to the other and usually results in an omitted film.

The bite-wing films are taken after maxillary periapicals, since the same head position and occlusal plane orientation are used. The mandibular periapical films are taken in the same order as the maxillary films.

Film holders

The use of film holders is strongly recommended. In the paralleling technique the film packet must be held in its proper position by one of a variety of film-holding devices all serving one purpose: to position the film parallel to the long axis of the tooth. Some of the devices, such as hemostats, Stabes, XCP, Precision, and Intrax holders, are pictured in Figure 7-8. Localizing rings align the PID with the film in both the horizontal and vertical planes and help to reduce the incidence of "cone cutting." The localizing rings are a great aid with some contour dental chairs which make it

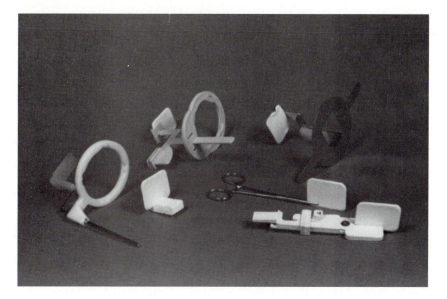

FIGURE 7-8   Film-holding (receptor) devices for use in paralleling technique. *Left to right:* XCP, Stabe, Intrax, Precision paralleling device, hemostat, Snap-A-Ray.

difficult to position the patient so that the occlusal plane is parallel to the floor. As long as the open-ended PID can be brought into flat contact with the localizing ring, strict adherence to occlusal plane orientation is not necessary.

Film holders are either disposable (e.g., styrofoam bite blocks) or nondisposable (e.g., XCP). Nondisposable film holders must be sterilized and not just disinfected.[5] As described in Chapter 5, the accepted methods of sterilization include steam autoclave, dry heat, chemical vapors, and ethylene oxide.[6] Some holding devices have plastic or vinyl parts that are not considered autoclavable.

METHOD

There are six factors that must be considered in any periapical projection: exposure time, chair position, film position and placement, point of entry of the beam, vertical angulation, and horizontal angulation.

Exposure time

Exposure time is determined by the area being radiographed, film speed, kVp, milliamperage, and FFD. Exposure charts are readily available, and most x-ray film packages contain them. It is customary to post such a chart near the machine so that exposure times need not be committed to memory. The timer always should be set before placing the film in the patient's mouth.

Chair position: occlusal and sagittal plane orientations

The patient is positioned so that when the mouth is open and the film packet is in position, the occlusal plane of the jaw being radiographed is parallel to the floor. In the maxilla this plane corresponds to the ala-tragus line on the face. When the maxilla is radiographed, the headrest is positioned high on the back of the patient's head, forcing the chin down (Figure 7-9). When the mandible is filmed, the headrest is placed below the occipital eminence, in what would be the normal dental chair position (Figure 7-10). For both upper and lower jaws the patient's head is positioned so that the sagittal plane is perpendicular to the floor (Figure 7-11).

Film position

The film packet is held with its long dimension vertical for anterior projections and horizontal for posterior periapical and bite-wing projections. The edge of the film always should extend evenly either ⅛ inch below (maxillary) or above (mandibular) the occlusal plane. This ensures adequate film at the apical area to record the image. The film should be placed in the patient's mouth so that the mounting orientation button is toward the occlusal surface (Figure 7-12). This helps in mounting and

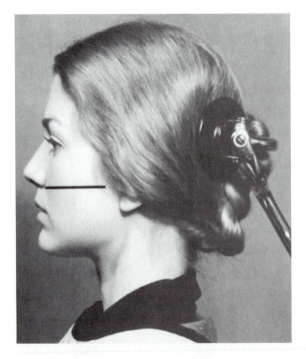

FIGURE 7-9   Proper patient position for maxillary periapical radiographs and bite-wing films. Note that occlusal plane of maxillary teeth, or ala-tragus line, is parallel to the floor.

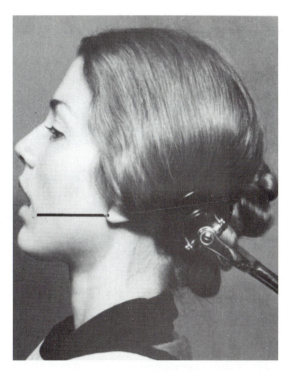

FIGURE 7-10   Proper patient position for mandibular periapical radiographs. Note that when mouth is open, occlusal plane of lower teeth is parallel to the floor.

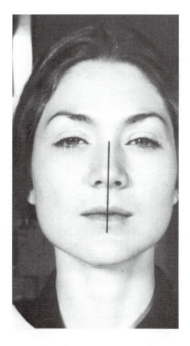

FIGURE 7-11   Proper patient position for orientation of sagittal plane of head perpendicular to the floor.

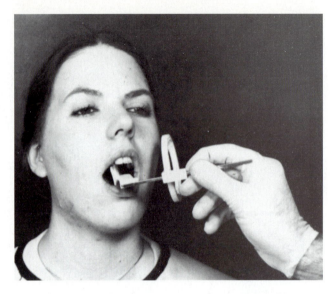

FIGURE 7-12   Placement of film-holding device in patient's mouth by operator. Note that correct side of film packet faces tube head and mounting dot is toward incisal edge.

precludes the possibility of the dots being superimposed over the apex of a tooth. The film is held in position by the patient with a bite block or other film-holding device.

Point of entry

The point of entry is the anatomic position on the patient's face at which the central ray of the x-ray beam is aimed. It corresponds to the middle of the film packet in the patient's mouth. The operator should know these anatomic points but also should align the beam with the film as viewed in the patient's mouth. The localizing ring, when used, determines the point of entry by its predetermined relationship to the film packet.

Vertical angulation

In the paralleling technique the vertical angulation is set to make the central ray perpendicular to the film. In the bisecting technique (see Chapter 8), the vertical angulation is determined by the bisection of the angle. The vertical angulations for the bisecting technique given in this text and elsewhere should be used only as guide angles. These angles can be strictly adhered to if film is positioned accurately. However, not all mouths allow this type of film positioning. Some mouths have crowded arches, misplaced teeth, and tight muscle attachments. In these cases the bisection of the film-tooth angle results in different vertical angulations than those listed. Vertical angulation of the x-ray beam is set according to the dial on the side of the tube head (Figure 7-13).

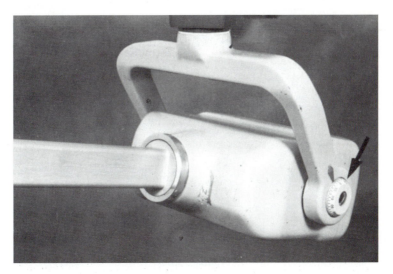

FIGURE 7-13   Photograph of tube head of x-ray machine, with arrow pointing to setting for vertical angulation.

Horizontal angulation

The central ray is directed so that it is perpendicular to the film in the horizontal plane. The central ray is directed through the interproximal spaces to avoid overlapping of structures. It may be easier for the operator to sight on the horizontal axis of the tube head and make this parallel to the film in the horizontal plane.

THE FULL-MOUTH SERIES
Maxillary central and lateral incisors (Figure 7-14)

Chair position.   The maxillary occlusal plane is positioned parallel to the floor, and the sagittal plane of the patient's face is perpendicular to the floor.

Film position.   The film is held vertically and positioned in the palate away from the lingual surfaces of the teeth so that the long axis of the film packet is parallel to the long axis of the teeth. The center of the film packet is between the central and lateral incisors. The film is positioned in the palate so that the entire length of the teeth is shown. This parallel placement of the film is held in position by one of the devices previously mentioned.

Point of entry.   The central ray is directed at the center of the film. If a localizing ring is used, the open face of the PID contacts the ring; this determines the point of entry and vertical and horizontal angulation of the x-ray beam.

Vertical angulation.   The central ray is perpendicular to the film packet.

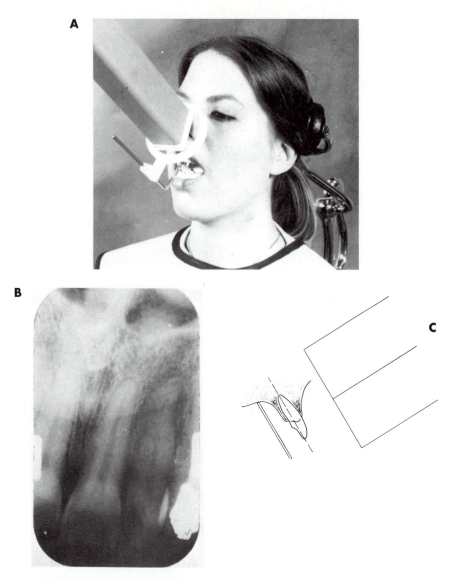

FIGURE 7-14   Maxillary central and lateral incisors. **A,** Film holder and position-indicating device (PID). **B,** Radiograph. **C,** Diagram.

Horizontal angulation. The central ray is perpendicular to the film in the horizontal plane.

If one film is to be used for the maxillary right and left central and lateral incisors, the center of the film is placed between the central incisors and the central ray is directed perpendicular to the center of the film packet (Figure 7-15).

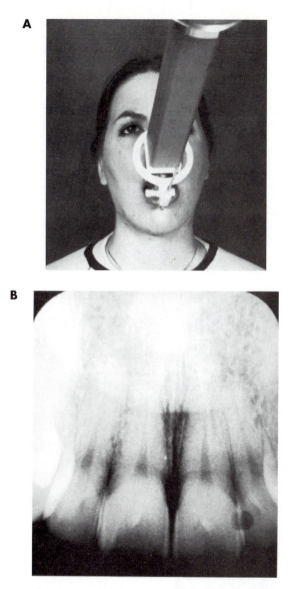

FIGURE 7-15   Right and left maxillary central and lateral incisors. **A,** Film-holding device and PID. **B,** Radiograph.

Maxillary canines (Figure 7-16)

Chair position. The maxillary occlusal plane is parallel to the floor, and the sagittal plane of the patient's face is perpendicular to the floor.

Film position. The film is held vertically, away from the lingual surface of the canine and parallel to its long axis. The center of the film packet is behind the canine

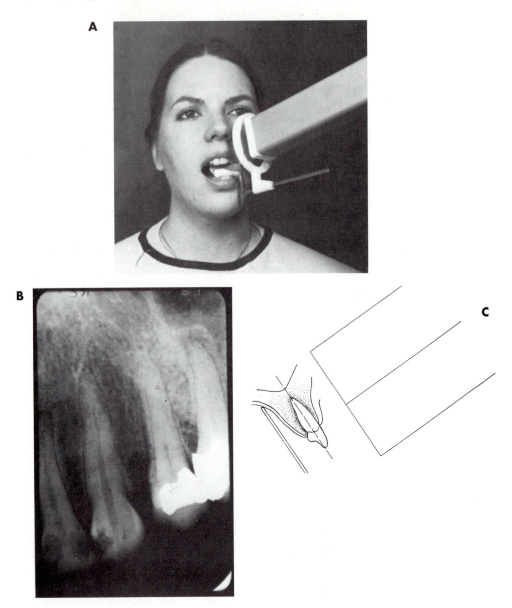

FIGURE 7-16 Maxillary canine. **A,** Film-holding device and PID. **B,** Radiograph. **C,** Diagram.

and positioned in the palate so that the entire length of the canine is shown. The film packet is held in position by a holding device.

Point of entry. The central ray is directed at the center of the film packet, or if a localizing ring is used, it is brought into flat contact with the open-ended PID.

Vertical angulation. The central ray is perpendicular to the film packet.

A

C

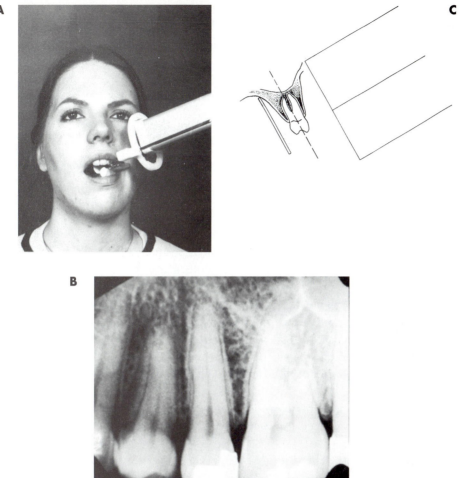

B

FIGURE 7-17 Maxillary premolars. **A,** Film-holding device and PID. **B,** Radiograph. **C,** Diagram.

Horizontal angulation. The central ray is perpendicular to the film in the horizontal plane.

Maxillary premolars (Figure 7-17)

Chair position. The maxillary occlusal plane is parallel to the floor, and the sagittal plane of the patient's face is perpendicular to the floor.

Film position. The film is held horizontally and positioned away from the lingual surfaces of the premolar so that its long axis is parallel to the long axis of the premolar. In the maxillary premolar and molar region this may position the film in the middle of the palate. The center of the film aligns with the second premolar. The packet is positioned in the palate so that the entire length of the teeth is shown on the film. The packet is held in position by a holding device.

Point of entry. The central ray is directed at the center of the film, or if a localizing ring is used, it is brought into flat contact with the open-ended PID.

Vertical angulation. The central ray is perpendicular to the film.

Horizontal angulation. The central ray is perpendicular to the film in the horizontal plane.

Maxillary molars (Figure 7-18)

Chair position. The maxillary occlusal plane is positioned parallel to the floor, and the sagittal plane of the patient's face is perpendicular to the floor.

Film position. The film is held horizontally and positioned away from the lingual surfaces of the molars so that the long axis of the film lies parallel to the long axes of the molars. The center of the film packet aligns to the middle of the second molar, and the packet is positioned in the palate so the entire length of the teeth is shown. The film packet is held in position by a holding device.

Point of entry. The central ray is directed at the center of the film, or the localizing ring is brought into flat contact with the open-ended PID.

Vertical angulation. The central ray is perpendicular to the film.

Horizontal angulation. The central ray is perpendicular to the film in the horizontal plane.

BITE-WING FILMS

The technique for bite-wing films is the same in the paralleling and bisecting angle technique except for the use of the 16-inch FFD and thus increased exposure time. Bite-wing films are always parallel films, no matter what technique is used for the periapical films. The film is positioned by the bite tab parallel to the crowns of both upper and lower teeth, and the central ray is directed perpendicular to the film.

Premolar and molar bite-wing projections (Figure 7-19)

Chair position. The maxillary occlusal plane is positioned parallel to the floor, and the sagittal plane of the patient's face is perpendicular to the floor.

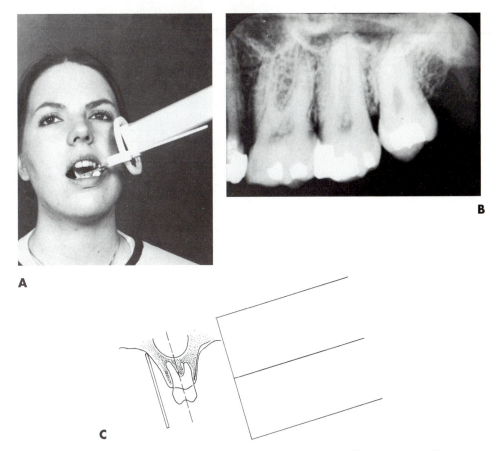

FIGURE 7-18   Maxillary molars. **A,** Film-holding device and PID. **B,** Radiograph. **C,** Diagram.

Film position. When the premolars are radiographed, the bite tab is placed on the occlusal surfaces of the first and second mandibular premolars. This depresses the film packet into the floor of the mouth. While the operator holds the tab down with thumb and forefinger, the patient is instructed to bite on the tab. The operator should be sure that the patient is biting on the back teeth and not just bringing the incisors together. If the back teeth are not moved to centric occlusion, the film packet is not secure; it may move and not be oriented correctly. The procedure for radiographing the molars is the same as that previously mentioned, except that the bite tab is centered over the occlusal surface of the second molar.

Point of entry. The central ray is directed at the bite-wing tab, which is held in position by the patient's teeth. If a localizing ring and film holder are used, the open end of the PID is placed against the ring.

Vertical angulation. The central ray is perpendicular to the film.

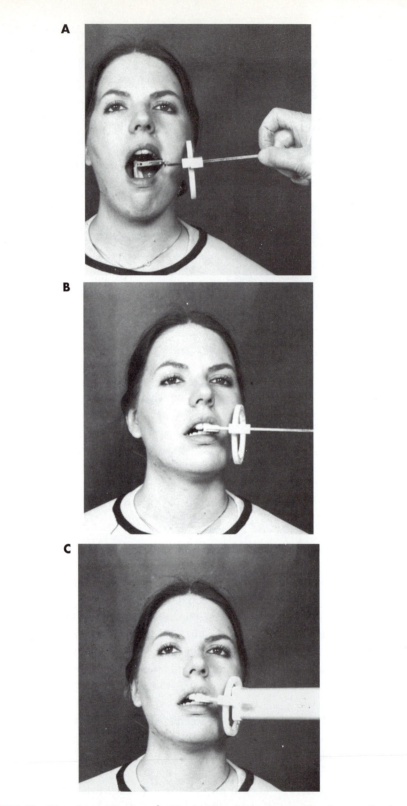

FIGURE 7-19 Bite-wing projection. **A,** Film-holding device being placed on occlusal surfaces of lower teeth. **B,** Patient bites on bite block. **C,** PID positioned.

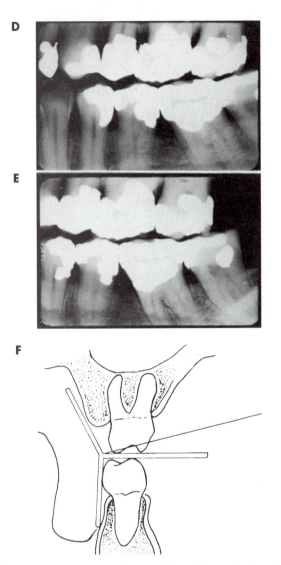

FIGURE 7-19   D, Radiograph of premolar area. E, Radiograph of molar area. F, Diagram.

Horizontal angulation. Horizontal angulation is a critical factor in the bite-wing film, and utmost attention should be paid to horizontal position. An overlapping image on the bite-wing film is useless. The central ray should be perpendicular to the film packet in the horizontal plane and should go through the contact points of the premolars or molars.

VERTICAL BITEWINGS (Figure 7-20)

Vertical bite-wings are used when the desired area would not be seen on the film with normal bite-wing placement; this could be the case in advanced bone loss or root

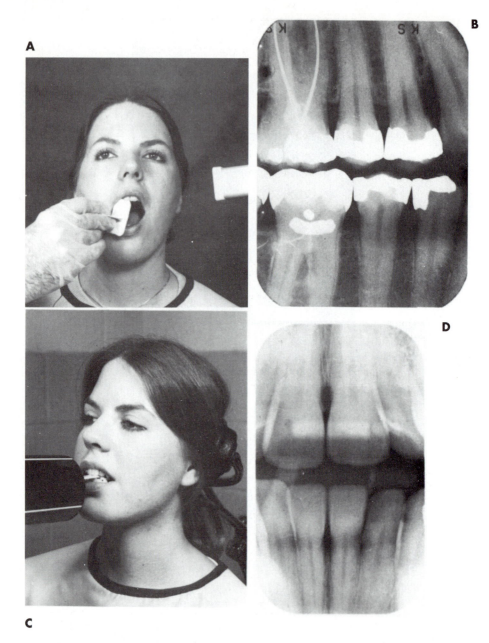

FIGURE 7-20 Vertical bite-wing. **A,** Posterior film position. **B,** Posterior radiograph. **C,** Anterior film position. **D,** Anterior radiograph.

caries. The film is placed in the patient's mouth with the longer side vertically positioned. All other exposure factors remain the same. It is necessary to use the paste-on tabs and not the loops or the preformed bite-wing packets in this technique. The vertical bitewing can be used in a posterior or anterior region.

Mandibular incisors (Figure 7-21)

Chair position. The patient is positioned so that when the mouth is open the mandibular occlusal plane is parallel to the floor and the sagittal plane of the patient's face is perpendicular to the floor.

Film position. The film is held vertically and positioned away from the lingual surfaces of the incisors so that the long axis of the film is parallel to the long axes of the incisors. The center of the packet is positioned at the midline so that all four incisors appear on the film. The film is depressed into the floor of the mouth so that the entire length of the teeth is shown. It may be necessary to displace the tongue distally as well as to depress the floor of the mouth to achieve this. The film packet is held in position by a holding device.

Point of entry. The central ray is directed at the center of the film, or the localizing ring is brought into flat contact with the open-ended PID.

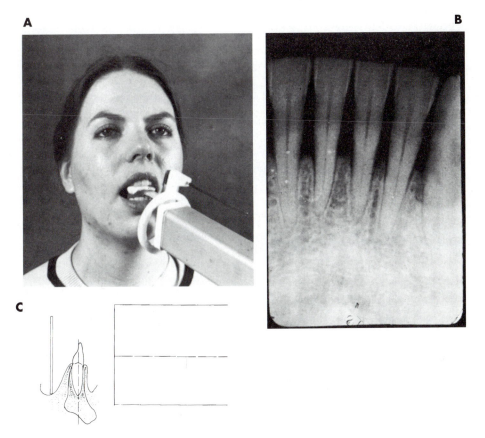

A

B

C

FIGURE 7-21 Mandibular incisors. **A,** Film-holding device and PID. **B,** Radiograph. **C,** Diagram.

Vertical angulation. The central ray is perpendicular to the film.

Horizontal angulation. The central ray is perpendicular to the film in the horizontal plane.

Mandibular canines (Figure 7-22)

Chair position. The patient is positioned so that when the mouth is open the mandibular occlusal plane is parallel to the floor and the sagittal plane of the patient's face is perpendicular to the floor.

Film position. The film is held vertically and positioned away from the lingual surface of the canine so that its long axis is parallel to that of the canine. The packet is positioned so that the canine is in the center of the film. The packet is depressed

A   B

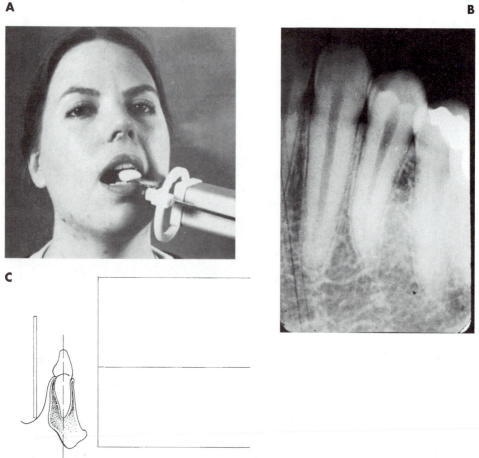

C

FIGURE 7-22 Mandibular canine. **A,** Film-holding device and PID. **B,** Radiograph. **C,** Diagram.

into the floor of the mouth so that the entire length of the tooth is shown on the film. The packet is held in position by a holding device.

Point of entry. The central ray is directed at the center of the film, or the localizing ring is brought into flat contact with the open-ended PID.

Vertical angulation. The central ray is perpendicular to the film.

Horizontal angulation. The central ray is perpendicular to the film in the horizontal plane.

Mandibular premolars (Figure 7-23)

Chair position. The patient is positioned so that when the mouth is open the mandibular occlusal plane is parallel to the floor and the sagittal plane of the patient's face is perpendicular to the floor.

Film position. The film is held horizontally and positioned so that it is parallel to the long axis of the premolar. The object-film distance in both the mandibular premolar and molar regions is almost minimal since the anatomy allows the film to be positioned very close to the tooth and still be parallel. The second premolar is

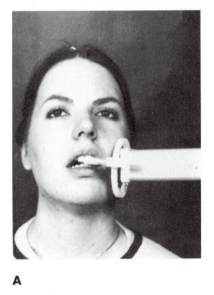

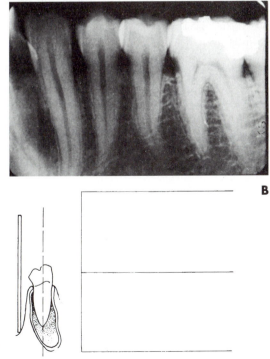

FIGURE 7-23 Mandibular premolar. **A,** Film-holding device and PID. **B,** Radiograph. **C,** Diagram.

centered behind the center of the film packet. The packet is depressed into the floor of the mouth so that the entire length of the teeth shows on the film. The film is held in position by a holding device.

Point of entry. The central ray is directed at the center of the film, or if a localizing ring is used, it is brought into flat contact with the open-ended PID.

Vertical angulation. The central ray is directed perpendicular to the film.

Horizontal angulation. The central ray is perpendicular to the film in the horizontal plane.

Mandibular molars (Figure 7-24)

Chair position. The patient is positioned so that when the mouth is open the mandibular occlusal plane is parallel to the floor and the sagittal plane of the patient's face is perpendicular to the floor.

Film position. The film is held horizontally and positioned lingually to the molar so that the long axis of the film is parallel to the long axes of the molars. The film is centered behind the second molar and depressed into the floor of the mouth so that the entire length of the teeth appears on the film. The packet is held in position by a holding device.

Point of entry. The central ray is directed at the center of the film, or if a localizing ring is used, it is brought into flat contact with the open-ended PID.

Vertical angulation. The central ray is directed perpendicular to the film.

Horizontal angulation. The central ray is perpendicular to the film in the horizontal plane.

COMMON ERRORS

All the errors mentioned and illustrated in this chapter also are possible in the bisecting technique, but the incidence differs. Whereas elongation and foreshortening are the most common bisecting errors, they are not that common in the paralleling technique. The most common error in the paralleling technique, even with the use of positioning devices, is in film placement. If the film packet and film holder are not placed correctly in the patient's mouth, the paralleling technique does not work. The most common error is to not place the film packet deep enough in the floor of the mouth or high enough in the palate, thus cutting off the apices of the teeth.

With the use of the localizing ring, which is aligned with the center of the film packet, cone cutting can be practically eliminated.

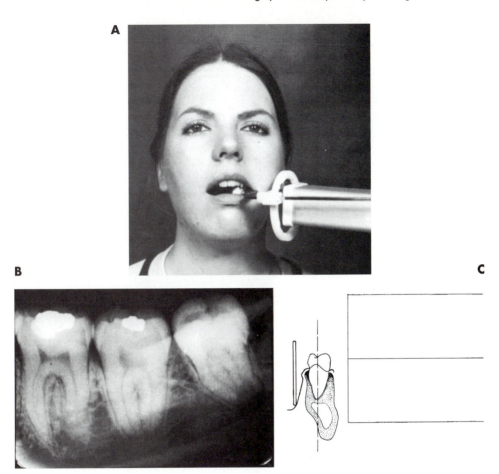

FIGURE 7-24   Mandibular molars. **A,** Film-holding device and PID. **B,** Radiograph. **C,** Diagram.

Occlusal plane and sagittal plane orientation of the patient's head is not important if the localizing ring on the film-holding device is used, as long as the open end of the PID is brought into flat contact with the localizing ring.

Horizontal overlapping of the images also is eliminated with the proper use of the positioning device and localizing ring.

The rest of the errors mentioned in this chapter (i.e., film reversal, overbending, crescent marks, overexposing and underexposing, double exposure, and failure to remove dental appliances) are all possible with the bisecting technique, and their remedies are the same.

Cone cutting (collimator cutoff) (Figure 7-25). An unexposed area on the radiograph occurs when the x-ray beam is not centered on the film packet. This is called *cone cutting* and is caused by improper x-ray beam film alignment.
Remedy. The central ray of the x-ray beam should be aligned carefully with the center of the film packet. With circular collimation the aperture of the diaphragm

A

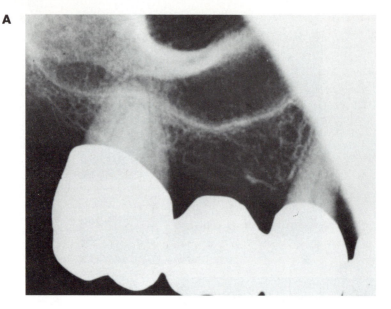

B

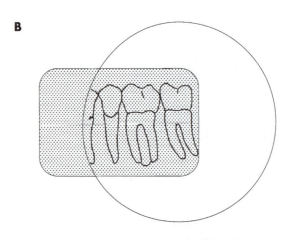

C

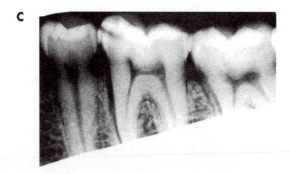

FIGURE 7-25 **A,** Collimator cutoff ("cone cutting"). Central ray positioned too far distal. **B,** Diagram of "cone cutting." Central ray positioned too far mesial. **C,** "Cone cutting" with rectangular collimation.

allows for a beam diameter, measured at the face, of 2¾ inches. Size #2 adult film is 1¼ × 1⅝ inches, which leaves almost ½-inch leeway for error in all directions. It is not sufficient to identify collimator cutoff; it should be analyzed to pinpoint the error. If it is always the distal part of a radiograph in a projection that is cut off, then the point of entry must be moved mesially. A localizing ring, with a film-holding device, aligns the beam and the film and eliminates collimator cutoff with both circular and rectangular collimation.

Film reversal (Figure 7-26). Film reversal is sometimes referred to as the "herringbone effect" because the herringbone pattern embossed on the lead foil backing is transferred to the processed, reversed radiograph. The "herringbone" light film results from placing the film packet backward in the patient's mouth. The x-rays are attenuated by the lead foil before striking the film. The pattern embossed in the lead that appears on the film distinguishes this light film from other underexposure errors.

Remedy. The front and back of the film packet should be noted. Some manufacturers color code or change the texture of the back of the packet. Operators should develop the habit of looking for these aids.

Film placement (Figure 7-27). The film has been poorly positioned if the whole tooth does not show on the film and the image is not elongated; there is no film behind the apex of the tooth to record the image.

Remedy. Only ⅛ inch of film should project above or below the occlusal or incisal edges of the teeth. If a bite block is used, the teeth being radiographed must bite firmly on the block.

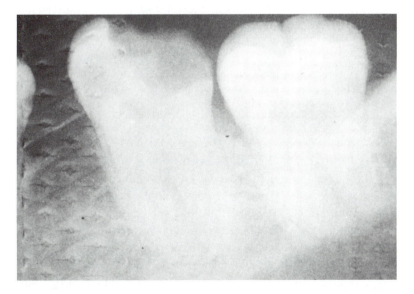

FIGURE 7-26   Film reversal. Film packet placed in mouth with the wrong side toward the tube.

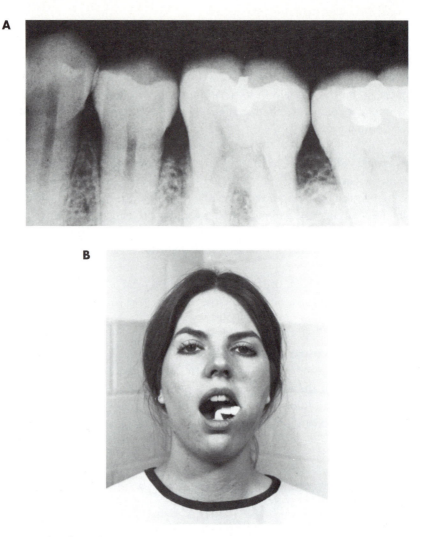

FIGURE 7-27 **A,** Nondiagnostic due to poor film packet placement. Note that apices of teeth are not seen. **B,** Poor film placement. Note how much film is visible above occlusal plane of tooth.

Overlapping (Figures 7-28 and 7-29). Overlapping of the images of the teeth will result if the central ray is not perpendicular to the film and teeth in the horizontal plane.

Remedy. The film should be aligned with some part of the tube head that is perpendicular to the central ray. There is usually a horizontal bar with the manufacturer's name on it. Standing in front of the patient, the operator should retract the patient's cheek and check the horizontal alignment. As in cone cutting, a positioning device with a localizing ring can be used to prevent overlapping. If the film is placed parallel to the teeth, the localizing ring aligns the beam perpendicular to the film.

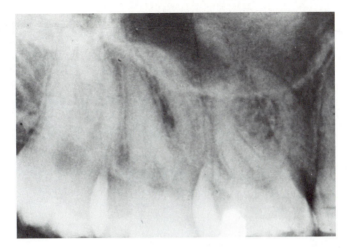

FIGURE 7-28   Overlapped images.

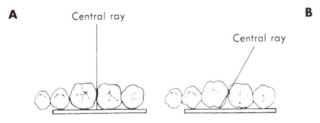

FIGURE 7-29   Proper **A**, and improper **B**, horizontal angulation of x-ray beam.

Crescent marks and bent films (Figures 7-30 and 7-31). Black crescent-shaped marks can be caused by excessive bending of the film packet, which cracks the emulsion. The crescent marks show when the film is developed. A film may be overbent to such a degree that the x-rays cannot strike it at all.

Remedy. Films can be made more pliable by rolling them slightly against one's index finger, which also may allow them to fit better in the patient's mouth. Films should not be bent to adapt to anatomic surfaces. X-rays travel in straight lines; they do not turn corners to expose bent films.

Light films (Figure 7-32). Light films or thin films without adequate density can result from underexposure or underdevelopment, assuming that the proper kVp has been used. If not enough kVp has been used, the dental structures are not adequately penetrated and the film, although light, does not differentiate structures of different density.

Remedy. For underexposure all settings on the machine should be checked before making an exposure (mA, time, kVp).

A very common error that leads to underexposure is unwittingly increasing the FFD by failing to bring the open end of the PID close to the patient's face. The exposure

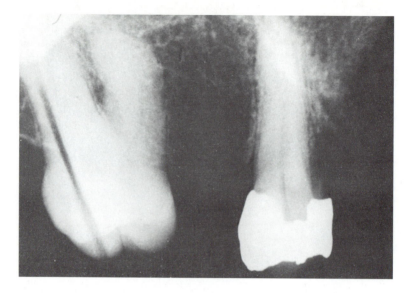

FIGURE 7-30   Black line due to cracking of film emulsion.

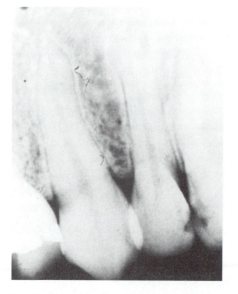

FIGURE 7-31   Result of overbending film packet. Note upper-right corner.

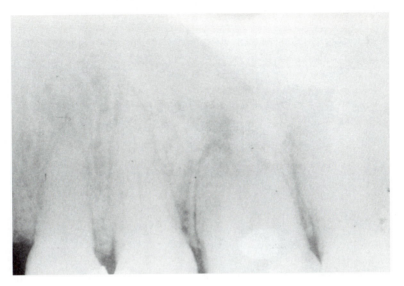

FIGURE 7-32   Underexposed radiograph.

times are calculated for an FFD that assumes a PID placement close to the face. If the PID is carelessly positioned away from the face, the inverse square lawintensifies the error, not just by the increased distance but the square of that distance (Figure 7-33). For a discussion of underdevelopment, see Chapter 6.

Dark film (Figure 7-34). Dark film is caused by overexposure or overdevelopment, the reverse causes of light films. The length of the PID prevents the possibility of decreased FFD. If a film is overpenetrated, it is black and none of the dental structures show or they are difficult to differentiate.
Remedy. To avoid overexposure operators should check all settings on the control panel before making an exposure. For a discussion of overdevelopment, see Chapter 6.

Double exposure (Figure 7-35). A double exposure results from using the same film packet twice. This is an unforgivable error and indicates lack of attention to detail.
Remedy. After the film packet has been exposed, it should be placed in a lead receptacle. The exposed and unexposed films should never be kept on the same shelf.

Blurred images (Figure 7-36). Blurred images are the result of patient, film, or tube head movement during the exposure.
Remedy. Tube heads and arms should be adjusted to prevent vibration and drifting. In most states drifting is a serious health code violation. Good chairside technique prevents film and patient movement.

A

B

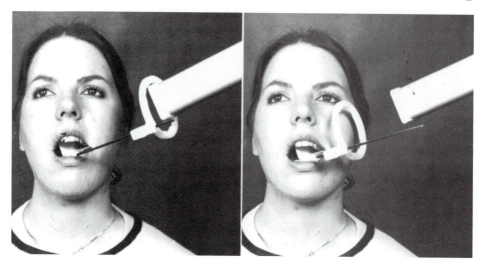

FIGURE 7-33 **A** and **B.** Light film can be caused by increased focal-film distance without compensatory increase in exposure time. Note distance between patient's face and PID.

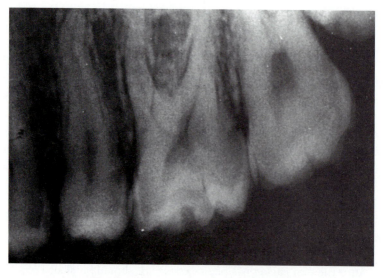

FIGURE 7-34   Overexposed radiograph.

Failure to remove dental appliances or facial jewelry (Figures 7-37 and 7-38). If dental appliances or pieces of facial jewelry are not removed, the metallic portions are superimposed on the tooth structure.

Remedy. It should be a part of the work routine to have patients remove all dentures, nose jewelry, and eyeglasses. For panoramic and extraoral projections patients also must remove earrings, hearing aids, and hair clips.

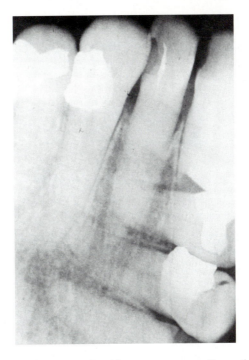

FIGURE 7-35   Double exposure on radiograph.

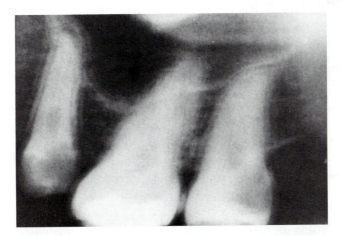

FIGURE 7-36   Blurred image caused by patient movement.

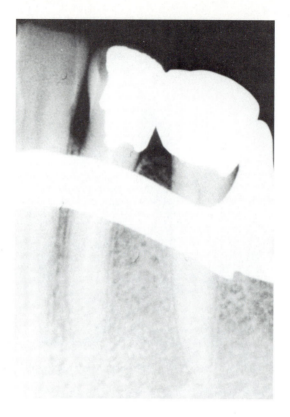

FIGURE 7-37 Patient's partial denture was not removed.

Poor bite-wings (Figure 7-39)

The three most common errors seen on bite-wing radiographs are overlapping, collimator cutoff, and film placement.

Overlapping (Figure 7-39, *A*). Overlapping results from improper horizontal beam alignment.
Remedy. The beam should be aligned in the horizontal plane so that it is at right angles to the film packet.

Collimator cutoff (cone cutting) (Figure 7-39, *B*). Collimator cutoff is failure to align the central ray with the center of the film packet. It occurs most often because the operator loses sight of the bite tab when the patient closes the mouth.
Remedy. The bite tab should be kept visible by asking the patient to smile while biting. If this is not possible, the operator can touch the tab with one hand while aligning the beam with the other. The central ray is directed at the tab. A localizing ring also can be used to help center the x-ray beam.

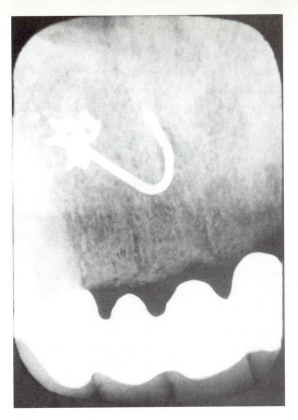

FIGURE 7-38 Facial jewelry (nose ring) was not removed.

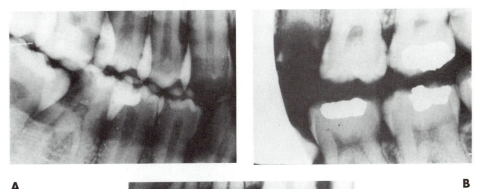

A

B

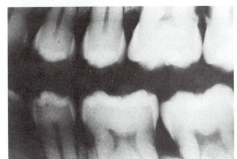

C

FIGURE 7-39 A, Overlapped bite-wing. B, Collimator cutoff on bite-wing. C, Improper film placement.

Poor film placement (Figure 7-39, *C*). Poor film placement occurs in bite-wing films when either the patient is allowed to bite the film into position after the operator has let go of the tab or the patient bites in protrusive instead of centric relation, allowing the film to float free and be repositioned by the tongue.

Remedy. The operator should not let go of the film tab until the patient is biting on it in centric occlusion.

REFERENCES

1. Department of Health and Human Services: The selection of patients for x-ray examinations: dental radiographic examinations, HHS Pub No (FDA) 88-8273, Rockville, Md, 1987, US Government Printing Office.
2. National Center for Health Care Technology: A summary of recommendations from the technology assessment forum, *J Am Dent Assoc* 103:423-425, Sept 1981.
3. Sikorski PA and Taylor KW: The effectiveness of the thyroid shield in dental radiology, *Oral Surg* 58:225-236, 1984.
4. Bean LR: Comparison of bisecting angle and paralleling methods for intraoral radiology, *J Dent Educ* 33:441-445, 1969.
5. American Academy of Oral and Maxillofacial Radiology: Infection control guidelines for dental radiographic procedures, *Oral Surg* 73:248-249, 1992.
6. American Dental Association, Council on Dental Materials, Instruments and Equipment, Council on Dental Practice, and Council on Dental Therapuetics: Infection control recommendations for the dental office and dental laboratory, *J Am Dent Assoc* 116:241-248, 1988.

Chapter

eight

Accessory Radiographic Techniques

BISECTING TECHNIQUE

Another method for taking intraoral periapical radiographs is the bisecting technique. In the bisecting technique the film packet is placed as close to the tooth as possible without bending the film. Because of the anatomy of the mouth, the long axis of the tooth is not parallel to the plane of the film with this placement. The vertical angulation of the tube head is directed so that the central ray is perpendicular to a line that bisects the angle formed by the long axis of the tooth and the plane of the dental film (see Figure 2-12). With this film placement, the object film distance is at a minimum. No compensation for image enlargement is necessary, and the technique usually calls for an 8-inch FFD. Although a "short cone" is used, this is not the determining factor in the technique.

ADVANTAGES AND DISADVANTAGES

Before listing the supposed advantages of the bisecting technique, we must note again that the consensus of opinion now among dental radiologists is that the paralleling technique is the technique of choice for periapical radiography. The bisecting technique should be considered an ancillary method that can be used in special circumstances when it is not possible to use the paralleling technique. It is in this context that the bisecting technique is presented in this textbook.

Advantages

The bisecting-angle technique is said to be easier to perform and is still used by many dentists in practice at this time. The use of the patient's finger or simple bite blocks for holding the film packets in position avoids the use of the paralleling instruments. For patients with small mouths, for children, and for patients with low palatal vaults, paralleling devices may be extremely difficult to use.

Since the film is held close to the tooth, it is possible to use an 8-inch FFD, and the objectionable, bulky, extension cylinder necessary in the paralleling technique can be avoided. This objection is not valid in the newer machines with the extended FFD within the tube head. Another argument is that a well-designed office should have room for the extra 8 inches of the PID.

Shorter exposure times can be used in the bisecting technique because of the shorter FFD; hence there is less chance for patient movement. In reality, this may not be a valid objection; with the use of faster film, we are comparing exposure times of 1/10 versus 4/10 second (inverse square law). Previously, with the use of slower films, the possibility of movement with a 4-second exposure compared with a 1-second exposure was greater, and the advantage was clear.

Disadvantages

The major disadvantage of the bisecting technique is that the image projected on the film is dimensionally distorted (see Chapter 7).

The bisecting technique is difficult to perform with the patient in a contour chair or in the supine position, as used in four-handed dentistry. In the newer dental chairs it is very hard to place the patient in the correct position so that the occlusal plane of the jaw being radiographed is parallel to the floor. All vertical angulations used in the bisecting technique are measured from this line.

Other disadvantages of the bisecting technique are related to the use of an 8-inch FFD. The 8-inch FFD when compared to the extended 16-inch FFD causes greater image enlargement and distortion (see Figure 2-6). There is also more tissue volume exposed with an 8-inch FFD than with a 16-inch FFD (see Chapter 4).

If the patient's finger is used to support the film, as is common in this method, then the patient's finger and hand are exposed unnecessarily to primary radiation. A bite block always should be used instead of the patient's finger.

METHOD

In this periapical technique the film is held as close to the tooth as possible without bending the film. The long axis of the film therefore is not parallel to the long axis of the tooth. An imaginary line is drawn to bisect the angle formed by the long axis of the tooth and the plane of the film. The central ray of the x-ray beam is directed perpendicular to this bisecting line; this determines the vertical angulation of the x-ray beam (see Figure 2-12). For the maxillary teeth, positive angulation (PID pointing down) is used, and for mandibular teeth, negative angulation (PID pointing up) is used. At zero-degree angulations, the PID is parallel to the floor; this becomes the reference point from which vertical angulations are measured. Therefore it is crucial to have the occlusal plane of the jaw being radiographed positioned parallel to the floor for predetermined angulations to be valid.

THE FULL-MOUTH SERIES
Maxillary central and lateral incisors (left or right) (Figure 8-1)

Chair position. The maxillary occlusal plane is positioned parallel to the floor, and the sagittal plane of the patient's face is perpendicular to the floor.

Film position. The film packet is held vertically so that it extends evenly ⅛ inch below the incisal edge of the incisors. The midpoint of this ⅛-inch border should be between the lateral and central incisors. The film packet is positioned as close to the lingual surface of the incisors as possible without bending it.

Point of entry. The central ray is directed just below the midpoint of the nares, aimed at the center of the film packet.

A   **B**

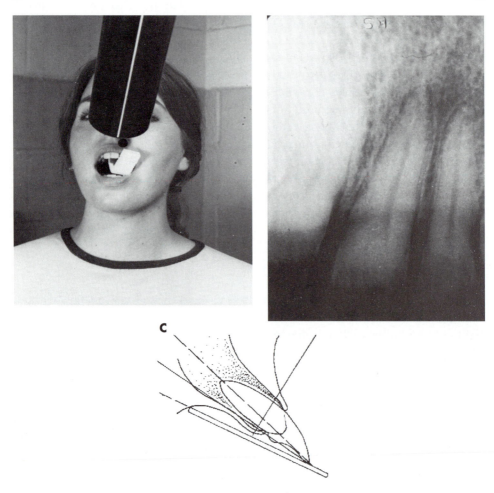

C

FIGURE 8-1 Maxillary central and lateral incisors. **A,** Film packet and PID. Dot represents point of entry. **B,** Radiograph. **C,** Diagram.

Vertical angulation. +50 degrees.

Horizontal angulation. The central ray is perpendicular to the film packet in the horizontal plane.

If only one film is to be used for the right and left maxillary central and lateral incisors, the center of the film packet is placed between the central incisors, and the central ray is directed just below the tip of the nose (Figure 8-2).

Maxillary canines (Figure 8-3)

Chair position. The maxillary occlusal plane is positioned parallel to the floor, and the sagittal plane of the patient's face is perpendicular to the floor.

Film position. The film packet is held vertically and extends ⅛ inch below the tip of the canine. The canine is in the center of the film packet, which is held firmly against the lingual surface of the canine.

Point of entry. The central ray is directed at the base of the lateral nasal grove, aimed at the center of the film packet.

Vertical angulation. +50 degrees.

A   **B**

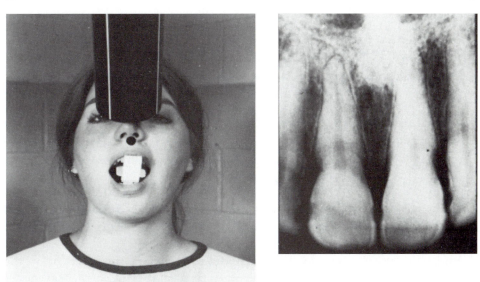

FIGURE 8-2 Right and left central and lateral incisors. **A,** Film packet and PID. Dot represents point of entry. **B,** Radiograph.

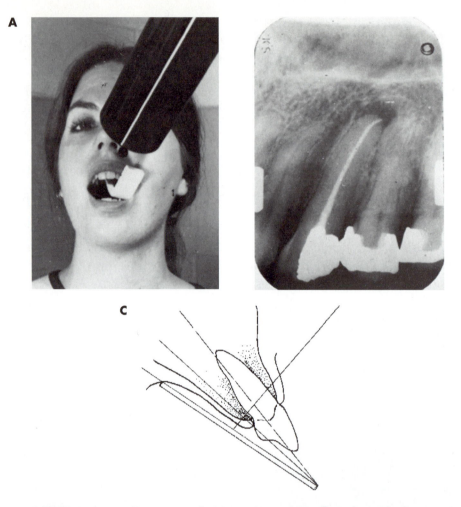

FIGURE 8-3 Maxillary canine. **A,** Film packet and PID. **B,** Radiograph. **C,** Diagram.

Horizontal angulation. The central ray is perpendicular to the film packet in the horizontal plane.

Maxillary premolars (Figure 8-4)

Chair position. The maxillary occlusal plane is positioned parallel to the floor, and the sagittal plane of the patient's face is perpendicular to the floor.

Film position. The film packet is held horizontally and extends ⅛ inch below the occlusal surfaces of the teeth. The second premolar is in the center of the film packet. The packet is held in position against the lingual surfaces. The operator should avoid shaping the packet to the arch.

A

B

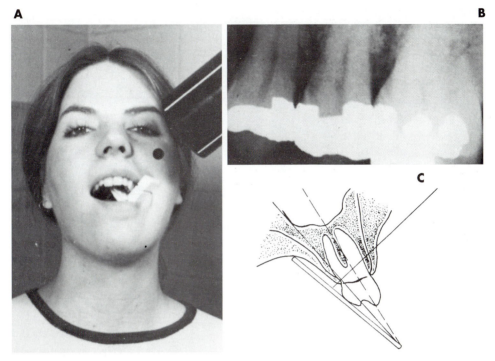

C

FIGURE 8-4   Maxillary premolars. **A,** Film packet and PID. **B,** Radiograph. **C,** Diagram.

Point of entry. The central ray is directed at the most anterior part of the cheekbone, aimed at the center of the film packet.

Vertical angulation. +40 degrees.

Horizontal angulation. The central ray is perpendicular to the film packet in the horizontal plane and is directed through the interproximal spaces.

Maxillary molars (Figure 8-5)

Chair position. The maxillary occlusal plane is positioned parallel to the floor, and the sagittal plane of the patient's face is perpendicular to the floor.

Film position. The film is held horizontally and extends ⅛ inch evenly below the occlusal surfaces of the teeth. The second molar is in the center of the film packet. The film packet is held against the lingual surfaces of the teeth.

Point of entry. The central ray is directed through the zygomatic arch at the center of the film. The distal curvature of the open-ended "cone" should not be distal to the outer canthus (corner) of the eye.

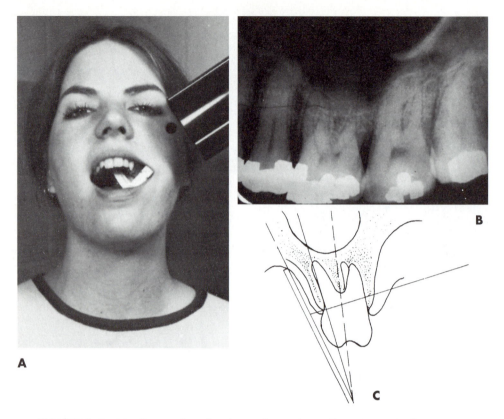

FIGURE 8-5   Maxillary molars. **A,** Film packet and PID. **B,** Radiograph. **C,** Diagram.

Vertical angulation. +30 degrees.

Horizontal angulation. The central ray is perpendicular to the film packet in the horizontal plane and is directed through the interproximal spaces.

Mandibular incisors (Figure 8-6)

Chair position. The patient is positioned so that when the mouth is open the mandibular occlusal plane is parallel to the floor and the sagittal plane of the patient's face is perpendicular to the floor.

Film position. The film packet is held vertically so that it extends ⅛ inch above the incisal edges of the incisors. The midpoint of this ⅛-inch border should be between the central incisors. All four lower incisors are shown on one film. The film is held against the lingual surfaces of the incisors.

Point of entry. The central ray is directed at the depression in the face just above the chin (mental groove), aimed at the center of the film.

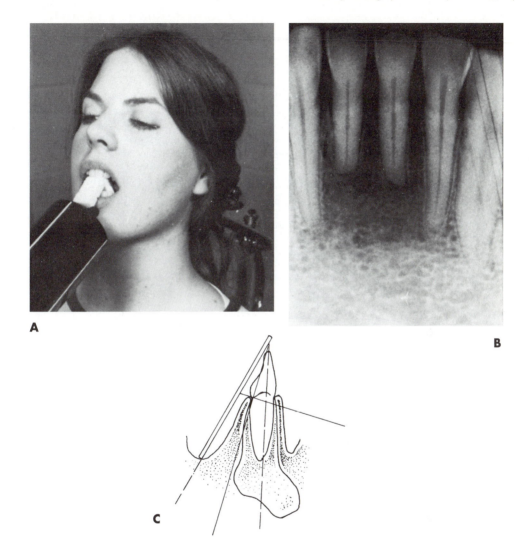

FIGURE 8-6   Mandibular incisors. **A,** Film packet and PID. **B,** Radiograph. **C,** Diagram.

Vertical angulation. −20 degrees.

Horizontal angulation. The central ray is perpendicular to the film in the horizontal plane.

Mandibular canines (Figure 8-7)

Chair position. The patient is positioned so that when the mouth is open, the mandibular occlusal plane is parallel to the floor and the sagittal plane of the patient's face is perpendicular to the floor.

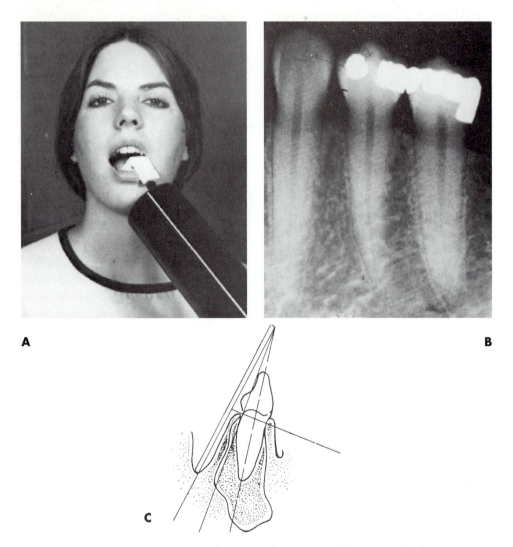

A

B

C

FIGURE 8-7   Mandibular canine. A, Film packet and PID. B, Radiograph, C, Diagram.

Film position. The film packet is held vertically and extends ⅛ inch above the tip of the canine, which is in the center of the film packet. The film packet is held against the lingual surface of the canine.

Point of entry. The central ray is directed at the root of the canine, aimed at the middle of the film packet.

Vertical angulation. –20 degrees.

Horizontal angulation. The central ray is perpendicular to the film in the horizontal plane.

Mandibular premolars (Figure 8-8)

Chair position. The patient is positioned so that when the mouth is open the mandibular occlusal plane is parallel to the floor and the sagittal plane of the patient's face is perpendicular to the floor.

Film position. The film packet is held horizontally and extends ⅛ inch above the occlusal surfaces of the teeth. The second premolar is in the center of the film. The film packet is held against the lingual surfaces of the teeth.

Point of entry. The central ray is directed at the mental foramen, aimed at the center of the film packet.

Vertical angulation. –15 degrees.

Horizontal angulation. The central ray is perpendicular to the film in the horizontal plane.

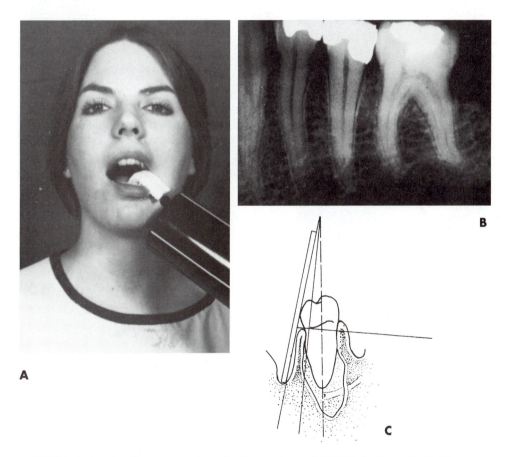

A

B

C

FIGURE 8-8   Mandibular premolars. **A,** Film packet and PID. **B,** Radiograph. **C,** Diagram.

Mandibular molars (Figure 8-9)

Chair position. The patient is positioned so that when the mouth is open, the mandibular occlusal plane is parallel to the floor and the sagittal plane of the patient's face is perpendicular to the floor.

Film position. The film packet is held horizontally and extends ⅛ inch above the occlusal surfaces of the molars. The second molar is in the middle of the film. The film is held against the lingual surface of the molars. Because of the anatomy of the area, the film packet is almost parallel to the long axis of the tooth, and most molar periapical films done in the bisecting technique are really parallel films.

Point of entry. The central ray is directed at the roots of the molars, aimed at the center of the film packet.

Vertical angulation. −5 degrees.

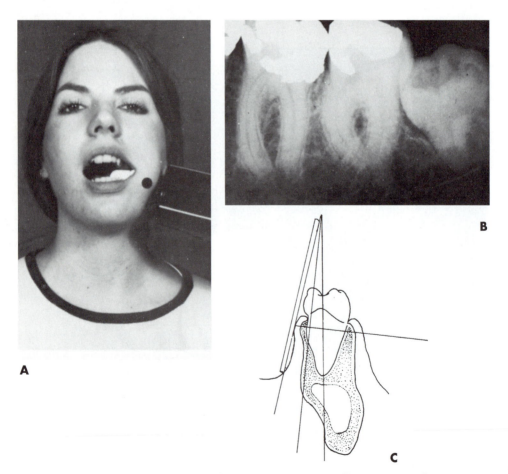

FIGURE 8-9 Mandibular molars. **A,** Film packet and PID. **B,** Radiograph. **C,** Diagram.

Horizontal angulation. The central ray is perpendicular to the film packet in the horizontal plane.

COMMON ERRORS

The following are the most common errors seen in the bisecting technique. Recognition and correction of occasional errors in technique are important. Not all patients are cooperative or have anatomically large mouths that are easy to radiograph. Remember that films retaken because of poor technique add unnecessarily to the patient's radiation burden (see Chapter 7 for a discussion of other chairside errors).

Elongation (Figure 8-10). *Elongation,* or lengthening of the image on the film, can be caused by inadequate vertical angulation, improper occlusal plane orientation because of patient position, or poor film placement.
Remedy. The film and the central ray must be in the correct relationship. In the bisecting-angle technique the vertical angulation should be increased to correct elongation. The occlusal plane of the jaw being radiographed should be parallel to the floor. Patients tend to move after a few exposures or lift their heads to watch the operator. Their movements disorient the occlusal plane. Check the patient's head position before making each exposure.

Foreshortening (Figure 8-11). *Foreshortening,* the shortening of the image on the film, is not as frequent an error as elongation. It can be caused by excessive vertical angulation or poor occlusal plane orientation.

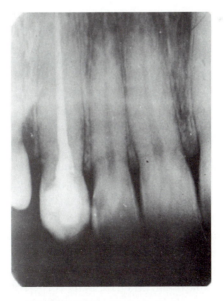

FIGURE 8-10   Elongated image.

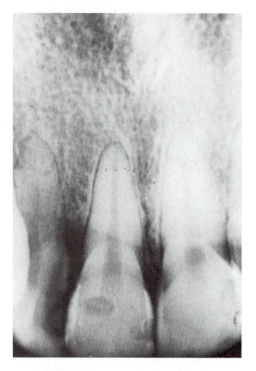

FIGURE 8-11 Foreshortened image.

Remedy. In the bisecting-angle technique, the vertical angulation should be decreased to overcome errors of foreshortening.

Sagittal plane orientation (Figure 8-12). When the periapical radiographs show the occlusal surfaces of the teeth, the patient's head has tipped away from the proper sagittal plane. This is accompanied by elongation of the image.
Remedy. The operator should make sure the patient does not tip his or her head away from the tube head as it is brought into approximation with the skin.

EDENTULOUS SERIES

A full-mouth series of radiographs is taken, even though the patient may be wholly or partially edentulous. The absence of teeth in an area of the mouth does not preclude the possibility of retained roots, impacted teeth, cysts, and other pathologic conditions present in the bone. The edentulous series is usually composed of 13 periapical films. The bite-wing films are not taken, since there are no teeth to support the tabs, and only one film is used in the maxillary central, lateral, and canine area (Figure 8-13). In small edentulous mouths an 11-film survey may suffice by using only one mandibular anterior periapical film and extending the premolar projection anteriorly to include the canine area.

A

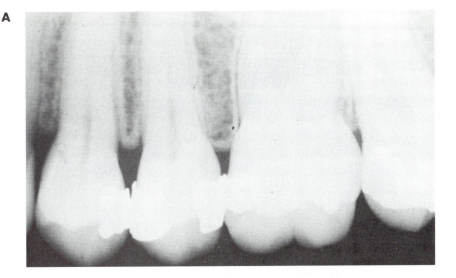

B

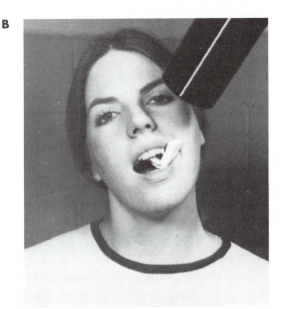

FIGURE 8-12 **A,** Elongated and distorted radiograph caused by poor sagittal plane orientation of patient's head. **B,** Poor sagittal plane orientation.

The films are positioned in the same way as a regular series, but with certain modifications. The crest of the edentulous ridge replaces the occlusal plane of the teeth as the plane of orientation. The film is positioned either ⅛ inch above or below the ridge. Since there are no teeth and there may be a great deal of ridge resorption, the film lies flatter against the palate or in the floor of the mouth, increasing the angle to be bisected. The vertical angulation then must be much greater. The best guideline

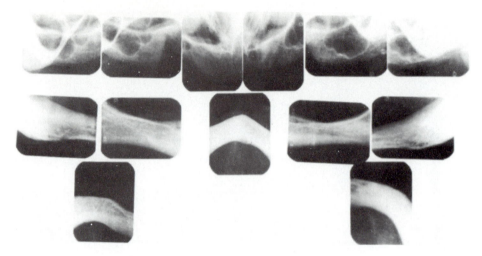

FIGURE 8-13　A 13-film edentulous survey.

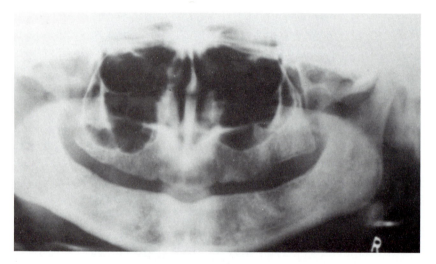

FIGURE 8-14　Edentulous panoramic survey.

in the edentulous series is to adjust the vertical angulation so that the central ray is almost perpendicular to the film. Any slight foreshortening that may result will not affect the diagnosis of any intrabony conditions. If the paralleling technique is used, extra cotton rolls may be necessary to support the holding device while the film is kept parallel to the edentulous ridge.

The exposure times are reduced by a factor of one fourth for the edentulous series.

There are two possible alternatives to the edentulous periapical survey. The first is a panoramic survey (Figure 8-14) which will be dicussed in Chapter 10; the second is the use of topographic occlusal film projections. The entire maxillary and mandibular ridges usually can be seen in their respective occlusal projections (Figure 8-15). Both

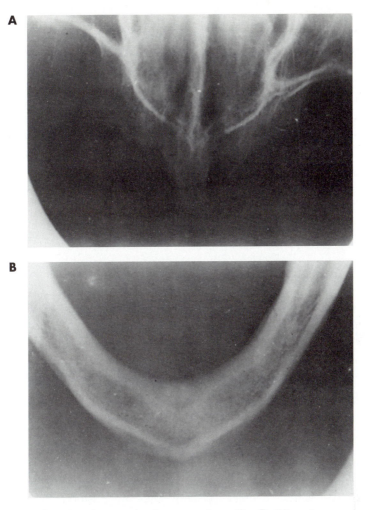

FIGURE 8-15 **A,** Edentulous occlusal survey of maxilla. **B,** Edentulous occlusal survey of mandible.

the panoramic and the occlusal are survey films, and if any suspicious areas are seen, a periapical projection of the area is done to make a definitive diagnosis.

OCCLUSAL FILM PROJECTIONS

Occlusal film projections are used to localize objects and pathologic conditions in the buccolingual dimension and to visualize areas that would not be seen on periapical films because of the insufficient field size. The right-angle occlusal technique is used for localizing in the buccolingual dimension; the topographic occlusal technique is used for the large pathologic areas. Occlusal films also are used when proper placement of periapical films is not possible in children or handicapped patients (see Chapter 11).

Right-angle projections

In right-angle projections the central ray is directed at an angle of 90 degrees to the film. For example, this technique would be used to locate an object such as an impacted tooth in the third dimension. We have mentioned that dental radiographs picture a three-dimensional subject in a two-dimensional plane, usually vertical and horizontal. The radiographs do not indicate depth. In the example of the impacted tooth, we might know from a conventional radiograph the impaction's mesiodistal location and its vertical height from the crest of the alveolar ridge, but we would not know its depth in the bone in a buccolingual dimension. One way to determine whether an impacted mandibular molar lies buccal or lingual to the alveolar ridge is to take a radiograph from another direction. In this example it would be an occlusal radiograph, with the central ray coming from underneath the mandible, directed at a right angle to a film placed on the occlusal surface of the mandibular teeth.

Topographic projections

The angulation of the topographic projection may vary from 45 to 75 degrees, depending on the anatomic area. Since the occlusal packet is approximately four times the size of the intraoral packet, it can record areas that would not be seen on the smaller film. The extreme vertical angulations are necessary to compensate for the lack of parallelism between the object and the film. This is a modification of the bisecting-angle technique.

Film packet

The occlusal film packet (size #4) is 2½ × 3 inches and is supplied in either single or double films (Figure 8-16), available in either film speed D or E. These films are sometimes called "sandwich films," because they are positioned in the patient's mouth with the teeth closed on the film packet, resembling the biting of a sandwich. Occlusal films are processed in the darkroom in the same way as other intraoral films.

Mandibular occlusal technique

In the mandibular occlusal technique the film packet is placed in the patient's mouth on the occlusal surfaces of the lower teeth. The back of the film packet faces the palate, with the front of the packet facing the tongue on the occlusal surfaces of the lower teeth. In patients with small mouths it is possible to get both right and left sides of the mandible on one film if it is inserted with the longer side extending across the patient's mouth. In patients with larger mouths it may be necessary to take separate film of each half of the mandible. In this instance the longest dimension of the film packet will run anteroposteriorly. The film is placed as far posterior on the mandible as possible so that the edge of the packet touches the ascending ramus of the

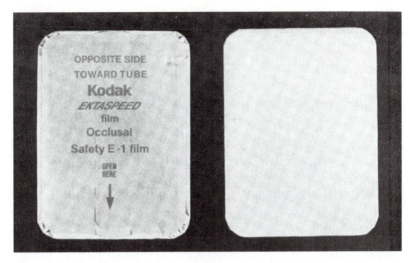

FIGURE 8-16   Front and back of occlusal film packet.

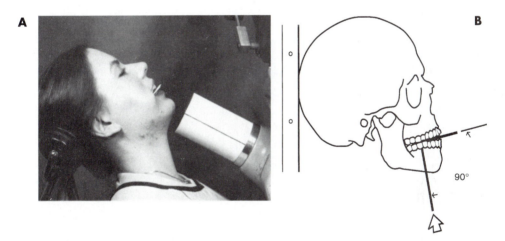

FIGURE 8-17   **A,** Film placement and PID position for mandibular right-angle occlusal film. Note that central ray is directed at 90 degrees to center of film packet. **B,** Diagram.

mandible. The patient is directed to bite gently on the film packet. For the right-angle projection, the central ray of the x-ray beam is directed from under the mandible, so that it is perpendicular to the center of the film packet (Figures 8-17 and 8-18). For the topographic view of the mandible, the central ray is directed at a point just above the mental eminence at a vertical angulation of 65 degrees. To accomplish these angulations the operator must tip the headrest of the chair back and have the patient extend his or her head and neck posteriorly (Figures 8-19 and 8-20).

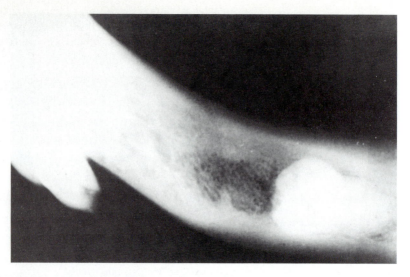

FIGURE 8-18 Right-angle occlusal radiograph of patient's mandibular posterior area. Note buccal and lingual cortex of bone and central position of the impaction.

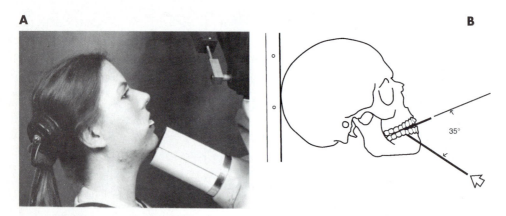

FIGURE 8-19 **A,** Topographic mandibular occlusal projection. **B,** Diagram.

Maxillary occlusal technique

In an anterior topographic occlusal view of the maxilla, the film packet is placed in the patient's mouth with the front of the film packet facing the palate and the long dimension of the packet running across the mouth. The packet is positioned as far posterior as possible so that the posterior edge of the film packet touches the ascending ramus of the mandible. With the patient's head positioned so that the film plane is parallel to the floor, the central ray is directed at a 50- to 65-degree vertical angulation through the bridge of the nose (Figures 8-21 and 8-22). In the right-angle occlusal view of the maxilla, the film is placed in the same position in the

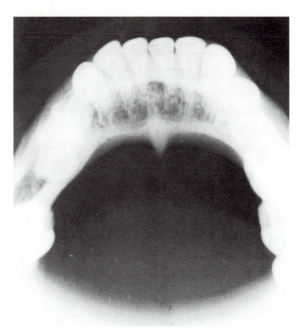

FIGURE 8-20   Topographic occlusal projection of mandible.

A   **B**

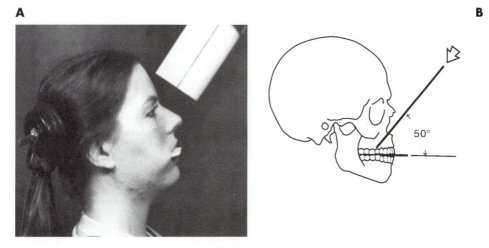

FIGURE 8-21   **A,** Film placement and PID position for topographic occlusal view of maxilla. Note that central ray is directed at 50 to 65 degrees to bridge of nose. **B,** Diagram.

patient'smouth but the central ray is directed perpendicular to the center of the film packet. To do this the PID must be positioned above the head of the patient at about the hairline. The vertical angulation is 90 degrees. Since there is an increased FFD when compared with the maxillary topographic view, this projection requires a longer exposure time (Figures 8-23 and 8-24).

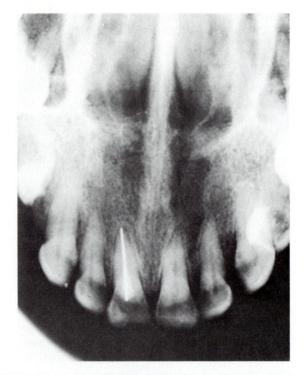

FIGURE 8-22   Occlusal radiograph of the maxilla, topographic view.

A

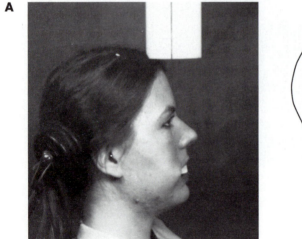

B

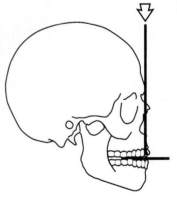

FIGURE 8-23   **A,** Film placement and PID position for a right-angle occlusal view of maxilla. Note that central ray is directed at 90 degrees to film packet. **B,** Diagram.

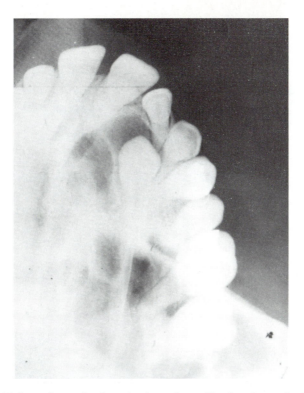

FIGURE 8-24   Right-angle occlusal projection of maxilla showing palatal relationship of impacted canine.

The posterior topographic view can be considered a topographic view of the maxillary sinus. The film packet is positioned either on the left or the right side of the patient's mouth, from the midline, laterally with the long side running anteroposteriorly. The central ray is directed to a point just above the apices of the premolars at a vertical angulation of 55 degrees (Figures 8-25 and 8-26).

A

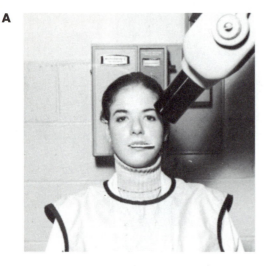

B

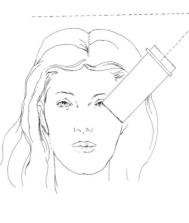

FIGURE 8-25   **A,** Posterior topographic occlusal projection. **B,** Diagram. The point of entry corresponds to the apices of the premolars, and vertical angulation is about 55 degrees.

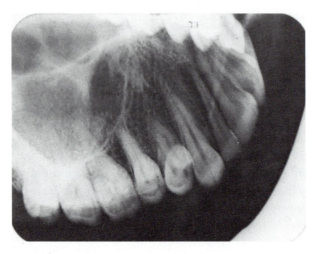

FIGURE 8-26   Topographic occlusal radiograph of maxillary sinus.

Chapter

Extraoral Radiographic Techniques

Dental radiography is not limited to the intraoral periapical, bite-wing, and occlusal films that have been previously described. There are many accessory techniques, intraoral and extraoral, using different imaging systems, film screen combinations, different projections, and other such types of x-ray machines as the panoramic unit. All of the extraoral techniques that are described in this chapter can be performed with the conventional dental x-ray unit in the dental office.

As with intraoral radiographs, the dental auxiliary should be knowledgeable and skilled in these accessory techniques. However, some states have laws that prohibit the dental auxiliary from performing certain extraoral techniques. Information about these restrictions is readily available from the appropriate agencies in individual states.

Newer imaging techniques such as CT scanning and magnetic resonance imaging (MRI) also are used by dentists to make complicated diagnoses, although this type of equipment is not found in the dental office. The dental auxiliary as an educated, aware professional should have some familiarity with these new imaging systems.

EXTRAORAL PROJECTIONS
Indications

There are two main categories of indications for the use of extraoral radiographs. The first is a situation in which a patient cannot or will not open his or her mouth to allow the film packet to be placed intraorally. Handicapped patients may be unable to open their mouths for film placement, and uncooperative patients may refuse (see Chapter 11). Patients with trismus or with temporomandibular joint ankylosis cannot open their mouths.

The second indication is when the area being radiographed is larger than or cannot be seen on intraoral films. There are many areas of the mandible and maxilla that cannot be seen on intraoral films. The scope of dental treatment is not limited to the teeth and alveolar bone; it may be necessary to radiograph such areas as the angle and ramus of the mandible, the temporomandibular joint, maxillary sinus, or lesions that grow so large they cannot be seen completely on periapical films.

Equipment

The equipment needed to do standard extraoral projections is minimal and not too costly. Extraoral techniques require a regular dental x-ray unit, film cassette, 8 × 10 or 5 × 7 inch film, intensifying screens, and cassette holders or angling boards. The use of grids is optional.

X-ray unit. Extraoral radiographs can be taken with a standard dental x-ray unit. The x-ray machine must be positioned in the operatory so that an FFD of 36 inches can be achieved. This is necessary to get a sufficiently large beam size at the patient's face. The kVp and mA of the dental x-ray machine are in the suitable range for extraoral radiography.

Cassettes. The films are contained in a carrier called a *cassette*. The cassette can be rigid or flexible and can come in varying sizes corresponding to the size of the film used (Figure 9-1). The rigid cassette may be cardboard, metal, plastic, or a combination of these. A cassette must be lighttight and yet allow the passage of x-rays to affect the x-ray film and intensifying screen contained within the cassette. The film packet wrapping in intraoral film also can be considered a cassette—a paper cassette—although it is never referred to as such.

Cassettes must be marked with lead letters to identify whether the film is of the left or right, or it will not be possible to orient the finished radiograph. Extraoral films have no raised dot to signify which side of the film should face the x-ray tube. Lead strips are available to imprint the patient's name and the date on the film.

A

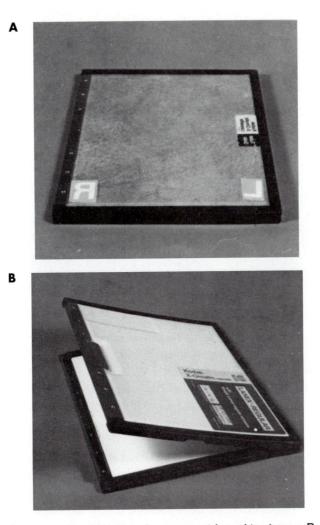

B

FIGURE 9-1   **A,** Front view of 8 × 10 inch cassette with marking letters. **B,** Cassette partially open.

Film screen combination

The imaging system used in extraoral radiography is a film screen system. The film is used in combination with intensifying screens. Previously in dentistry some extraoral projections were taken with film alone in the so-called nonscreen technique. Today, with the improved film quality and our concern for radiation safety, all extraoral films should be taken using intensifying screens. The screen film used is more sensitive to the light emitted by the intensifying screens than it is to radiation. However, the film used has to be sensitive to the type of light emitted by the particular screen (e.g., blue light or green light).

Extraoral film is available in 5 × 7 or 8 × 10 inch sizes as well as the panoramic sizes, 5 × 12 and 6 × 12 inches.

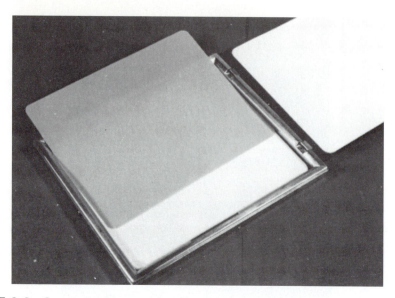

FIGURE 9-2   Cassette in open position, showing front and back intensifying screens and piece of film.

Intensifying screens. Metal and plastic cassettes usually contain intensifying screens (Figure 9-2). The rigid, nonflexible ones have the intensifying screens mounted on the inside of the front and back of the cassette. As the name implies, these screens intensify or increase the radiation and thus decrease the exposure time. The screens are coated with a substance that has the property of *fluorescence.* Such a substance emits light when struck by x-radiation and is called a phosphor.

The intensifying screens produce light in the same pattern as the x-rays that have penetrated the object so that the film sandwiched inside the cassette between the intensifying screens is affected by both x-rays and the light from the intensifying screen. However, a loss of image detail results from this intensification of the x-ray beam as the light produces a halo at the periphery of the field (Figure 9-3) that diffuses the borders of the image and thus decreases image sharpness.

Intensifying screens vary in their speed or exposure time requirements, just as film does. The speed of the screen depends on the type of phosphor and the size of the crystal. The larger the crystal, the faster the screen but the poorer the definition. Until a few years ago the most common type of phosphor was calcium tungstate, which produces blue light. A number of new phosphors, the rare earth elements, are now used in intensifying screens. The rare earth elements are four times more efficient in converting x-ray energy into light than calcium tungstate crystals, and thus the screens are faster and require less exposure time. Rare earth screens must be used with a compatible film that is sensitive to the light in the green portion of the light spectrum. It is recommended that the rare earth screens with their corresponding film be used in preference to the calcium tungstate screens. The appropriate film must be used with the intensifying screen.

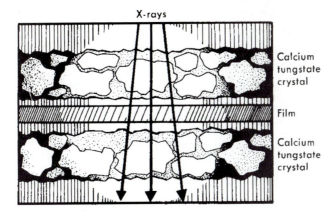

FIGURE 9-3   Diagram of effect of x-rays on intensifying screens. Note halo of light produced at periphery that reduces radiographic definition.

Fast screens usually are used for extraoral work, because the lesions we are looking for are marked by gross changes. An extraoral projection using intensifying screens would not be the procedure of choice when looking for recurrent decay or a thickened periodontal membrane.

When cassettes are loaded or unloaded in the darkroom, operators should take care not to scratch the intensifying screens with sharp objects such as film racks. If an intensifying screen is badly scratched and the phosphor removed, a white streak will appear on the film taken with this screen. Damaged screens and cassettes should be discarded. Maintenance and monitoring of screens is part of a quality control program.

Holding devices.   Extraoral film holders are available that can be wall mounted or used on a tabletop. If no device is available, the patient can hold the cassette. Holding devices have the disadvantage of standardizing techniques and preventing patient and film movement (Figure 9-4).

Grids.   The use of grids for extraoral radiography is not common in dental practice. The function of the grid is to decrease the amount of scatter radiation originating in the object (Figure 9-5). This scatter degrades the image by decreasing the contrast. The grid is a plate of radiotransparent and radioabsorptive strips that is placed in front of the cassette. The grid absorbs all radiation leaving the object that is not at right angles to the film. In doing so it decreases the effect of scatter on the diagnostic image. Grids are not used in intraoral radiography because the secondary radiation does not greatly degrade the image because of the small field size. The panoramic units, with their narrow field size, also do not need grids. Medical x-ray units use grids routinely. Extraoral radiographs taken with a medical x-ray machine have better quality density and contrast than similar films taken with a dental x-ray unit because of the grid.

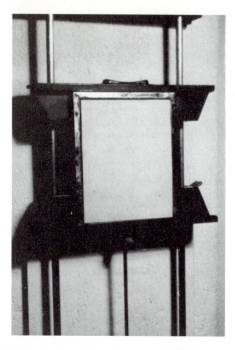

FIGURE 9-4   Cassette in wall-mounted, film-holding device.

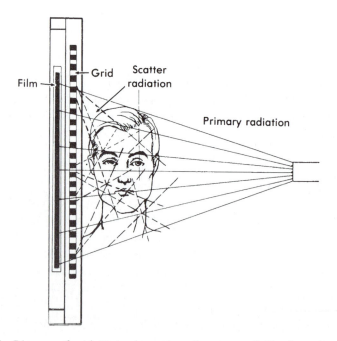

FIGURE 9-5   Diagram of grid. Note absorption of scatter radiation by radioresistant strips of grid.

Film sensitivity and processing

Extraoral screen films are more sensitive to light than are intraoral films. Therefore what would be acceptable safelight conditions in the darkroom for processing intraoral films might fog the extraoral films. The films used in panoramic radiography are especially sensitive to excessive safelighting and may be not merely fogged but ruined. Safelighting always should be checked before processing extraoral films.

Extraoral films are processed in the same manner as intraoral films, either manually or by automatic processors that can accommodate large-size film. The time-temperature method is used with the same fixation and washing time as with intraoral films. The only difference is that special sizes of film hangers are used. Operators should take special care when processing the large films because they are easier to scratch when more than one film is processed at a time (Figure 9-6).

Projections

As in intraoral radiography, certain factors must be known for every projection made: (1) the relationship of the film to the patient, (2) the relationship of the central ray of the x-ray beam to the patient and the film, (3) the FFD, (4) the point of entry of the x-ray beam, (5) the kVp, and (6) the mAs.

Suggested exposure times and mA and kVp settings are given, but these may vary, depending on the film speed, intensifying screen used, and size of the patient. The suggested exposure times assume the use of rare earth intensifying screens.

Lateral oblique projection of the mandible. The lateral oblique projection of the mandible is used for surveying one side of the mandible from the distal of the

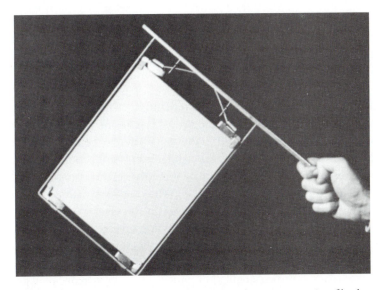

FIGURE 9-6   Piece of 8 × 10 inch film mounted on a processing film hanger.

canine to the angle, ramus, condyle, and coronoid process. It is not diagnostic anterior to the canine because of the superimposition caused by the anterior curve of the mandible. Before the advent of pantomography it was the most often used extraoral technique, because it is ideal for showing mandibular third molar impactions and other mandibular pathologic conditions.

An 8 × 10 or a 5 × 7 inch cassette may be used for this projection. The cassette is supported by the patient's shoulder or a holding device on the side of the mandible to be radiographed. The cassette is in contact with the cheekbone and mandible. The patient's head is inclined about 15 degrees away from the x-ray tube. The central ray is directed from under the opposite side of the mandible at right angles to the cassette. The FFD is 14 inches. An average exposure time at 65 kVp and 10 mA would be 5 to 10 impulses (Figure 9-7). This technique can be used with an occlusal film packet or in the reverse bite-wing (see Chapter 11).

Lateral skull projection. The lateral skull projection is used to survey the whole skull. The right and left sides of the skull are superimposed on each other, with the side nearer the tube magnified slightly more than the side nearer the film. It is used in dentistry to detect fractures and systemic pathologic conditions such as Paget's disease; it is the projection used in lateral cephalometric measurement in orthodontics.

An 8 × 10 inch cassette is used with intensifying screens. The cassette is held in position by the patient, supported on the patient's shoulder or by some supportive device. The cassette is positioned parallel to the sagittal plane of the skull. The central ray is directed at the external auditory meatus at an FFD of 36 inches. The vertical angulation is zero degrees. An average exposure time for an adult at 65 kVp and 10 mA would be 8 to 15 impulses (Figure 9-8).

If the lateral skull projection is to be used for cephalometric measurement, then a head positioning device (a cephalostat) must be used (Figure 9-9). The cephalostat ensures that the patient's head is accurately aligned with the sagittal plane and allows for reproducibility of patient position so that films taken during and after treatment are valid for comparison.

Posteroanterior projection. The posteroanterior projection is used to survey the skull in the anteroposterior plane and provides a means of localizing changes in a mediolateral direction. The left and right sides of the facial structures are not superimposed on each other as in the lateral skull projection. In dentistry this projection is used to detect fractures and their displacements, tumors, and large areas of disease. It is not effective for studying the maxillary sinus because of the superimposition of other cranial structures on the sinuses.

An 8 × 10 inch cassette is used with intensifying screens. The cassette can be held in position by the patient, but some type of cassette-holding device is preferable. The patient is positioned with the nose and forehead touching the cassette. The central ray is directed at a zero-degree vertical angulation, aimed at the external occipital protuberance

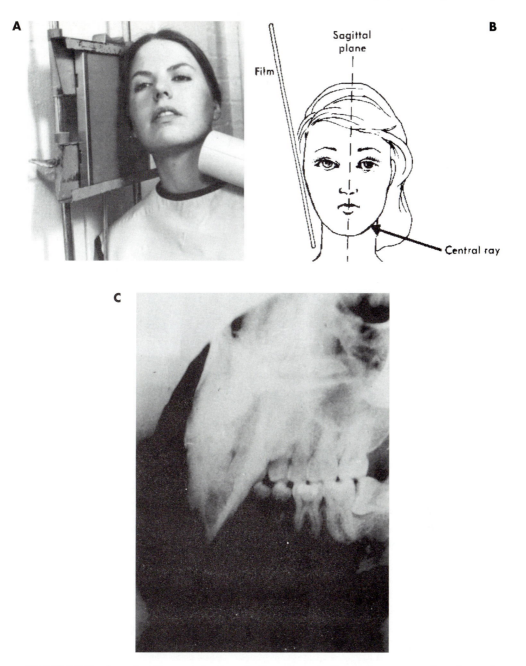

FIGURE 9-7   Lateral oblique projection. **A,** Central ray is directed at cassette from beneath opposite side of mandible. **B,** Drawing **C,** Radiograph.

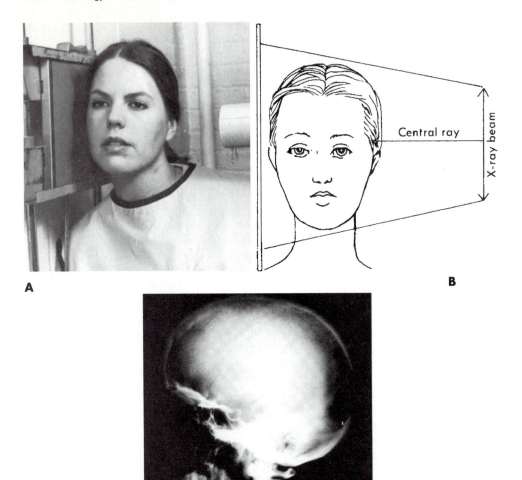

A

B

C

FIGURE 9-8 Lateral skull projection. **A,** Central ray is directed at external auditory meatus at a minimum FFD of 36 inches. **B,** Drawing. **C,** Radiograph.

(the prominent bump near the base of the skull). The FFD is 36 inches. An average exposure time at 65 kVp and 10 mA would be 8 to 15 impulses (Figure 9-10).

Posteroanterior (Waters') view of the sinuses. Waters' view is a variation of the posteroanterior projection that enlarges the middle third of the face and is useful in the diagnosis of maxillary sinus and other pathologic conditions occurring in the middle third of the face. It differs from the posteroanterior projection positioning in that the patient's mouth is kept open while the nose and chin are touching the cassette. The central ray is again directed at the external occipital protuberance, and

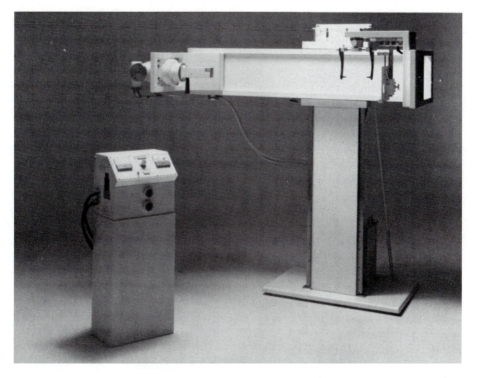

FIGURE 9-9   Cephalometric unit. Note cephalostat (head holder) and extended (6-foot) focal-film distance. *Courtesy Quint Sectograph Corp., Los Angeles.*

an FFD of 36 inches is used. An average exposure time at 65 kVp and 10 mA would be 15 to 20 impulses (Figure 9-11).

Temporomandibular joint.   The transcranial technique and modified pantomography are the best ways to visualize the temporomandibular joint using dental x-ray equipment. They can be used for screening when there are positive or questionable findings. Tomography, CT scanning, or MR imaging should be used for a definitive diagnosis.[1]

Transcranial projection.   The temporomandibular joint (TMJ) is difficult to radiograph well because of its anatomic location. It is bordered medially by the petrous portion of the temporal bone and laterally by the zygomatic arch. Yet it is necessary to examine the condyle to look for such conditions as calcifications, ankylosis, arthritic changes, fractures, and tumors. The transcranial technique positions the cassette and the central ray so as to avoid most of the superimposition of these structures.

A 5 × 7 inch cassette can be used if only one exposure is to be made. Usually, radiographs are taken of both the left and right condyles in both the open and closed positions. Since the diagnostic area is relatively small, the four views can be placed on an 8 × 10 inch film if appropriate lead shielding is used on the cassette. The patient's

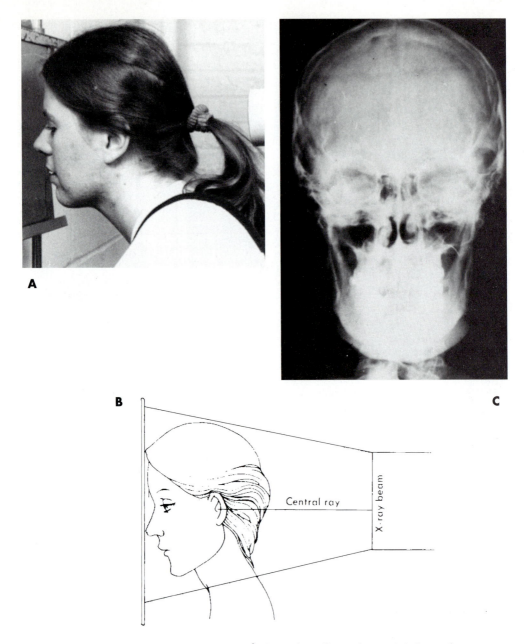

FIGURE 9-10   Posteroanterior projection. **A,** Central ray directed at occipital protuberance at minimum FFD of 36 inches. **B,** Drawing. **C,** Radiograph.

head is positioned parallel to the cassette with the side to be radiographed closest to the cassette. The cassette can be supported on the patient's shoulder or on a positioning device. The point of entry for the central ray of the x-ray beam is on the opposite side of the head from the condyle being radiographed, approximately 2½ inches above and ½ inch in front of the external auditory meatus. The x-ray beam is

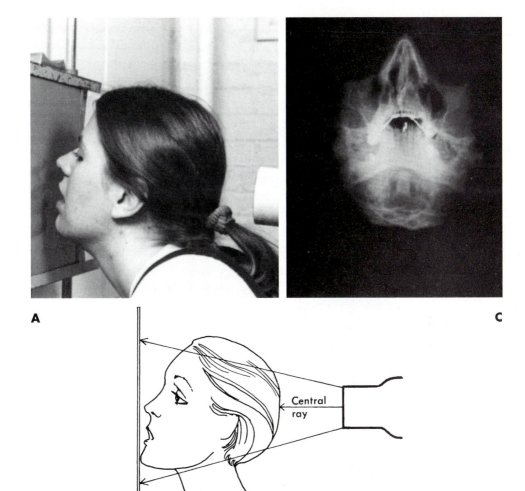

FIGURE 9-11   Posteroanterior projection of the sinuses (Waters' view). **A,** Central ray is directed perpendicular to cassette at occipital protuberance using 36-inch FFD. **B,** Drawing. **C,** Radiograph.

directed at a vertical angulation of 25 to 30 degrees. The end of the PID approximates the skin. An average exposure time at 65 kVp and 10 mA using fast film and screens would be 7 to 15 impulses (Figure 9-12).

Temporomandibular joint positioning boards are available to use with the transcranial technique that also incorporate means to hold the patient in a fixed position while allowing for movement of the cassette to give up to three exposures for each condyle (open, closed, and at rest) on an 8 × 10 inch film (Figure 9-13).

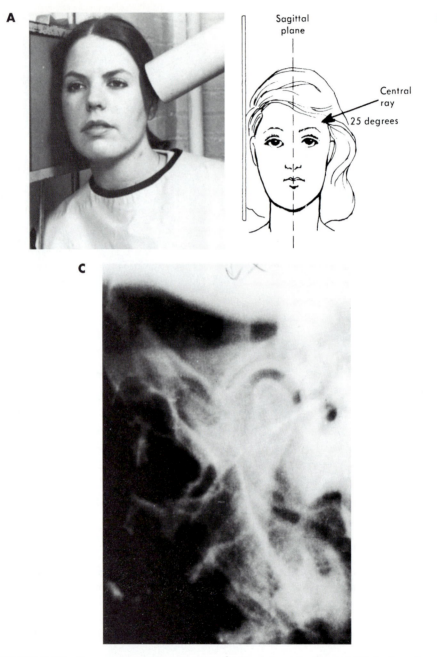

FIGURE 9-12 Transcranial TMJ projection. **A,** Central ray is directed 2½ inches above and ½ inch forward of external auditory meatus with vertical angulation of 25 to 30 degrees. **B,** Drawing. **C,** Radiograph.

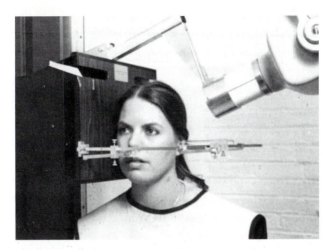

FIGURE 9-13   TMJ angling board. *Courtesy Margraf Dental Mfg. Inc., Jenkintown, Penn.*

XERORADIOGRAPHY

Xeroradiography was introduced to the dental market more than 15 years ago as an alternative to intraoral film packets. It was greeted at the time with great enthusiasm but did not capture the share of the market that was necessary for commercial viability. With the introduction of digital imaging the xerox unit is not used by many dentists. It is mentioned here because it remains an interesting, but probably not practical, alternative to film as an imaging system.

Xeroradiography is an imaging system that had been used in medical radiology for some time. The system uses the xerographic copying process to record images produced by x-rays from a standard dental x-ray machine. The system does not replace the conventional x-ray unit; it replaces film as the image receptor. Instead of conventional film, a photoreceptor plate covered with a uniform charge is used as the image receptor. The charged plate is held in a plastic cassette the size of either #0 or #2 film. The reusable cassette is covered with a plastic bag and exposed intraorally in the routine manner with a dental x-ray machine. The x-rays dissipate the charge on the photoreceptor plate in a pattern that corresponds to the absorption of the x-rays by the object radiographed. A latent electrostatic image is thus formed (Figure 9-14). The exposed receptor plate then is placed back into the processing machine, and the latent image is transformed into a real image on opaque paper that can be viewed directly or by reflected light on a viewbox. This transformation uses specifically charged pigmented powder. The copying process takes 20 seconds. After the photoreceptor plate is sterilized, reconditioned, and recharged, it is ready to be used again (Figures 9-15 and 9-16).

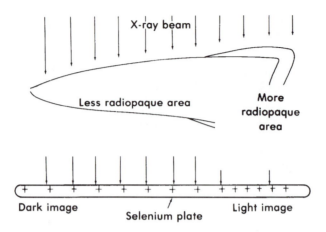

FIGURE 9-14 X-ray beam selectively penetrating the tooth and discharging the photoreceptor plate. *Courtesy Xerox Medical Systems, Pasadena, Calif.*

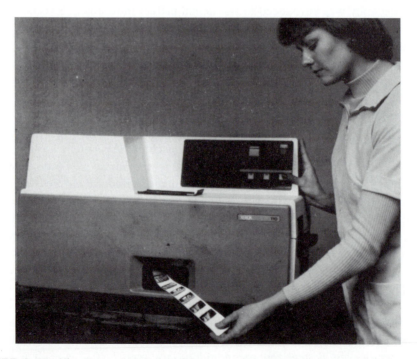

FIGURE 9-15 The Xerox 110 Dental Diagnostic Imaging System. *Courtesy Xerox Medical Systems, Pasadena, Calif.*

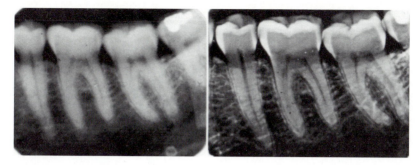

FIGURE 9-16 Conventional dental radiograph *(left)* and xeroradiograph *(right)* of same area. *Courtesy Xerox Medical Systems, Pasadena, Calif.*

REFERENCES

1. Griffiths RH: Report on the president's conference on the examination, diagnosis, and management of temporomandibular joint patients, *J Am Dent Assoc* 106:75-77, January 1983.

Chapter

ten

Panoramic Radiography, New Imaging Systems

Panoramic radiography refers to a technique, which produces a radiograph that shows the patient's mandible and maxilla on one film. Two techniques are currently available which produce such films. The first of these involves the use of an intraoral x-ray source in which the x-ray tube is placed within the patient's mouth and emits a 180 degree x-ray beam that hits a film wrapped externally around the patient's jaws. This technique, although theoretically interesting and innovative, is not commonly used, and the radiographs produced show a great deal of distortion; however the radiation exposure is significantly decreased (Figure 10-1). The second technique, by far the more extensively used, employs curved surface tomography.

Tomography

Tomography is a radiographic technique that allows radiographing in one plane of an object while blurring or eliminating images from structures in other planes. *Tomo* is the Greek word for section. These projections also could be called *laminograms,* from the word *lamina* (layer), as this is a layered radiographic technique. Tomography is used extensively in medicine and is the basis for computer tomography (CT) scanning.

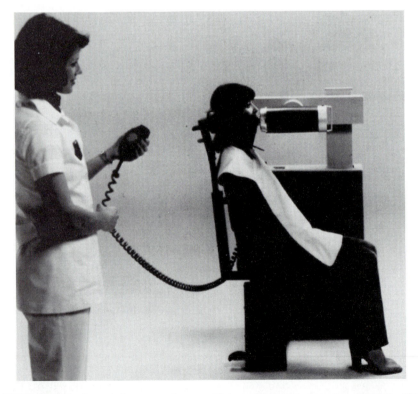

FIGURE 10-1   Intraoral source. *Courtesy Siemans Medical Systems Inc., Charlotte, N.C.*

A tomogram is made by moving the x-ray source and the film in opposite directions in a fixed relationship through one or a series of rotation points, while the patient remains stationary (Figure 10-2). The plane of the object that is not blurred on the radiograph is called the *plane of acceptable detail* or *focal trough*. It is also called the image layer. Clinically this concept is very important, because many of the errors in technique that we will discuss later in the chapter are caused by improper patient positioning; the result is not having the desired area in the image layer. The points of rotation around which the tube head travel can be either inside or outside of the focal trough. The width or thickness of the focal trough is governed by many factors, including the angle of movement of the x-ray beam, the width of the x-ray beam, and the size of the focal spot. Any object that lies in the focal plane is shown clearly, and objects above and below it appear blurred. By varying the focal-object distance—the distance between the tube head and the patient—on a tomographic series, different focal troughs or "cuts" can be achieved. A tomographic series is usually composed of multiple cuts, 0.5 cm apart, with the number of cuts varying according to the thickness of the object (Figure 10-3).

Some tomographic units now on the market are made specifically for use in the head and neck region. These units enable certain dentists to do tomography in their own offices. Indications for dental office tomography include implant planning, TMJ tomography, and diagnosis of pathologic lesions. Some of these new tomographic units are computer driven (Figure 10-4). This means that the computer controls the motion of the tube head and film and other exposure parameters from choices and information entered by the operator. This use of the computer should not be

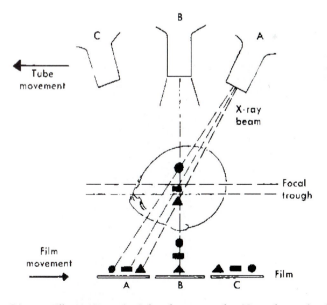

FIGURE 10-2 Diagram illustrating principle of tomography. Note that only objects in focal trough *(square)* project onto the same area of the film and are not blurred out.

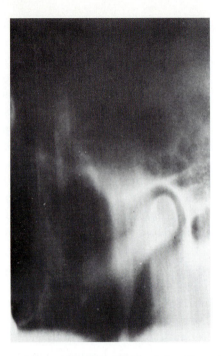

FIGURE 10-3   Tomogram of the temporomandibular joint. Note the clarity of the condyle and the blurring of the rest of the image.

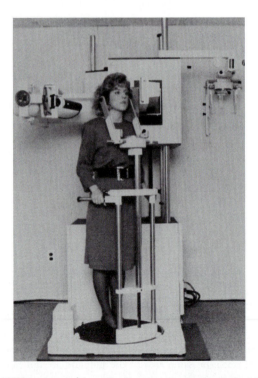

FIGURE 10-4   TOMAX tomographic unit. *Courtesy Incubation Industries Inc., Ivyland, Penn.*

confused with the computer imaging described later in this chapter. In the computer-directed units the imaging system is still a film screen combination, not the electronic sensors to be described. The computer does not produce or store the image as in digital imaging, it simply directs the patient exposure, and then the film is processed to produce the diagnostic image.

Pantomograph. A panoramic radiograph of the maxilla and the mandible produced by using tomography is properly called a *pantomogram*. The pantomogram is a curved-surface tomogram, in contrast to the plane-surface or straight line tomogram illustrated in Figure 10-2. In common usage the term *panoramic radiograph* is usually substituted for pantomogram. The term "panorex" should never be used as a substitute for panoramic radiograph unless the Panorex unit is being used. Panorex is not a generic term but the manufacturer's name for the first panoramic unit introduced in the dental market.

Many pantomographic units are available on the market today. They differ primarily in the number and locations of the centers of rotation, the choice of a fixed or adjustable focal trough, and the type and shape of the film transport mechanism. All units use intensifying screens, with a film size of either 5 × 12 or 6 × 12 inches. Design differences include head positioning devices, bite blocks, kVp and mA range, standing or sitting patient position, and wall-mounted or freestanding units.

Individual manufacturers use trade names such as Panorex, Orthopantomograph, Panelipse, and Panoral for their own panoramic units. Each manufacturer's machine has its own technique for operation, which can be learned easily from the instruction manual (Figures 10-5 and 10-6). With any of the pantomographic units, positioning the patient and maintaining that position during movement of the tube head are critical. Without correct positioning, the structure to be radiographed may not be or remain in the plane of focus and will appear blurred on the radiograph.

Pantomographic image. The image on a panoramic film shows the entire dentition and supporting bone from condyle to condyle on one film. The image, however, does not have the same definition seen on an intraoral periapical or bite-wing film. This factor is inherent in the pantomographic process and the use of intensifying screens. These images also have a significant amount of horizontal distortion but less vertical distortion.

All objects in the field of the x-ray beam, even those out of the plane of focus, are projected onto the film but most are not seen. The objects that have the greatest density (e.g., bone or metal objects), are shown on two places on the panoramic film. One place is the intended image or the usable image, and the other is referred to as the "ghost image" (Figure 10-7). The ghost image always has less sharpness and is seen at a point higher on the film than the desired image. The ghost image is always reversed; that is, the left appears on the right and vice versa.

Some panoramic units can be used to take tomograms of the TMJ (Figure 10-8). To accomplish this the unit must have an adjustable focal trough. The focal trough is set for the position of the condyle instead of the usual focal which is through the body of the mandible. By stopping the rotation and rewinding the film carrier, an open and closed view can be taken on each side with one piece of film.

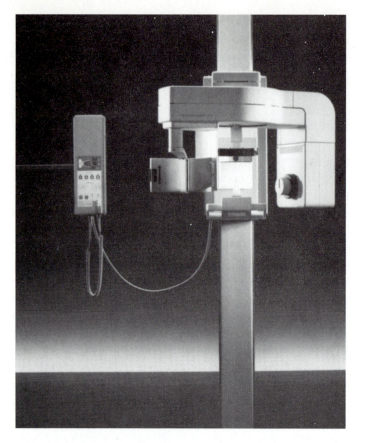

FIGURE 10-5 Orthopantomograph 10E. *Courtesy Siemans Medical Systems Inc., Charlotte, N.C.*

Advantages and disadvantages

Like any technique, panoramic tomography has its advantages and disadvantages when compared with conventional intraoral techniques. The pantomographic unit is expensive, approximately four times the cost of a regular x-ray tube head, which is still necessary even with the panoramic unit. The full-mouth series, composed of periapical and bite-wing films, has been and still is the norm for routine dental radiography, and any other technique should be judged in comparison.

Advantages.

Size of the field. Field size is one of the major advantages of the pantomogram. The full-mouth series is not composed of radiographs of the entire mouth but only of the teeth, alveolar ridges, and part of the supporting bone. The pantomogram covers an area that includes all of the mandible from condyle to condyle and the maxillary regions extending superiorly to the middle third of the orbits (Figure 10-9). Such areas as the condyles, inferior border, angle, ascending ramus and coronoid process of the mandible, and the entire maxillary that are not visualized on intraoral surveys are

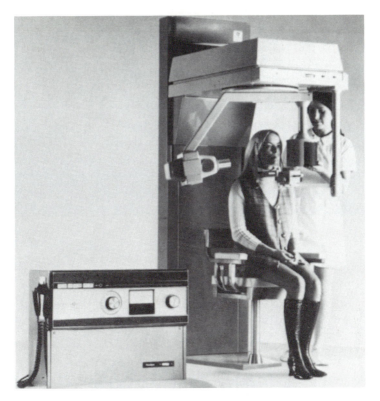

FIGURE 10-6   Panelipse panoramic x-ray system. *Courtesy Gendex Corp., Milwaukee.*

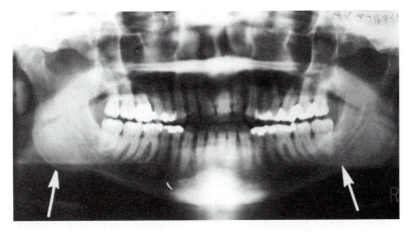

FIGURE 10-7   Ghost images of the opposite sides of the mandible, outlined by the arrows.

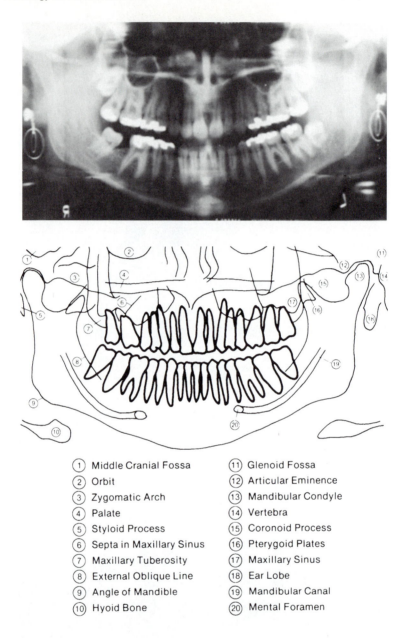

1 Middle Cranial Fossa
2 Orbit
3 Zygomatic Arch
4 Palate
5 Styloid Process
6 Septa in Maxillary Sinus
7 Maxillary Tuberosity
8 External Oblique Line
9 Angle of Mandible
10 Hyoid Bone

11 Glenoid Fossa
12 Articular Eminence
13 Mandibular Condyle
14 Vertebra
15 Coronoid Process
16 Pterygoid Plates
17 Maxillary Sinus
18 Ear Lobe
19 Mandibular Canal
20 Mental Foramen

FIGURE 10-8   Panoramic radiograph and tracing showing numbered anatomic landmarks. *Courtesy Gendex Corp., Milwaukee.*

seen routinely on pantomograms. Lesions that might go undetected on intraoral surveys show up on pantomograms.

Quality control. In maintaining quality control, good chairside technique is essential so that the undistorted complete image is seen. Full visualization of all the teeth and surrounding bone, including the third molar area, is of prime importance. This is

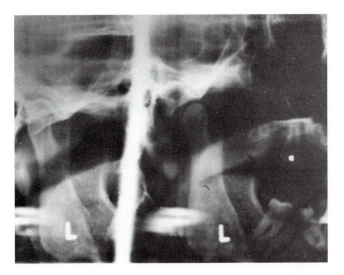

FIGURE 10-9   Pantomography of the temporomandibular joint. This is done using a pan-oramic unit with an adjustable focal trough. The focal trough is set for the plane of the condyle instead of the body of the mandible.

more easily done with a pantomographic unit than an intraoral full-mouth series, because the technique, though not simple, is not as demanding as intraoral radiography. There are fewer retakes and quality control is easier to maintain.

Simplicity. Pantomographic procedures, as just mentioned, are relatively simple to perform. With a minimum amount of training and strict attention to detail, the dentist or dental auxiliary can become very proficient in taking these films.

Patient cooperation. Since pantomography is an extraoral procedure, it requires a minimum amount of patient cooperation when compared with intraoral techniques. No film packet is placed in the patient's mouth. The patient is asked to bite on a rod and is only required to sit or stand still for the 12 to 22 seconds of exposure. Most units can be operated without radiation to demonstrate to an apprehensive patient what the procedure will be like. Pantomography practically eliminates problems with intractable gaggers, patients with trismus, and fearful or uncooperative children.

Time. Less time is required to do a pantomographic examination than an intraoral survey. The most skilled operator requires at least 10 to 15 minutes to do an intraoral survey; pantomograms can be taken in less than 5 minutes.

Dose. There seems to be general agreement that the radiation dose to the patient is less than or at most equal to intraoral radiography, depending on technique and how and where measurements are made.[1,2] The panoramic radiograph gives a bone marrow dose that is 20% or less than that received from a full-mouth intraoral series.[3] The panoramic dose is about equivalent to that received from four bite-wing films. This dose can be reduced even further by using rare earth intensifying screens in the panoramic cassettes. It should be noted, however, that the patient dose is relatively higher in the regions of the centers of rotation. Significant thyroid dose during the panoramic procedure also has been reported.[4,5]

Disadvantages.

Image quality. Tomograms inherently show magnification, geometric distortion, and poor definition.[6] Compared with an intraoral radiograph, the pantomogram does not give comparable definition. Besides the tomographic process, other factors that tend to degrade the images as compared with intraoral films are (1) external placement of the film with resulting increased object-film distance, (2) the use of intensifying screens, and (3) faster film with large grain size.[7]

Many diagnostic problems in dentistry require a high degree of radiographic definition. Early detection of such conditions as interproximal caries, disruption of the lamina dura, loss of crestal alveolar bone, and a thickened periodontal membrane all require the maximum amount of radiographic definition. Because of these factors, pantomographs have very limited value in the diagnosis of periodontal disease[8] and the detection of early periapical lesions. These are common diagnostic problems that comprise the bulk of diagnostic problems for practitioners, and the pantomographic technique is lacking in these areas. If a pantomogram is used instead of a full-mouth series, it must be augmented with bitewings and selected periapical films where indicated.

Focal trough (image layer). Areas that lie outside—either in front of or behind— the focal trough may be seen poorly or not at all. The focal trough or plane of acceptable detail is not as wide as either the mandible or maxilla, and only structures or changes that lie within the trough are visualized clearly. Pantomographic units that have adjustable focal troughs have far greater diagnostic capabilities than those that do not.

Overlap. Pantomographic units have a tendency to produce overlapping images, particularly in the premolar area.

Superimposition. Frequently superimposition of the spinal column shows up on the anterior portion of the pantomogram. If the patient is positioned properly, this should not happen. However, all patients are not perfect, and some have physical problems that make proper positioning difficult. The anterior teeth and periapical bone are the most difficult to interpret on pantomograms.

Distortion. The amount of vertical and horizontal distortion varies from one part of the film to another, resulting in an uneven magnification of the image; structures, spaces, and distances may appear larger than they actually are. This is a critical factor as some dentists use panoramic radiographs for case planning utilizing implants.

Overuse. This is one of the prime concerns regarding patient exposure. The ease and convenience in obtaining the pantomograph might lead to carelessness by substitution for other projections that yield better results. The pantomogram might be taken instead of one periapical film of an area because it is easier to do.

Technique

The following are general rules of technique for preparing and positioning the patient for panoramic radiography. These rules are valid for all units, but some slight technique changes may be necessary for individual units, depending on the manufacturer's specific instructions.

1   Explain the procedure to the patient, pointing out the importance of not moving during the procedure. Point out the movement of the film cassette and tube around the patient's head and the possibility that the film cassette may touch the shoulder or ear gently during the exposure rotation.

2   Have the patient remove a jacket or any other bulky piece of clothing that might interfere with movement of the cassette holder.

3   Ask the patient to remove any dentures, eyeglasses, earrings, nose rings, hearing aids, and hairpins to avoid their appearance on the film.

4   Seat or stand the patient in the most erect position possible so that the spinal column is straight.

5   Align the patient's head so that the midsagittal plane is perpendicular to the floor.

6   Place the patient's chin on the chin rest (if present) so that the ala-tragus line is tilted slightly down, about 5 degrees, from a parallel line to the floor.

7   Drape the patient's abdomen with the lead apron. Do not use a thyroid collar or a bib chain, because it would be superimposed on the image.

8   Place a cotton roll or a bite stick, if the unit has one, between the patient's upper and lower incisors.

9   Have the patient close the lips and place the tongue against the roof of the mouth. This prevents the formation of an airspace that is represented as a radiolucent area above the apices of the upper teeth.

10   Take any readings or measurements called for and set exposure factors.

11   Make the exposure. Since the exposure can be as long as 22 seconds as the tube and film cassette travel around the patient, it is a good idea to talk and remind them not to move.

Processing

Panoramic films are processed with regular dental solutions either by hand or automatically, if the processor can accommodate the panoramic-size film. The time-temperature method is used with the same fixation and washing times as with intraoral films. The film used in panoramic radiography is especially sensitive to excessive safelighting and may be not merely fogged but ruined. Make sure that the film screen combination used is compatible with the intensity and type of safelight used.

One of the most common artifacts seen on panoramic films is caused by static electricity. Multiple black linear streaks resembling tree branches without leaves appear on the radiograph (Figure 10-10). This artifact can be caused by pulling a piece of film quickly and forcefully out of a tightly packed full box of film or when loading or unloading film between the intensifying screens of a flexible cassette. Static electricity is produced most often on cold, dry days.

Common errors

Patient too far forward (Figure 10-11). If the patient is positioned in front of the focal plane, the upper and lower anterior teeth appear blurred and narrow. The spinal column is superimposed on the ramus and the premolars are overlapped.

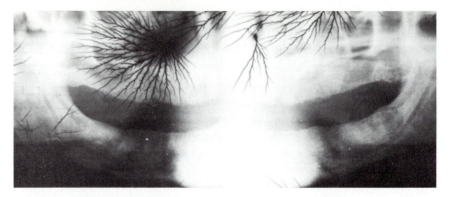

FIGURE 10-10   Panoramic radiograph showing static marks.

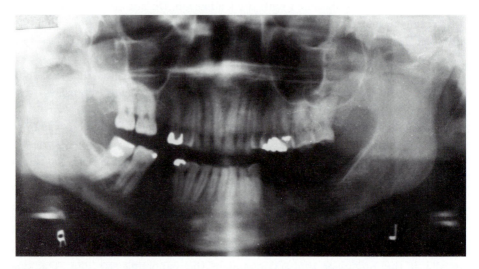

FIGURE 10-11   Patient positioned too far forward. Anterior teeth appear blurred and narrow. The spinal column is superimposed on the ramus, and premolars are overlapped.

Remedy. The patient's teeth or edentulous ridges must be in the proper position in the anterior-posterior plane. Check the position of the teeth on the bite block or bite stick and the position of the patient's chin on the rest. Make sure the distance setting is correct.

Patient too far back (Figure 10-12). If the patient is positioned in back of the focal plane, the upper and lower anterior teeth appear blurred and widened. Increased ghosting of the mandible also appears.

Remedy. The patient's teeth or ridges must be in the proper position on the bite block or bite stick. Check the position of the chin rest and the chin for the correct distance in the posterior-anterior plane.

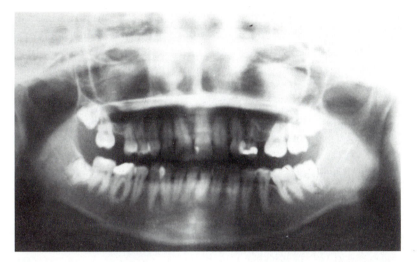

FIGURE 10-12   Patient positioned too far back. Upper and lower anterior teeth appear blurred and widened.

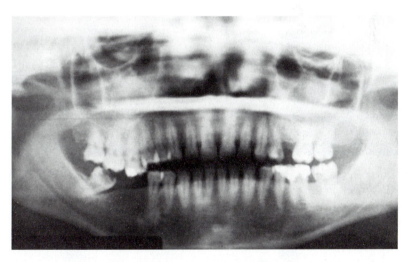

FIGURE 10-13   Patient's head tilted up. Hard palate (radiopaque band) is superimposed on apices of upper teeth.

Patient's head tilted up (Figure 10-13). If the patient's head is tilted up, the forehead is too far back and the chin too far forward. This causes the upper incisors to be out of focus, and the radiopaque hard palate is superimposed over the apices of the upper teeth. The condyles may be off the film.

Remedy. The reference lines on the patient's face, the Frankfort plane or the ala-tragus line, should be aligned parallel to the floor.

Patient's head tilted down (Figure 10-14). If the patient's head is tilted down, then the chin is back and the forehead forward. This causes the lower incisors to be blurred. The radiopaque image of the hyoid bone is superimposed on the anterior part of the mandible. The superior portions of the condyles may be cut off the film, and the premolars are overlapped.

Remedy. The reference lines on the patient's face, the Frankfort plane or the ala-tragus line, should be aligned parallel to the floor.

Patient moved during exposure (Figure 10-15). If the patient moves anytime during the exposure, the part of the film that was being exposed at that time appears blurred. This differs from intraoral radiography in which patient movement blurs the entire film.

Remedy. Talk to patients during the exposure, reminding them not to move.

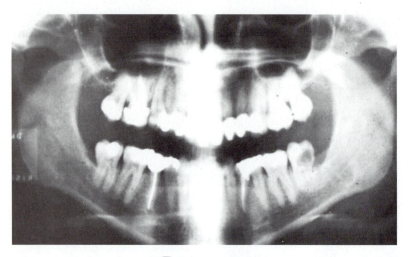

FIGURE 10-14 Patient's head is tilted down. Lower incisors are blurred, and image of the hyoid bone is superimposed on the mandible.

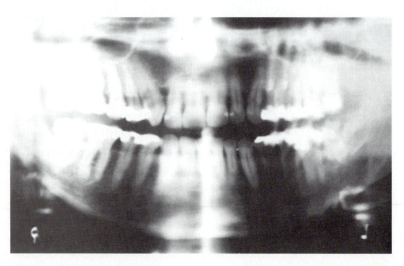

FIGURE 10-15 Patient movement during exposure. Note the blurred and sharp areas.

Large radiolucent area below the palate (Figure 10-16). If patients do not hold their tongue against the roof of the mouth, an airspace is created that produces a black shadow on the radiograph.

Remedy. Remind patients during the exposure to keep the tongue against the roof of the mouth.

Patient does not sit or stand erect (Figure 10-17). If the patient slumps, either standing or sitting, the spinal column causes a triangular-shaped radiolucency to be superimposed on the anterior teeth.

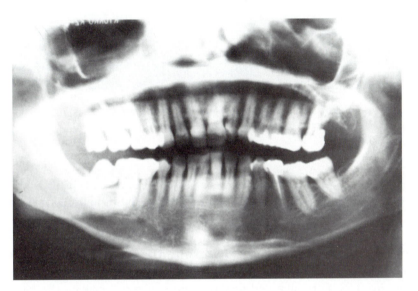

FIGURE 10-16   Tongue not against roof of the patient's mouth. Note the large radiolucent band superimposed over apices of the maxillary teeth.

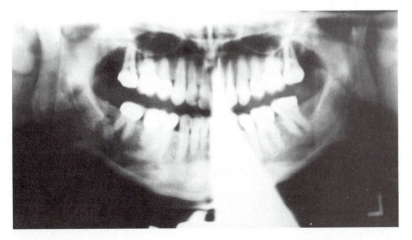

FIGURE 10-17   Patient slouching. Note superimposition of triangular-shaped radiopacity representing the spinal column.

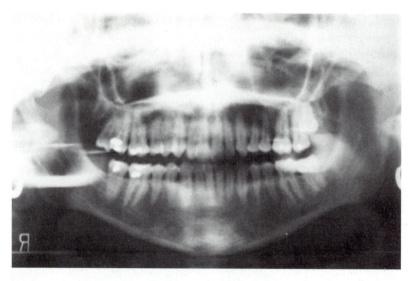

FIGURE 10-18   Failure to remove metal objects from the patient's face (large earrings). Note ghosting effect of the metal.

Remedy. When positioning patients, keep their spines erect. If patients are seated, the operator can place a cushion or support in the small of the back to help them to sit upright.

Failure to remove metal objects from the face, head, and mouth (Figure 10-18). These metal objects, if not removed, cause radiopaque ghosting on the opposite side of the film and may obscure structures, making the film undiagnostic.
Remedy. Remove all dentures from the patient's mouth as you would in intraoral radiography. All objects must be removed from the face as well.

Lead apron placed too high on the patient (Figure 10-19). The lead apron cannot be placed on the patient above the level of the clavicles, because it will create a large radiopacity on the film.
Remedy. Keep the lead apron low on the patient and never use a thyroid collar when taking a panoramic radiograph.

Film cassette slowing down because of patient contact (Figure 10-20). If the film cassette is slowed down or stopped for an instant during the exposure travel around the patient, black vertical bands show up on the film as a result of the localized overexposure.
Remedy. Position the patient carefully. With large-framed patients the operator should run the machine first without radiation to acquaint the patient with the procedure and to check on the patient's position.

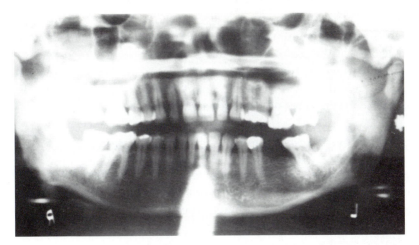

FIGURE 10-19   Placing lead apron too high on the patient.

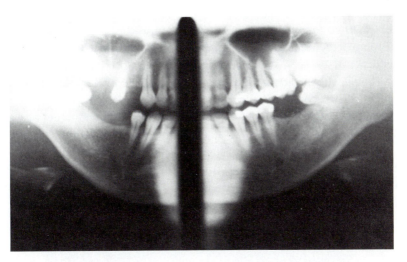

FIGURE 10-20   Film cassette slowed because of patient contact. Note radiolucent band where the overexposure took place.

NEWER IMAGING SYSTEMS

With the introduction and now common use of such new imaging techniques as CT scanning (computerized tomography), MRI (magnetic resonance imaging), and digital radiology, the field of dental radiography has expanded. These new techniques are used by dentists to image structures in ways that were heretofore unobtainable. Using CT scans for diagnosing lesions and planning implant cases and MRI to visualize the soft tissue components of the temporomandibular joint are now accepted as standard procedures in dentistry. Although the CT scanners and MRI units are not found in dental offices, the dental auxiliary as an educated, aware, interested professional should have some familiarity with these newer imaging systems; therefore an overview is included in this chapter. In the case of digital radiography, the placing of the image sensor in the patient's mouth uses the same principles as intraoral film placement so it is very likely that the use of digital radiography will become more widespread.

The common theme in these imaging techniques is the absence of x-ray film as the sensing device and the use of electronic detectors that feed electrical impulses into a computer which then stores or generates an image on a screen.

COMPUTED TOMOGRAPHY (CT SCANNING)

CT was introduced into radiology in the mid-1970s. In contrast to conventional radiographic techniques where film and/or film screen combinations are used to produce images, CT images are computer generated. However, CT still uses ionizing radiation as the energy source.

CT scanners produce digital data measuring the extent of the x-ray transmission through the patient. The patient is placed in the CT unit, and the x-ray source and image detector rotate around the patient, who remains stationary (tomographic principle). Multiple tomographic images are taken of the patient. They are recorded by a radiation detector, fed into a computer, and reconstructed to form the final image, which can be seen on a viewing monitor or printed out as a film (Figure 10-21). Although the image may have been taken in one plane (e.g., the axial plane), the computer can reconstitute the image from stored data to produce an image in another plane such as the frontal or sagittal plane. This technique was originally called the CAT scan (computerized axial tomography), but since studies are not limited to the axial plane, the more accurate name *CT scan* is used.

Special software programs have been written for CT scanners that are specific for dental use in implant planning (Figure 10-22). This software directs the computer in obtaining the desired images just as any software would direct a computer.

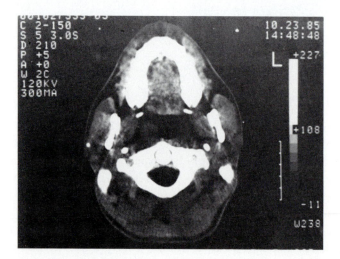

FIGURE 10-21   CT scan of a skull in the coronal plane. Note the gray soft tissue imaging that would not be seen on a conventional radiograph.

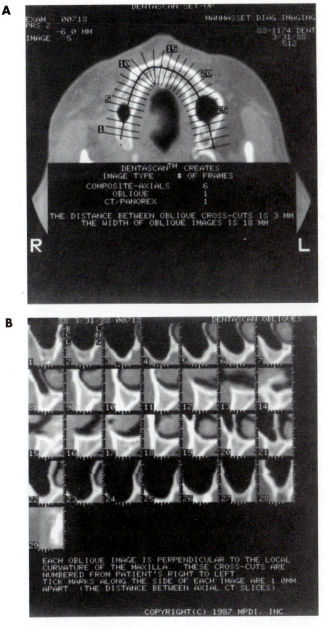

FIGURE 10-22   CT scan programmed specifically for dental implants. **A** is axial cut with orientation numbered planes that are seen in corresponding vertical cuts in **B.**

MRI (Magnetic Resonance Imaging)

This imaging technique does not use ionizing radiation as the energy source, and hence there is no radiation dose to the patient. The patient is placed in a large, extremely powerful magnet— 10,000 times more powerful than the earth's magnetic field. The magnetic field temporarily changes the alignment and orientation of the protons in the patient's body. Radio frequency waves are applied to the realigned protons, and this radio frequency energy is absorbed. When the radio frequency signal ends, the protons release the absorbed energy, and this signal is received by a sensor, and the information is transmitted to a computer and processed to generate an image. Since MRI is actually measuring proton density and 70% of the human body is water, of which protons are the major component, the MRI is better for visualization of soft tissues and not as good for bone which has little water. The image produced shows a strong signal (white area) for soft tissue with many water molecules and a weak signal (black area) where there are few water molecules. To date the main application of MRI in dentistry has been in imaging the articular fibrous disc of the temporomandibular joint (Figure 10-23).

DIGITAL IMAGING

Now or certainly in the future all dental health care professionals likely will be making digital images. Instead of placing film packets in the patient's mouth, we will place a nonfilm sensor electronically connected to a computer (Figure 10-24). The computer will receive the digitized penetration information and produce an instantaneous

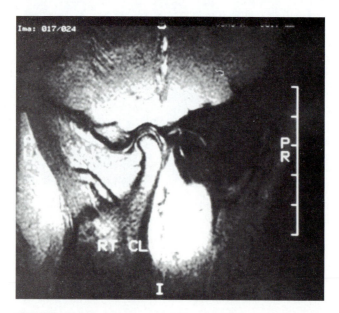

FIGURE 10-23   MRI image of the temporomandibular joint.

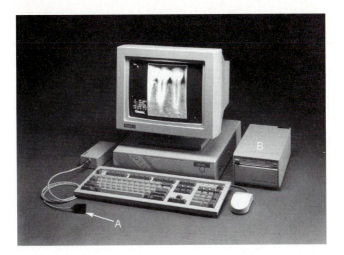

FIGURE 10-24   Intraoral digitizing unit. **A,** Intraoral sensor. **B,** printer for hard copy. *Courtesy of Gendex Corp., Milwaukee, WI.*

image on the monitor. The image can be stored, converted to a hard copy, or transmitted to a remote site. The image itself can be altered by darkening or lightening, enlarging or zooming in on a particular area. Digital imaging, when compared to intraoral film imaging, has the advantage of instant imaging, decreased patient exposure as the electronic sensors require less radiation, and the possibility of image enhancement.

REFERENCES

1. Van Aken J and Vander Linden LW: The integral absorbed dose in conventional and panoramic complete examination, *Oral Surg* 22:603, November 1966.
2. Valachovic RW and Lurie AG: Risk-benefit considerations in pedodontic radiology, *Pediatr Dent* 2:128, 1980.
3. White SC and Rose TC: Absorbed bone marrow dose in certain dental radiographic techniques, *J Am Dent Assoc* 98:553-558, April 1979.
4. Block AJ, Goep RA, and Mason EW: Thyroid radiation dose during panoramic and cephalometric dental x-ray examinations, *Angle Orthod* 47:17-24, January 1977.
5. Antoku S et al: Doses to critical organs from dental radiography, *Oral Surg* 41:251-260, 1976.
6. Brueggeman LA: Evaluation of a panoramic unit, Oral Surg 24:348, September 1967.
7. Reports of Councils and Bureaus, *J Am Dent Assoc* 94:147, January 1977.
8. Dental radiology: a summary of recommendations from the technology assessment forum, *J Am Dent Assoc* 103:423-425, September 1981.

Chapter

eleven

Patient Management and Special Problems

MANAGEMENT

Patient management is as important to the dental auxiliary as it is to the dentist. Patient psychology is a valuable tool to help dental hygienists perform their chairside duties. Dental auxiliaries may be responsible for other patient management assignments.

such as scheduling appointments, handling and screening telephone calls, and collecting fees. These duties also demand the use of patient psychology to manage patients successfully.

The dental health professional encounters all types of personalities in the dental office. Some patients may be very apprehensive and tense about dental treatment, whereas others are calm and matter-of-fact. Some reveal their anxieties through behavioral and speech patterns; others may hide their anxieties.

Even with modern equipment, techniques, and attitudes, dentistry remains a stressful procedure for most patients. As a profession, dentistry is still plagued by the image of the unpleasant experience. This image problem is reinforced in the public's mind by unfortunate representations on television and other media. Jokes and cartoons about dentistry raise the level of apprehension of our patients. It is within this societal context that we must endeavor to serve our patients.

One of the important roles of the dental auxiliary—which when performed successfully makes the work easier—is to try to relax the patient. The dental auxiliary may be the first member of the office staff to greet the patient in the reception area. Patients like to be recognized and greeted by name. This is especially important for new patients. It is helpful to say, "We will be with you shortly" rather than "The dentist or hygienist will be with you shortly." "We" implies the team concept of treatment and stresses the importance of the dental auxiliary in the office, indicating that the auxiliary takes part in the active treatment.

In performing dental radiography, the dental auxiliary also must develop a chairside manner. Patients must be made to feel comfortable and confident about the auxiliary's ability to perform the radiographic examination.

It is routine in most dental offices for the auxiliary to do radiographic surveys. However, some patients may have never had dental auxiliaries perform services for them. They are accustomed to having the dentist do all their work. These patients may be apprehensive and even object to the auxiliary performing any service for them. Auxiliaries should not take this attitude personally; they should regard it as a lack of patient orientation to new modes of treatment. If the patient objects strenuously, the dentist should be called in to reassure the patient. The dental auxiliary should then perform the procedures.

We are striving for high clinical proficiency with efficient and confident work patterns. The auxiliary can achieve these objectives through experience and critical evaluation by oneself, co-workers, and the dentist. The quality of the finished radiograph should be the same regardless of who performs the procedure. Dentist and auxiliary should be held to the same standard of quality control.

When the dental auxiliary is seating patients and draping them with the lead apron, some small talk may help to relax them. Patients want to know that you are interested in them and not just performing a mechanical procedure. This is not wasted time, because a relaxed, confident patient is much easier to work with.

Appearance is very important. The dental auxiliary should wear a clean uniform and be well groomed. Fingernails should be kept short to avoid trauma to patients' oral tissues. Hands should be washed, gloves worn, and the prescribed infection control procedures followed after the patient is seated in the dental chair so that the patient can take note of these procedures. If one sneezes, coughs, picks up something from the floor, or has to leave the treatment room, regloving is mandatory before starting work again.

The dental auxiliary should never chew gum while working with patients. If one must smoke (and as a health professional you should not), remember that tobacco odor on the breath or hands can be very offensive to patients. Mouthwash and hand lotions should be used to mask the tobacco residue before seeing patients.

One should always explain to the patient what procedures are to be performed and how many films will be taken. Any questions the patient has should be answered if the dental auxiliary feels capable of doing so. If the question involves diagnostic judgments or treatment planning that cannot be answered with confidence, it should be referred to the doctor. Patients often ask about the need for radiographs and the potential radiation risk. Since these questions are usually asked before work begins, a well-answered question will give the patient confidence and lessen apprehension about having the radiographs taken. Answers to questions of this type will be found in this text, and the fears and concerns of the patient can be allayed by intelligent, meaningful answers.

The "light touch" of certain dentists and dental auxiliaries is really nothing more than good technique and confidence developed with experience and respect for the oral tissues. No one is born with a "heavy hand"; and thus there is no excuse for clumsy, uncomfortable, intraoral radiographic technique.

Films must be placed in the patient's mouth and directions given to the patient in a manner that indicates self-confidence. A patient likes to feel that the operator is in full control of the situation at all times. Instructions to the patient should be given in a firm but polite tone. Auxiliaries should encourage and praise patients for their cooperation. If a patient is not following instructions—for example, raising the head and altering occlusal plane orientation—the patient should be corrected. An auxiliary should not accept improper patient position because of reticence about reminding patients about their movements.

Every patient is different, both in the anatomic configuration of the mouth and in psychologic makeup. This is the challenge of the profession: to perform one's duties and to maintain standards of excellence even as the clinical situation changes. Through study, practice, and self-evaluation, these goals can be met.

SPECIAL PROBLEMS

Gagging

Of all the problems one may encounter in intraoral radiography, gagging is probably the most troublesome. Gagging, more properly called the *gag reflex,* is a body defense mechanism. The coughing and retching produced in the gag reflex are meant to expel any foreign body from the throat and thus protect the airway from obstruction. An anesthesiologist never leaves a patient after surgery with a general anesthetic until the patient is awake and the gag reflex restored. At this point the patient can expel any mucus or other material that might obstruct the air passage because of the action of the gag reflex. All patients have gag reflexes; some are more active than others. The areas that are most sensitive to stimuli producing the gag reflex are the palate, base of the tongue, and posterior wall of the pharynx. It is making the maxillary molar projection that gagging will occur most frequently. The level of excitation of these reflexes varies from person to person. The patient with a low threshold for stimulation of the gag reflex presents the problem in intraoral radiography.

Very few patients, probably less than 0.1%, have a gag reflex so active that intraoral radiography is impossible. With this in mind, how do we deal with the remaining 99.9%? Following are a set of generally accepted suggestions and techniques that can be used to prevent gagging and to overcome it when it occurs. Not all techniques are applicable, nor will they succeed with every patient. One must be able to determine which technique best suits the individual patient. Studies have shown that technique, authority, and self-confidence of the operator are major factors in preventing and suppressing gag reflexes in dental radiography.[1]

Attitude. Always maintain the appearance of being in control of the situation. The patient wants to believe that the operator is so competent that it would be impossible for the film to slip and lodge in the throat. Firm positioning of the film holder with decisive instructions to the patient and proper body language are all necessary.

Think positively: never mention the possibility of gagging. The worst thing you can say to a patient is, "This won't make you gag." The patient may never have thought of gagging until reminded of the possibility.

Film order and technique. When taking a full-mouth radiographic survey, start in the maxilla, taking the anterior films first and working posteriorly. The film placement in the maxillary molar area is the one most likely to excite the gag reflex. Once the reflex is excited, the patient may continue to gag even on anterior films.

When placing the film in the patient's mouth for maxillary molars and premolars, do not slide the film along the palate. Place the film in the desired position near the lingual surface of the teeth, and then with one decisive motion bring the film into contact with the palate.

Always set the exposure timing dial for the desired exposure before you place the film in the patient's mouth. Have the tube head on the side of the patient's face that is to be radiographed, with the PID at the approximate vertical angulation. The object is to minimize the amount of time the film packet has to remain in the patient's mouth. Preparations like these can save valuable seconds and lessen the likelihood of the patient's gagging. Generally, the longer the film stays in the mouth, the more likelihood of gagging.

Deep breathing. It is often helpful to instruct the patient to take deep breaths through his or her nose as the film packet is placed in a gag-sensitive area such as the palate. Why this works is debatable, but it may be that breathing through the nose avoids the rush of air across the sensitive tissues of the palate. Another explanation is that it gives patients something to do and distracts them from thinking about gagging. Use a firm tone of voice when instructing the patient to take these deep breaths. The operator also may take some audible deep breaths to encourage the patient to do likewise.

Bite blocks and film-holding devices. Any film-holding device that requires the patient to bite and maintain pressure also may help in avoiding gagging. Again, the patient is given something positive to do. Another tactile sensation, that of biting and the pressure of the bite block against the teeth, may distract the patient from thoughts of gagging. Finger holding film techniques, which are not recommended for other reasons, tend to excite the gag reflex more than film-holding devices.

Lozenges, gargles, and sprays. All of these may be of some help in certain situations. The key is that the patient be made to believe that the medication will have an effect. In some instances a patient was given a vitamin pill as an "antigag pill." The patient was told in advance what the pill would do, and the rate of success was very high. This placebo effect is seen also in many other areas of dental practice. Note, however, that the patient was told what the effect of the placebo medication would be.

Many viscous topical anesthetics are available for rinsing the mouth, gargling, or spraying the palate to produce a numbing sensation, intended to block the gag reflex.

An undiluted mouthwash also may have some anesthetic effects on the palate. Many cough lozenges contain some local anesthetic; having the patient suck on a lozenge before radiography may be helpful.

In all these cases it may not be so much the anesthetic vehicle used as the manner of presentation to the patient that produces the desired results.

Hypnosis. Although the practice of hypnosis is out of the province of the dental auxiliary, its use in dentistry should be mentioned. In intractable gaggers hypnosis by trained, competent practitioners may be necessary to permit intraoral radiography.

Convincing a patient that something (like gagging) may not occur can be considered a form of hypnosis. An application of this principle is to tell gagging patients that you are going to press the antigag nerve located in their neck. We know that there is no antigag nerve, but the patient may not. If the area in the neck is pressed hard, some sensation will result and patients may become convinced that gagging will not occur.

Salt. One of the more amusing techniques described in the literature to stop gagging is to place ordinary table salt on the tip of the tongue of the gagging patient. The salt is placed in the palm of the patient's hand and he or she is asked to touch the tip of the tongue to the salt and then raise the tongue to touch the palate. It may be a method worth trying at least once in one's professional career.

For the intractable gagger, where all else fails, one must then resort to accessory techniques. Panoramic films and extraoral projections, previously discussed, because of their extraoral film placement, will circumvent the gag reflex.

Localization

Standard intraoral periapical and bite-wing films show the teeth and bone in only two dimensions—the superoinferior and anteroposterior plane. However, many clinical situations require a proper radiographic diagnosis to establish the position of structures in the buccolingual plane. Clinical examples include localization of impactions, foreign bodies, and areas of pathology, as well as differentiating buccal and palatal roots in endodontic procedures (Figures 11-1 and 11-2). This information is essential to the dentist before any treatment can be instituted.

The four techniques that can be used for localization are (1) definition evaluation, (2) tube shift, (3) right-angle technique, and (4) pantomography.

Definition evaluation. Structures that lie closer to the x-ray film have better radiographic definition than those that are farther from the film. This is true for both intraoral and extraoral films. It is sometimes possible, depending on the quality of the radiograph, to determine the relative position of superimposed structures by determining which has better radiographic definition. Because intraoral film is positioned lingually in the patient's mouth, the superimposed structure that is more sharply

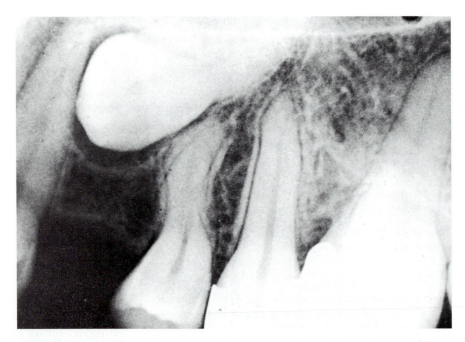

FIGURE 11-1   Impacted maxillary canine. Is the tooth positioned buccally or palatally to the alveolar ridge?

defined is positioned lingually in relation to the other structures (Figure 11-3). An advantage of this technique, when compared with the others that follow, is that it requires no further x-ray exposures of the patient. It is, however, the least reliable of the techniques mentioned.

Tube shift. The tube shift method uses what is referred to as Clark's rule, or the *buccal-object rule.* Its advantage to the practitioner is that it can be accomplished by using standard periapical technique. To determine the relative buccolingual relationship between two structures that appear radiographically superimposed, a second radiograph is taken. All factors remain the same for the second exposure, except that the tube is shifted about 20 degrees either mesially or distally. The point of entry, film position, and vertical angulation remain the same as in the previous film. When the

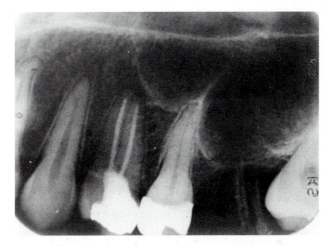

FIGURE 11-2   Maxillary first bicuspid with endodontic filling. Which canal is buccal, and which is palatal?

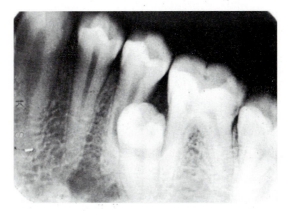

FIGURE 11-3   Localization by definition. Is the impacted supernumerary tooth more clearly defined than the rest of the teeth? If not, it is probably positioned buccally.

two radiographs are compared, the buccal object will appear to have moved in the opposite direction from the tube shift when compared to other structures on the radiograph (Figures 11-4 and 11-5). If the tube is shifted mesially by changing the horizontal angulation, the buccal object will appear to have moved distally. Conversely, a distal shift will result in the more buccal object moving mesially. This can be demonstrated on your fingers. Hold your hand so that the second and third fingers are superimposed when you are sighting them from the side. Move your head either to the left or to the right (mesially or distally) and imagine the images of the fingers being recorded on the film. You now can see two distinct fingers and not the fingers superimposed. Now apply the buccal object rule. The key phrase is "same lingual, opposite buccal"; the acronym is SLOB.

Right-angle technique. The right-angle technique uses two projections taken at right angles to each other—first a periapical film and then an occlusal film of the same area, for example. The planes radiographed are at right angles to each other. The occlusal techniques and examples are discussed in Chapter 8.

Pantomography. The redundant images produced in the anterior region by some older-model pantomographic units, such as the Panorex, can be used to localize objects in repeated areas. In viewing the film, the object in question will be seen twice, once on each half of the film. A recommended technique is to compare the relative movement of the object with adjacent structures from one side of the film to the other with the direction that the clinician reads the film (for example, left to right).[2] The object will seem to have moved in the same direction as the clinician's viewing movement if it is lingually positioned and in the opposite direction if it is on the buccal side (Figure 11-6).

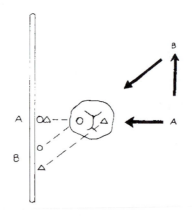

FIGURE 11-4 Buccal-object rule. As the tube position is shifted mesially (position B), the buccal object is seen to move relatively in the opposite direction, distally.

A

B

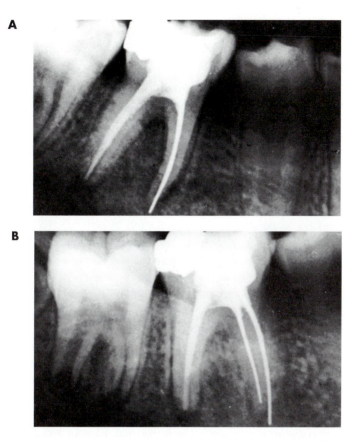

FIGURE 11-5   Radiographs illustrating the buccal-object rule. The tube in **B** was shifted to the mesial, indicating that the short endodontic point is in the mesiobuccal canal.

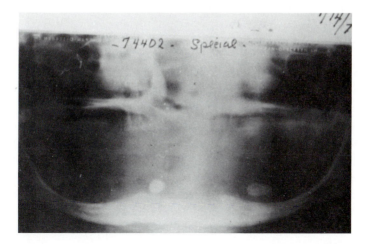

FIGURE 11-6   Localization of an object by pantomographic redundant image.

Third molars

The third molars are in an area of the mouth difficult to radiograph. In many cases it may not be possible to position the film packet intraorally to visualize these areas adequately on radiographs. This is especially true if the teeth are impacted. In these cases it may be necessary to use the extraoral and panoramic techniques described in Chapters 9 and 10. The third molar area must be seen to make a complete diagnosis. If it cannot be seen on periapical films, other methods must be used.

Maxilla. As the film is placed more and more distally toward the patient's throat, the likelihood of exciting the gag reflex increases. It may be helpful to hold the film packet with a hemostat to maintain a minimum of contact with the palate. The film packet should be kept as parallel to the palatal vault as possible. To avoid distortion the vertical angulation must be increased, with the resulting relationship of the central ray to the film packet looking very much like an occlusal projection.

Mandible. The most common difficulty in radiographing lower third molars is the inability to place the film packet distal enough to record the image of the whole tooth and root structure. This placement is prevented by the muscles of the floor of the mouth and tongue. To overcome this problem the tongue can be deflected to the opposite side of the mouth by the operator's finger or a mouth mirror. The floor of the mouth is gently depressed, almost massaged, to relax the mylohyoid muscle. While this is being done, the film packet is slid along the lingual surface of the mandible as far distally as possible. In certain horizontal impactions of the mandible it may be necessary to distort the image in the horizontal plane in order to visualize the entire tooth with intraoral radiography. This is done by changing the horizontal angulation of the x-ray beam so that it is not at right angles to the film packet, which is the usual procedure. Instead, the beam comes from the distal side, and the central ray makes an acute angle with the film.

Narrow arch

In some mouths it may be impossible to place anterior film packets properly without excessive bending, with resultant distortion of the radiographic image. The best way to overcome this problem is to vary the film size. The #1 narrow anterior film is recommended, although it may be possible to use #0. No rule states that you cannot use different-sized intraoral packets in the same full-mouth series. The only possible problem is in mounting the films. The smaller or narrower films must be attached to the mount by cellophane tape or staples so they do not slip from the window in the mount. Pedodontic or narrow film may be used as the situation dictates (Figure 11-7).

If radiographs show overlapping teeth, especially in the anterior region, it does not necessarily indicate that the films were taken improperly. If the teeth are overlapped in the mouth, they appear overlapped radiographically.

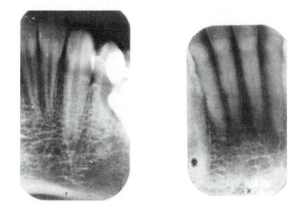

FIGURE 11-7   Periapical radiographs of lower anterior region using narrow anterior (#1) film seen on left and pedodontic size (#0) film seen on right.

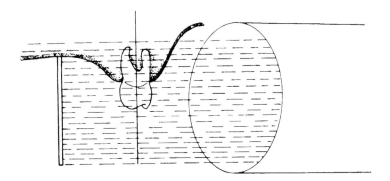

FIGURE 11-8   Problem of film placement in paralleling technique with patients with low palatal vaults. Note that film cannot be placed high enough to record image of root apices.

Shallow palate

The shallow palatal vault presents a problem in the paralleling technique. Fortunately this does not occur so frequently and severely that the bony structures make it impossible to place the film packet parallel to the long axis of the tooth and high enough to record the radiographic image (Figure 11-8). In these rare cases the bisecting-angle technique may be the better choice. Before changing techniques one should always check to see that the film is in the midline where there is the greatest palatal height. The number of times that the paralleling technique cannot be used is quite small.

The bisecting-angle technique compensates for the shallow palate by increasing the vertical angulation. The film packet must be in the patient's mouth with a 3-mm border projecting beneath the incisal or occlusal edge of the teeth and the central ray bisecting the angle formed between film packet and the long axis of the tooth (Figure 11-9).

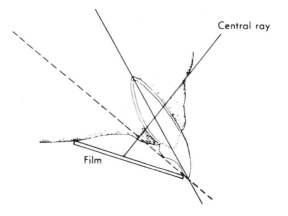

FIGURE 11-9   How to overcome the problem of a low palatal vault in bisecting-angle technique. Note increase in vertical angulation.

Lingual frenulum

It is extremely difficult to radiograph patients who have a large, tight, lingual frenulum, attached close to the tip of the tongue. These patients are sometimes referred to as "tongue-tied" because they cannot protrude their tongues very far out of their mouths.

The paralleling technique is not the method of choice for these patients because the tight frenulum does not allow placement of the film packet deep in the floor of the mouth. Relaxing the muscle as recommended for the mylohyoid still does not produce enough room. The best choice is to use the bisecting technique. Since the film cannot be placed very deep in the mouth, negative vertical angulations in the range of minus 40 degrees to minus 60 degrees can be expected.

Tori

The maxillary torus (torus palatinus), if present, usually causes no problems in periapical radiography. It is located posteriorly in the midline of the palate and does not hinder periapical film placement. The best way to radiograph a torus palatinus is by use of an occlusal projection.

The mandibular tori, or torus as the case may be, are located on the lingual aspect of the mandible in the premolar area. Their presence prevents the placement of the film packet in its usual position. This difficulty is more accentuated in the bisecting-angle technique than in the paralleling technique. The film packet cannot be depressed into the floor of the mouth and still kept close to the lingual surface of the teeth. The only possible solution is to place the film over the torus. This increases the angle between the film packet and the long axis of the tooth; increasing the vertical angulation to bisect the angle compensates for the change. In the paralleling method with its increased object-film distances, the film is positioned behind the tori.

Canine overlap

Overlapping the image of the mesial portion of the maxillary first premolar with the image of the distal surface of the canine is a common problem. The overlapping is caused by the large palatal cusp of the first premolar. The problem can be solved by changing the horizontal angulation so that the central ray comes more from the distal side, as in a premolar periapical projection (Figure 11-10). Then the palatal cusp is not superimposed. Overlapping does not occur in the mandible, because the first premolar has a very small lingual cusp.

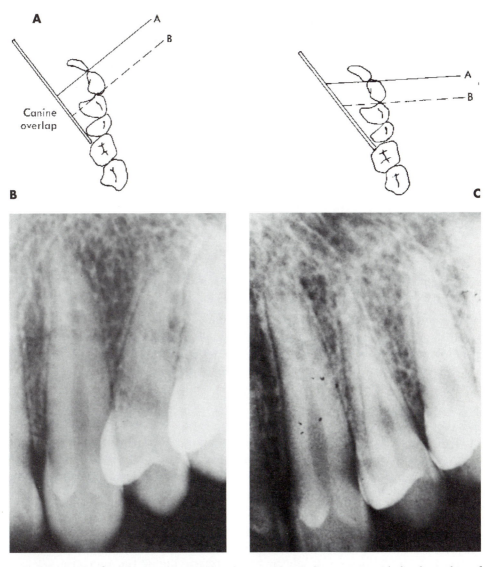

FIGURE 11-10 A, Diagram of changing horizontal angulation to avoid distal overlap of maxillary canine. **B,** Overlapped canine. **C,** Overlapping eliminated.

Trismus

Trismus is the condition in which a patient is unable to open the mouth. It may be partial or complete and is usually caused by infection or trauma. To make an adequate diagnosis and identify the infected tooth or area, radiographs are necessary. If the patient's mouth cannot be opened at all, extraoral or panoramic films are necessary. If there is partial opening, it may be possible to place an intraoral film by modifying the usual technique. A hemostat is used to hold the film packet, since it is much narrower than a finger or any other film-holding device. The film packet is placed in the mouth by sliding it between the partially opened anterior teeth in the horizontal plane. Once beyond the teeth, the film can be turned to its proper vertical orientation. If possible, the patient then holds the hemostat with the film packet attached to it in position while the exposure is made.

Handicapped patients

The problems of treating the handicapped patient in the dental office vary according to the degree of disability. With patients confined to wheelchairs, it may be easier to radiograph them in the wheelchair than to transfer them to the dental chair. This presents no problem as long as the x-ray machine and patient can be maneuvered into the proper relationship. Panoramic and extraoral projections are useful in this type of patient.

The patient who has no digital control cannot hold film packets in place, so a bite block or other film-holding device is used.

The spastic patient with uncontrollable movements presents the greatest problem. A parent, friend, or care provider may need to hold the patient's head steady while the radiograph is taken. This person can wear lead gloves and a lead apron for radiation protection. The dental auxiliary or the dentist, who constantly works with radiation, should not hold the patient and stand in the direct x-ray beam.

For a totally unmanageable patient, radiographs may have to be taken with the patient under general anesthesia. These films are usually developed immediately and the necessary dental procedures performed while the patient is still anesthetized.

Bedridden patients

Some patients in hospitals and nursing homes cannot be brought to the dental suites; their dental procedures and radiographs must be done at the bedside. Mobile dental x-ray units can be brought to the bed and radiographs taken. For the patient in the supine position, it is easier to use a film-holding device with a localizing ring. In treating a patient at home or at a site that does not have a dental x-ray unit, portable x-ray units can be adapted for dental use and assembled on site (Figure 11-11). A small, portable, rapid processing tank also should be brought along so that the radiographs can be processed and the patient treated during the same visit.

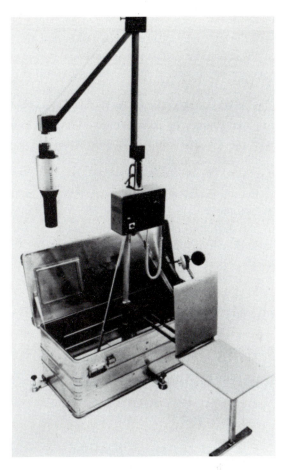

FIGURE 11-11 Siemens Portaray transportable x-ray examination unit. *Courtesy Siemens Medical Systems Inc., Charlotte, N.C.*

Children

Dental radiography requires the complete cooperation of the patient. If the patient moves, the radiographic image is blurred and the film rendered useless. In no other area of dentistry is this absolute cooperation so necessary. If a child moves during an operative dentistry procedure, the dentist can compensate. In radiography the patient must hold still while the exposure is made.

The unknown is frightening to any child, and very few children know anything about x-rays. In fact, the dental radiograph may be their first introduction to any radiography. The procedure must be explained to the child in terms the child can understand. One should talk of taking a "picture" of the tooth with a "camera." Remind children that they must hold still when the picture is taken. Show children the film packet and let them put it in their mouths. Taking a picture of the child's thumb is a good way to introduce the concept of holding still and to assure the child that he or she will feel nothing when the tooth is radiographed. Of course, the x-ray machine is off when these thumb exposures are made.

Children like to see pictures, and it is sometimes helpful to show them what a radiograph of a tooth looks like. The auxiliary should follow up with a promise to show them what their teeth look like on the finished radiograph. We have in certain instances even taken children into the darkroom and let them help process the films. Children are fascinated by the darkroom with its tanks and chemicals. Any effort expended to relax children and make them feel at ease will reap benefits at later appointments.

Children usually tolerate periapical films, and the film can be held in place with a bite block or any film holding device. If they resist periapical film placement, have the children bite on the film and increase the vertical angulation to bisect the angle so that the procedure resembles an occlusal projection (Figure 11-12). This type of film is not as desirable as the regular technique, but it is better than no film at all. This method will work for any area of the child's mouth, and a full-mouth series can be taken this way if necessary. Either adult-size or occlusal film can be used for this technique (Figure 11-13).

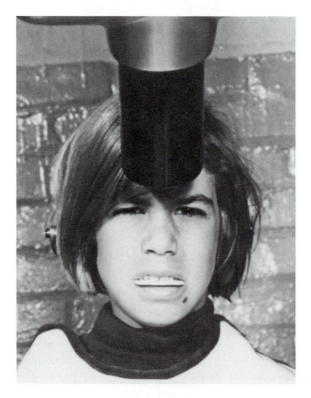

FIGURE 11-12   Technique for periapical films that allows child to bite on film. Note increase in vertical angulation.

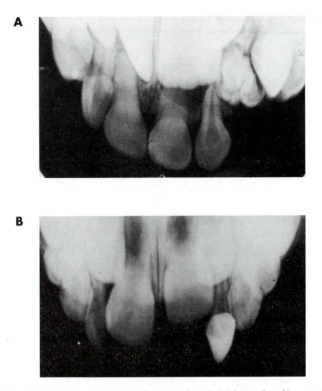

FIGURE 11-13   Radiographs taken by having the child bite the film packet. **A,** Adult-size periapical film packet. (Note odontoma blocking tooth eruption.) **B,** Occlusal film.

Reverse bitewings. Some children will not tolerate placement of the bite-wing film. When instructed to close on the tab, they push the lower part of the film out of the floor of the mouth with their tongue and then close their teeth on the film. If after repeated attempts proper placement meets with failure, a reverse bite-wing technique can be substituted. In this method, the film packet is placed on the cheek side of the teeth in the buccal sulcus (Figure 11-14). The child bites on the tab to hold the film packet in place. The x-ray beam is directed extraorally from under the opposite side of the mandible as in a lateral oblique projection (Figure 11-15). The exposure time must be increased by a factor of 4 or 5 because of the increased FFD. The resulting film will not have the detail of an intraoral bite-wing radiograph but will be a useful substitute (Figure 11-16).

   If intraoral film placement is not possible for the child, an extraoral film can be substituted. The view that is most diagnostic is also a slight variation of the lateral oblique technique. The cassette is positioned in the usual way, but the central ray is directed from behind the angle of the mandible on the opposite side (Figure 11-17). Again the radiograph is not as diagnostic as an intraoral film but is better than none (Figure 11-18).

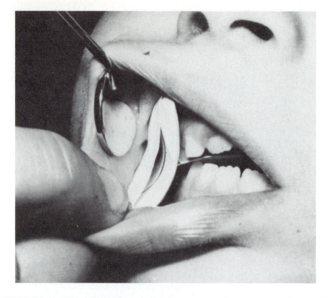

FIGURE 11-14   Film placement for reverse bite-wing radiograph.

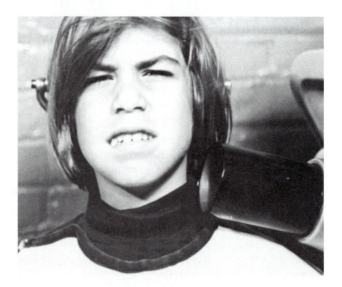

FIGURE 11-15   Tube position for reverse bite-wing radiograph. Note that central ray is directed from underneath mandible of opposite side while being aimed at bite-wing film.

If there is no extraoral cassette in the office, a piece of occlusal film can be substituted (Figure 11-19) but with the resulting increase of radiation exposure to the patient. An exposure time of nearly 2 seconds will be necessary because of the increased FFD. The radiograph produced will be of some diagnostic value (Figure 11-20).

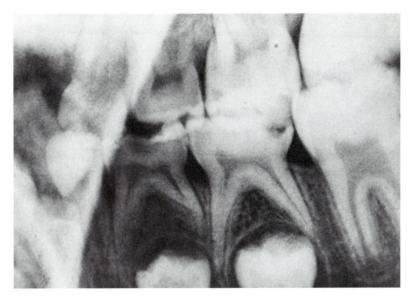

FIGURE 11-16   Reverse bite-wing radiograph.

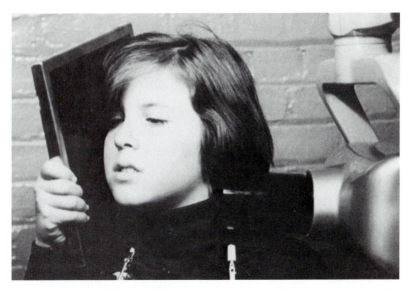

FIGURE 11-17   Lateral oblique technique for caries and pathology detection in children. Note that central ray is aimed from behind angle of mandible on opposite side.

Endodontic radiographs

In patients undergoing endodontic treatment it is necessary to take working and measurement films while the rubber dam is in place. The bisecting method can be used, with the patient supporting the film packet under the rubber dam with a finger or bite block, but it is not recommended. It is difficult to use the paralleling method

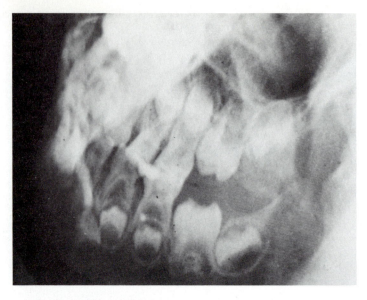

FIGURE 11-18 Radiograph taken by lateral oblique technique.

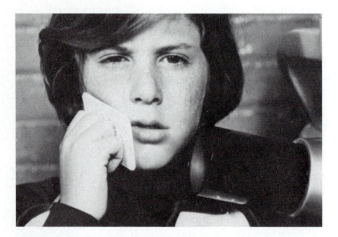

FIGURE 11-19 Occlusal film packet used as extraoral film.

with the dam in place because of the lack of working space in the mouth and the patient's inability to bite on any film-holding device because of the rubber dam clamp and protruding endodontic files from the tooth. The best course is to disengage the rubber dam frame, keeping the saliva ejector in place, and position the film packet in a hemostat or "Snap-a-Ray," parallel to the tooth and held by the patient.

Plastic rubber dam frames and saliva ejectors should be used to avoid superimposition of their images on the radiograph (Figure 11-21). Punching a hole in a predetermined corner of the dam will make it easier to reorient the dam in the frame once the exposure has been made.

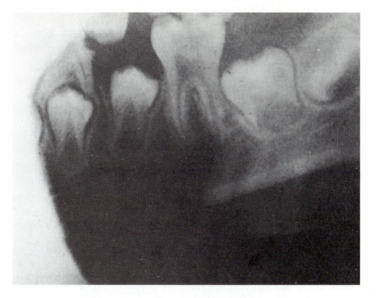

FIGURE 11-20   Radiograph made by using occlusal film packet extraorally.

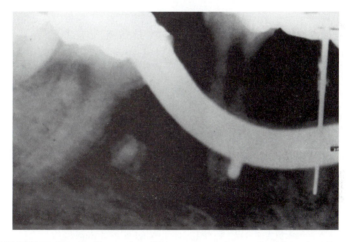

FIGURE 11-21   Radiograph with superimposition of rubber dam frame.

   Rapid processing discussed in Chapter 6 minimizes working time and can be adequately diagnostic in endodontic working films.

Grid measurement

Intraoral measurement grids are available that superimpose thin radiopaque or radiolucent lines in the vertical and horizontal planes in 1-mm gradations. The marking grid is affixed to the front of the film packet when the exposure is made. One manufacturer makes film packets with the grid markings incorporated into the film

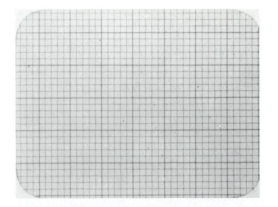

FIGURE 11-22   Photograph of intraoral grid placed on dental film packet.

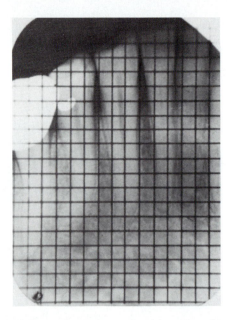

FIGURE 11-23   Radiograph with grid markings.

packet. No increase in exposure is necessary with the use of the marking grid, and the films are processed in the usual manner. The measurement or marking grid should not be confused with the grid used in extraoral projections (Chapter 9) to absorb object scatter (Figures. 11-22 and 11-23).

Radiopaque media

The use of radiopaque media has many applications in dental practice. It is used routinely in endodontics, with the radiopaque file, to determine root length. Gutta-percha or silver points can be placed in periodontal soft tissue pockets to

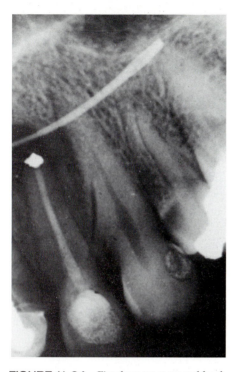

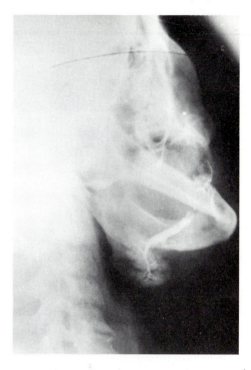

FIGURE 11-24 Fistulous tract traced back from palatal opening to its origin by insertion of gutta-percha point.

FIGURE 11-25 Sialograph outlining submandibular duct and gland.

determine pocket depth and direction. Fistulous tracts can be traced to their origin using thin, flexible wire or gutta-percha points (Figure 11-24).

The technique of sialography involves injecting radiopaque media into salivary ducts and glands and then visualizing these soft tissues radiographically. This method is used in diagnosing ductal and glandular obstructions, salivary stones, infections, and tumors of the major salivary glands. The contrast medium used is usually an iodine-containing formula in either an aqueous or oil suspension (Figure 11-25).

REFERENCES

1. Sewerin I: Gagging in dental radiography, *Oral Surg* 58:725-728, 1984.
2. Langlais RP, Langland OE, and Morris CR: Radiographic localization techniques, *Dent Radiogr Photogr* 52:4, 1979.

Chapter

Film Mounting and Radiographic Anatomy

The mounting of processed dental radiographs is another important function of the dental auxiliary. It is much easier to view and diagnose radiographs when the films are placed in mounts in their proper anatomic orientation than it is to look at them on a film hanger or sort them from an envelope. Properly mounted films make charting and examination a much more orderly procedure. The mounted films are kept with the patient's chart, and at each subsequent visit the radiographs are placed on the viewbox for the dentist to refer to.

Radiographs are identified and oriented as to position in the mouth by the tooth and bony structures visible on each film. A thorough understanding of radiographic anatomy will make mounting an interesting and challenging procedure, not one that is done automatically. Mistakes are made when the auxiliary has no basic understanding and work becomes tedious.

DESCRIPTIVE TERMINOLOGY

Since we now are dealing with the processed radiograph in mounting and interpretation, we need certain terms to describe the shades of black, white, and gray that appear. The appearance of any area is determined by the density of the area and the quality, and hence, the penetration of the x-ray beam that reaches the film. With these terms we can more accurately describe the radiographic findings. The black areas, where there is greater penetration on the radiographs, are called *radiolucent,* and the white areas, where there is little or no penetration, are called *radiopaque.* All structures are either radiolucent or radiopaque, but each category includes gradations. For instance, metallic fillings are more radiopaque than enamel, but both are still radiopaque. Caries appears radiolucent, because the decay causes a lessening of density when compared with enamel and dentin.

One should never refer to a radiograph as an x-ray. One may say x-ray film, but the term *x-ray* should be used only when referring to the beam of energy that is aimed at the film packet in the patient's mouth. The film then is processed to produce a radiograph.

MOUNTS

Various types of dental film mounts are available. Mounts are made for both pedodontic and adult surveys and come with a full range of numbers of windows (Figure 12-1). In addition to full-survey mounts, single film, double film, and bite-wing survey mounts are also available (Figure 12-2). Film mounts usually are made of either a cardboard or a celluloid-like material. The overall size and shape of the mount are made to fit the various types of viewboxes found in dental offices. The area around the film windows may be either clear or opaque. The opaque mounts are preferred because the light is concentrated behind the radiographs and viewing is easier and more diagnostic. If the number of radiographs taken does not fill the mounts, the unused windows should be covered so as not to allow the light to distract the viewer. The black opaque wrapper from the periapical film packet is ideal for this because it is the correct color and size and is easily attached to the mount.

The patient's name, date, and number of films taken must be recorded on each mount.

A   **B**

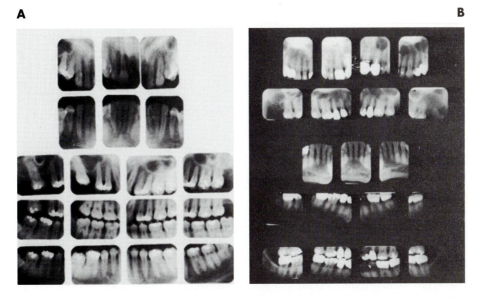

FIGURE 12-1   Full-mouth series mounted in clear celluloid **A,** and opaque mounts **B**.

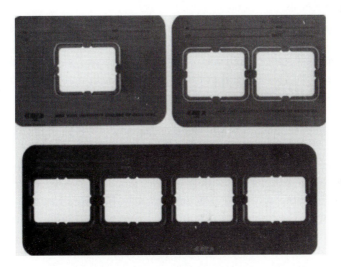

FIGURE 12-2   Bite-wing and single film mounts.

MOUNTING

Placement of the radiographs in their correct position in the mounts may seem baffling at first. However, if auxiliaries develop a system based on understanding, they can master this problem in a short time. Auxiliaries must always work on a light-colored tabletop so they can see the radiographs easily when they are laid out. The radiographs are viewed on an illuminator or viewbox placed on or in front of the surface where the mounting is being done.

Lingual mounting view
↓

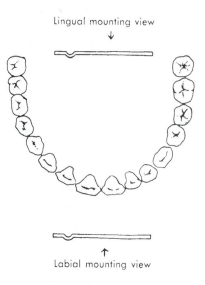

↑
Labial mounting view

FIGURE 12-3   Raised dot on x-ray film and its orientation in film mounts for labial or lingual viewing.

Every radiograph has an embossed or raised dot to help indicate the film orientation. The film packet is placed in the patient's mouth so that the side with the dot is always nearest the occlusal surface of the teeth. Manufacturers position the film in the packet so that the raised portion of the dot faces the x-ray machine when the exposure is made. If you mount the radiographs so that the raised portion of the dot is toward you, you are looking at the film as if you were facing the patient; the patient's left side is on your right (Figures 12-3 and 12-4). This is called *labial mounting.* If you mount the film so that the depressed side of the dot is toward you, you are looking at the films as if you were viewing them from a position on the patient's tongue; the patient's left side is on your left. This is called *lingual mounting.* Both mounting systems are used in dentistry today, but the trend has been to adopt labial mounting as the universal system. The American Dental Association recommends labial mounting for use by all dental offices.

PROCEDURE

The films from the patient's full-mouth series are laid out on the tabletop and the empty mount placed on the viewbox. The films are placed so that the dots are all one way, either up or down. The films are then divided into three groups: bitewings, anterior periapical, and posterior periapical. The bite-wing films are easily identified because the crowns of both the upper and lower teeth are seen. The anterior and posterior periapical films are differentiated by the vertical orientation on the film for anterior teeth and the horizontal orientation for posterior teeth.

Auxiliaries can differentiate the maxillary anterior films from the mandibular anteriors on the basis of root and crown shape and anatomic landmarks that will be discussed later. The films then are placed in their proper position in the mount.

A

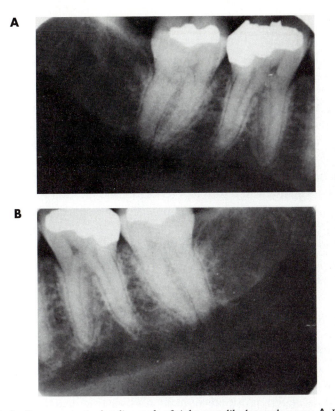

B

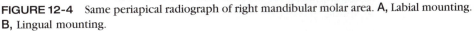

FIGURE 12-4   Same periapical radiograph of right mandibular molar area. **A,** Labial mounting. **B,** Lingual mounting.

The same routine is repeated for the posterior films. The bite-wing films are mounted last. Since they show only the crowns of the teeth, there are no root shapes and surrounding bony landmarks to aid in anatomic identification. Once the periapical films are mounted, fillings and missing teeth can be used to help identify and orient the bite-wing films.

Certain generalizations can be made about crown and root shapes seen on radiographs. The following hints will aid the novice in mounting films:

1 Crowns of upper anterior central and lateral incisors are wider and have longer roots than those of lower central and lateral incisors. Since they are wider, the maxillary anteriors do not fit on one film as the mandibular incisors do.

2 Maxillary premolars usually have two roots; mandibular premolars have one root.

3 Mandibular first and second molars usually have two divergent curved roots with bone clearly visible between them. This is particularly true of the first molar. Maxillary molars have three roots, two buccal and one palatal. The large palatal root obscures the interradicular bone.

4 Most roots curve distally.

5 The occlusal plane as it goes distally curves up.

These aids, along with the anatomic landmarks that will be described next, enable the dental auxiliary to properly orient radiographs in the x-ray film mount.

NORMAL RADIOGRAPHIC ANATOMY

To fully utilize and properly interpret radiographs, the dental auxiliary must be thoroughly familiar with normal radiographic anatomy. This includes all the structures seen on periapical, bite-wing, occlusal, panoramic, and extraoral projections. The first consideration in diagnosing a suspected lesion should be to differentiate it from a normal structure. This may often be difficult because there are wide variations of normal in the gross anatomy in regard to size, shape, and location that may be further modified by age, use, and disuse. Radiographically, these variations may be further exaggerated by the projection and angulation used. Not all landmarks are always demonstrated on every full-mouth survey or individual film. When confronted by a suspicious lesion, the first things to consider are the anatomic landmarks normally seen in that particular area. Normal anatomy should be ruled out first when making a differential pathologic diagnosis.

In interpreting radiographic landmarks dental staff should keep in mind the gross configuration of the structure. A thick, bony structure such as a ridge or muscle attachment appears more radiopaque because of increased object density. Any foramen, cavity, or concavity of bone produces an area represented on the film as a radiolucency because of decreased density. Radiographs, as two-dimensional representations, produce superimpositions of many normal structures that can be misleading, and dental staff should remember this as they interpret films.

Since radiographs are two-dimensional pictures of a three-dimensional object, they do not portray depth; teeth may be superimposed on anatomic structures in the mandible or maxilla or skull that may be millimeters in front of or in back of them. The best example is the roots of the maxillary molars and the maxillary sinus. Very few molar roots are actually in the sinus, although they may appear that way on almost all molar radiographs (see Figure 12-9).

RADIOGRAPHIC TOOTH ANATOMY

The component structures of the tooth and its supporting structures are well defined on the dental radiograph because of their differences in density (Figure 12-5).

Enamel is the densest and thus the most radiopaque of the natural tooth structures. It is seen as a radiopaque band that covers the crown of the tooth and ends in a fine edge at the cemento-enamel junction.

Dentin is the next layer of tooth structure. It is not as highly calcified as enamel and thus not as radiopaque. It comprises the major part of the tooth structure and is seen in both the crown and the root portions. On a radiograph with poor contrast it is difficult to see the border between enamel and dentin, the dentino-enamel junction.

Cementum is the thin, calcified covering on the surface of the root of the tooth. It is difficult to distinguish cementum from dentin because it is thin and its density is not

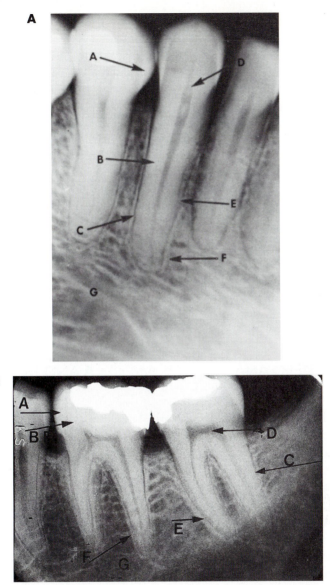

FIGURE 12-5 Normal radiographic tooth anatomy **A** anterior and **B** posterior tooth: **A,** enamel; **B,** dentin; **C,** periodontal membrane; **D,** pulp chamber; **E,** cementum; **F,** lamina dura; **G,** alveolar bone.

very different from that of dentin. Cementum is best seen in the pathologic condition hypercementosis, which is an overgrowth of cementum.

The *pulp chamber* and *pulp canal* are seen as a continuous radiolucent space in the center of the crown and root of the tooth. The fingerlike projections in the coronal portion are called pulp horns. They are seen most often in young patients, because the pulp chambers of teeth become smaller with age and in some cases may be totally obliterated by secondary dentin.

The *periodontal membrane* is seen as a radiolucent line about 0.5 mm wide between the cementum of the root of the tooth and the lamina dura. The periodontal membrane may not always be seen clearly on every root surface because of differences in horizontal angulation when the radiograph was taken.

The *lamina dura* is a radiopaque line of cortical bone that surrounds the periodontal membrane. It represents the bony wall of the tooth socket. It may not be seen on every surface because of angulation.

The *alveolar bone* is the bone that supports the tooth. It is composed of cancellous and cortical-compact bone. The cancellous bone is seen as a series of small radiolucent compartments called *medullary spaces.* These spaces are separated by a radiopaque honeycomb called *trabeculae.* The occlusal part of the alveolar bone is referred to as the *alveolar crest,* which is made of cortical bone. The mandible is a much denser bone than the maxilla; hence the medullary spaces are smaller and there is greater trabeculation in the mandible.

The *cortical bone* is seen as a dense radiopaque structure that comprises the buccal and palatal plates of the maxilla and the buccal and lingual plates, the inferior border of the mandible, the lamina dura, and the alveolar crest.

RADIOGRAPHIC ANATOMY OF MAXILLA AND MANDIBLE
Maxilla

Maxillary incisor area (Figure 12-6). The nasopalatine (incisive) foramen is seen as an oval radiolucency between the roots of the maxillary central incisors. In some radiographs the incisive canal can be seen leading to the foramen. The foramen is actually in the anterior portion of the palate, but superimposition makes it appear to be located between the roots of the central incisors. The position of the nasopalatine foramen on the radiograph may vary from just above the crest of the alveolar ridge to the level of the apices of the teeth because of anatomic variations and vertical angulation. In some cases, the shadow of the foramen may be superimposed on the apex of a central incisor and must be differentiated from periapical disease. This is done by taking another radiograph at a different horizontal angulation or by testing pulp vitality.

The median palatine suture is seen as a thin radiolucent line running vertically between the roots of the maxillary central incisors. It must be differentiated from a fracture line, nutrient canal, and fistulous tract.

The nasal fossa is the paired radiolucent structure superior to the apices of the incisor teeth. The fossa is also seen on the canine projection, where it may overlap or appear to adjoin the maxillary sinus. The radiopaque band that separates the left and right nasal fossa is called the median nasal septum. The septum ends inferiorly in the V-shaped radiopaque anterior nasal spine.

The radiopaque anterior nasal spine is near or superimposed upon the incisive foramen. The radiopacity that sometimes projects into the nasal fossa from its lateral

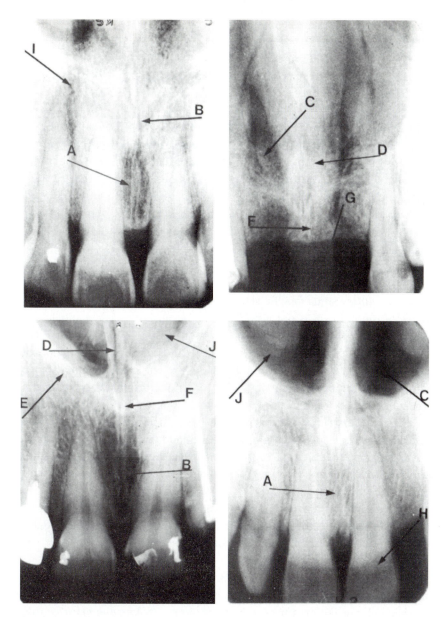

FIGURE 12-6   Maxillary central incisor area. **A,** Nasopalatine foramen. **B,** Median palatine suture. **C,** Nasal fossa. **D,** Median nasal septum. **E,** Floor of nasal cavity. **F,** Anterior nasal spine. **G,** Columella of nose. **H,** Lip line. **I,** Lateral fossa. **J,** Inferior concha.

wall is the inferior concha (turbinate). The concha is not calcified, so it does not appear as radiopaque as the walls of the nasal cavity.

The soft tissue and cartilaginous shadow of the tip of the nose as well as the soft tissue outline of the lip may be superimposed from the crest of the ridge to the crowns of the teeth. These soft tissue shadows are seen most clearly on edentulous films in which even the nares (openings) of the nose and the columella (separating column) are seen.

The lateral fossa is a depression in the labial plate in the lateral incisor region. It appears as a radiolucency between the lateral incisor and canine because it represents an area of thin bone.

Maxillary canine area (Figure 12-7). In the maxillary canine region two large radiolucent areas are seen. The more mesial area is the lateral aspect of the nasal fossa and the more distal is the anterior extent of the maxillary sinus. In edentulous film the radiopaque Y formed by the anterior and inferior border of the maxillary sinus as the arms and the floor of the nasal cavity as the stem is useful in mounting orientation.

The radiopaque soft tissue shadow of the nose may also show on canine area radiographs. In some projections a radiolucent area is seen distal to the canine and represents the nasolabial fold.

Maxillary premolar area (Figure 12-8). In the maxillary premolar area the radiolucent maxillary sinus may be seen either superimposed on, between, or above the apices of the teeth. It is not always visible because of vertical angulation of the x-ray beam and because the size and position of the maxillary sinus may vary from patient to patient. The floor of the maxillary sinus appears as a radiopaque line running horizontally at its lower border. The floor of the nasal fossa may be seen as a radiopaque line running horizontally at the superior portion of the maxillary sinus. Nutrient canals may be seen in the alveolar bone along with grooves for vessels in the walls of the maxillary sinus. Bony septum also may be seen in the maxillary sinus.

The edentulous premolar radiograph is identified by the presence of the maxillary sinus. It differs from the molar radiograph in the absence of the maxillary sinus in the mesial part of the film and the start of the radiopaque zygomatic arch band at the distal portion of the film.

In some edentulous films the shadow of the buccinator muscle is seen. This shadow makes part of the normally radiolucent area below the ridge appear radiopaque because of the increased density of the muscle.

Maxillary molar area (Figure 12-9). The maxillary sinus is a radiolucent area that always appears on periapical projections of the maxillary molar region. The sinus may be unilocular or compartmented by bony septa. Radiopaque spurs or ridges may project into the sinus; radiolucent tracts or grooves, representing blood vessel positions, may be seen in the walls of the sinus. The size of the maxillary sinus varies greatly because of age, morphology, radiographic projection, and vertical angulation used. A patient's sinuses may be asymmetrical and may tend to enlarge or grow into areas of the alveolar ridge where teeth have been extracted. This process is called pneumatization. Just distal to the third molar ridge area is the maxillary tuberosity. This area of cancellous bone also may contain the posterior extension of the maxillary sinus. The large, fibrous buildup of soft tissue above the tuberosity may cause a slightly radiopaque shadow on the radiograph and is called the tuberosity pad.

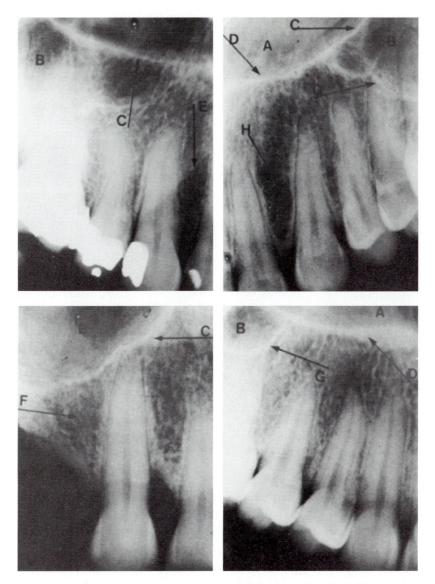

FIGURE 12-7 Maxillary canine area. **A,** Nasal fossa **B,** Maxillary sinus. **C,** Septum of bone separating maxillary sinus and nasal septum. **D,** Floor of nasal cavity. **E,** Shadow of the nose. **F,** Nasolabial fold. **G,** Floor of maxillary sinus. **H,** Lateral fossa.

The zygomatic process of the maxilla is seen as an inverted U-shaped radiopacity superimposed on the roots of the first and second molars and the maxillary sinus. The malar bone (zygoma), which is a continuation of the zygomatic process, appears as a broad, uniform radiopaque band that extends posteriorly. Together they make up the zygomatic arch.

The hamular process is the radiopaque projection that extends downward distal to the posterior surface of the maxillary tuberosity. It is the inferior end of the medial

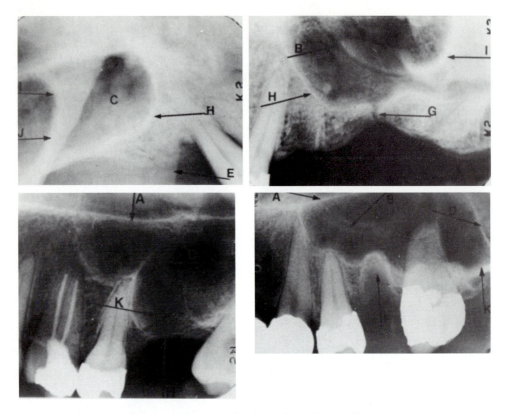

FIGURE 12-8 Maxillary premolar area. **A,** Floor of nasal fossa. **B,** Nutrient canals in sinus wall. **C,** Maxillary sinus. **D,** Sinus septum. **E,** Buccinator shadow. **F,** Extraction socket. **G,** Oral antral communication. **H,** floor of maxillary sinus. **I,** Zygomatic process of maxilla. **J,** Zygomatic arch. **K,** Pneumatization.

pterygoid plate of the sphenoid bone. The radiolucent area between the tuberosity and the hamular process is referred to as the hamular notch (Figure 12-10).

In the distal inferior portion of maxillary molar radiographs a large radiopaque structure may be seen. This is the coronoid process of the mandible. When an edentulous series is mounted, this landmark is helpful in determining which is the most distal of the maxillary radiographs.

The maxillary torus (torus palatinus) is a lobulated bony growth in the midline of the palate. On a periapical radiograph it appears as a dense, well-demarcated, radiopaque area (Figure 12-11).

Mandible

Mandibular incisor area (Figure 12-12). In the mandibular central incisor area, just below the apices of the central incisors in the midline, there is often a somewhat circular radiopacity. This is the genial tubercle, which represents a bony growth on the lingual surface of the mandible to which the genioglossus and the

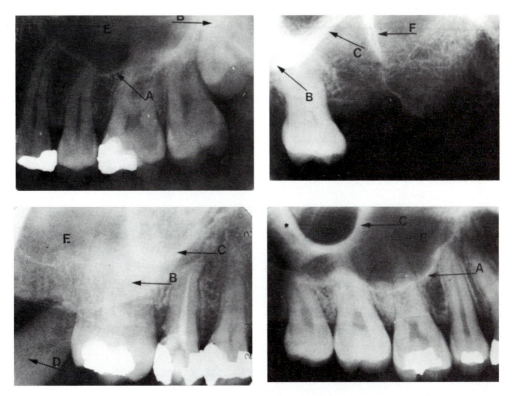

FIGURE 12-9 Maxillary molar area. **A,** Floor of sinus. **B,** Zygomatic arch. **C,** Zygomatic process of maxilla. **D,** Coronoid process of mandible. **E,** Maxillary sinus. **F,** Septum in sinus.

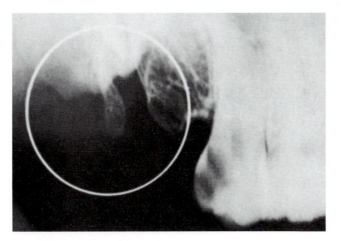

FIGURE 12-10 Posterior part of maxillary molar region. In circle are maxillary tuberosity, hamular notch, and hamular process.

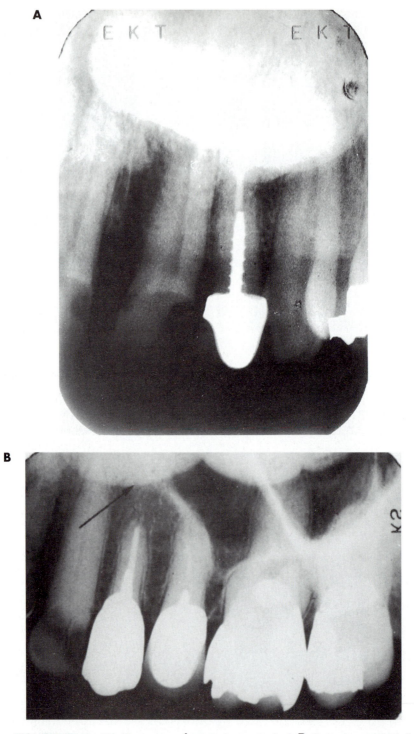

FIGURE 12-11   Maxillary torus. A, Anterior periapical. B, Posterior periapical.

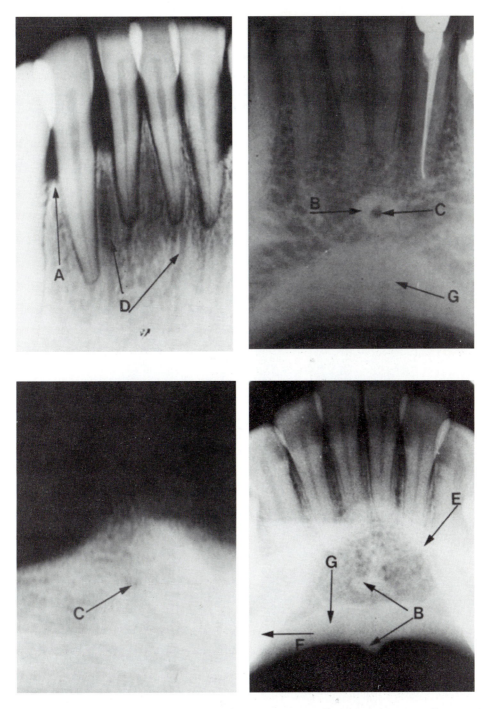

FIGURE 12-12   Mandibular incisor area. **A,** Alveolar ridge. **B,** Genial tubercles. **C,** Lingual foramen. **D,** Nutrient canals. **E,** Mental ridge. **F,** Mylohyoid ridge. **G,** Inferior border of mandible.

geniohyoid muscles are attached. In the middle of the genial tubercle a small circular radiolucency may be seen. This is the lingual foramen, which is the exit point from the mandible for the lingual branches of the incisive vessels. Nutrient canals, although found in all areas of the mandible and maxilla, are seen most easily in this area. They appear as radiolucent lines that run vertically in the alveolar bone and terminate in small circular radiolucent nutrient foramina. The nutrient canals are pathways for blood vessels and nerves.

The mental ridge is a broad radiopaque band that represents a ridge of bone on the labial aspect of the mandible. It arises bilaterally below the apical area of the canine

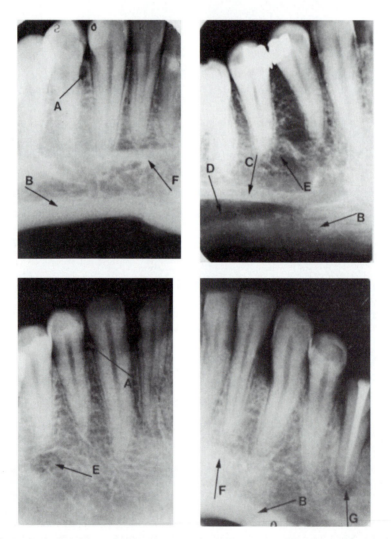

FIGURE 12-13   Mandibular canine area. **A,** Alveolar ridge. **B,** Inferior border of mandible. **C,** Internal oblique ridge. **D,** Submandibular fossa. **E,** Mental foramen. **F,** Mental ridge. **G,** Periapical pathology.

and incisors and runs medially and upward toward the mandibular symphysis. The ridge, if superimposed over the apices of the teeth, may hinder diagnosis. The ridge should be differentiated from the internal oblique ridge.

The shadow of the lip is seen on anterior radiographs. That portion of the film not covered by the lip appears darker than the rest of the film because there is no soft tissue attenuation in the area. The lip line, unless identified as such, can hinder radiographic interpretation.

The inferior border of the mandible is seen as a broad radiopaque band that represents the thick cortical bone of this area.

Mandibular canine area (Figure 12-13). The anterior extension of the internal oblique ridge and submandibular fossa can be seen in the canine area.

The edentulous mandibular canine may be difficult to orient in the mount. One should look for the genial tubercle on the mesial part of the film and possibly the mental foramen in the distal part. The edentulous alveolar ridge crest slopes downward as it goes distally.

Mandibular premolar area (Figure 12-14). The mental foramen is seen as a round or oval radiolucency near the apices of the premolars. The mental foramen may be found between, below, or even superimposed on the apices of the premolars. It is through this foramen that the mental nerves and blood vessels emerge. In some cases the radiolucent mandibular canal may be seen leading directly to the foramen. The mental foramen in many cases because of its superimposition on the apices of the premolar must be differentiated from periapical pathology.

The termination of the external oblique ridge can be seen in this area along with the internal oblique ridge, submandibular fossa, and inferior border of the mandible.

The mandibular tori (torus mandibularis), although not strictly considered normal landmarks, are included in this section because of their frequency. They are seen singularly or multiply, usually bilaterally on the lingual aspects of the mandible in or near the premolar region. They appear as clearly outlined radiopacities (Figure 12-15).

The edentulous premolar film is identified and oriented for mounting by the presence of the mental foramen and the ending of the external oblique ridge. The crest of the edentulous alveolar ridge tends to rise as it goes mesially.

Mandibular molar area (Figure 12-16). The mandibular canal is seen as a radiolucent band below the apices of the posterior teeth, originating at the mandibular foramen and running downward and forward to end at the mental foramen. It is bordered by thin, radiopaque lines.

The oblique ridges refer to the internal and external oblique ridges. The external ridge, a continuation of the anterior border of the ramus, is seen as a radiopaque line that passes diagonally down and forward across the molar region. The internal or mylohyoid ridge is a radiopaque line that runs from the medial and anterior aspect of the ramus downward and forward to end at the lower border of the symphysis. When

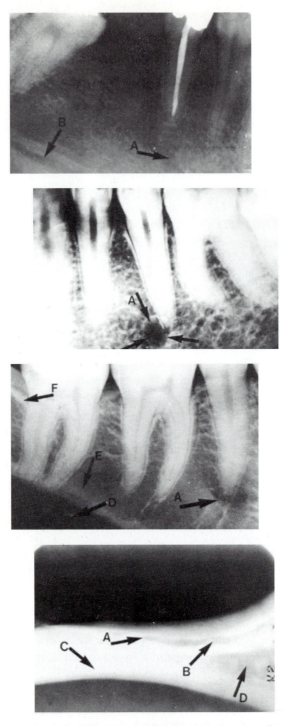

FIGURE 12-14 Mandibular premolar area. **A,** Mental foramen. **B,** Mandibular canal. **C,** Inferior border of the mandible. **D,** Submandibular fossa. **E,** Internal oblique ridge. **F,** External oblique ridge.

A

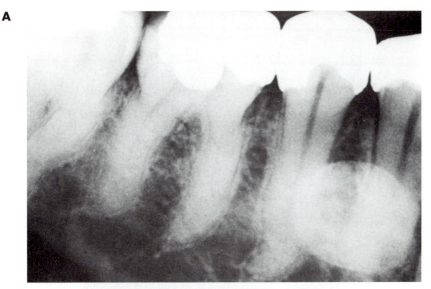

B

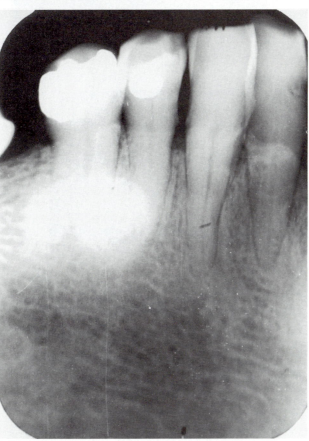

FIGURE 12-15 Mandibular tori. **A,** Premolar projection. **B,** Cuspid projection.

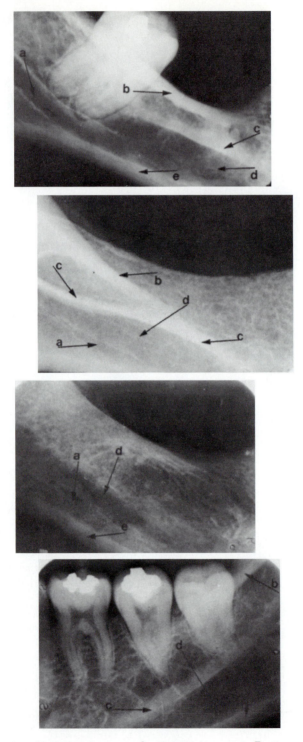

FIGURE 12-16 Mandibular molar area. **A,** Mandibular canal. **B,** External oblique ridge. **C,** Internal oblique ridge. **D,** Submandibular fossa. **E,** Inferior border of mandible.

these two ridges are seen together, the internal oblique ridge is the lower of the two radiopaque lines.

The submandibular fossa is seen as a radiolucent area below the internal oblique (mylohyoid) ridge. It represents an area of reduced thickness of bone caused by a depression on the medial surface of the mandible. This radiolucency may be accentuated by a prominent mylohyoid ridge and a thick, opaque, inferior border of the mandible.

Nutrient canals are seen commonly in the molar region, especially when it is edentulous.

RESTORATIONS

As with tooth and bone structure the density of the restoration determines its appearance on radiographs. Metallic restorations such as gold inlays, crowns, foils, posts, pins, or silver amalgam are the most radiopaque areas seen on radiographs (Figures 12-17 and 12-18). One can identify them only on the basis of size and shape, not on the degree of radiopacity. The synthetic restorations used in anterior teeth (e.g., glass ionomers, laminates, composites, and acrylics) (Figure 12-19) appear radiolucent and may be mistaken radiographically for caries. Manufacturers of some synthetic restorations now incorporate radiopaque particles in their preparations to distinguish the restorations from caries (Figure 12-20). Temporary or sedative fillings and cavity liners, such as zinc oxide, calcium hydroxide, and zinc oxyphosphate cement, appear radiopaque because they contain some metallic elements (see Figures 12-17 and 12-19). Porcelain jackets appear slightly radiopaque, as the silicate from which they are made

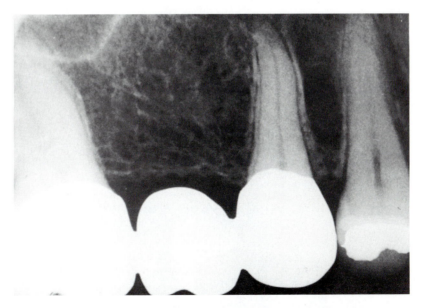

FIGURE 12-17   Fixed bridge and amalgam restoration. Note that acrylic facing of pontic does not appear on radiograph. Also note difference in radiopacities between amalgam and the cement base in the premolar.

A

B

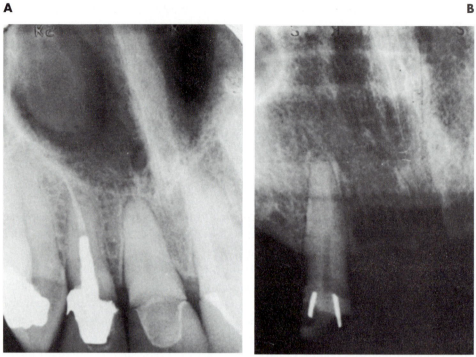

FIGURE 12-18 **A,** Gold post and core under porcelain jacket. **B,** Metallic pins under synthetic restoration.

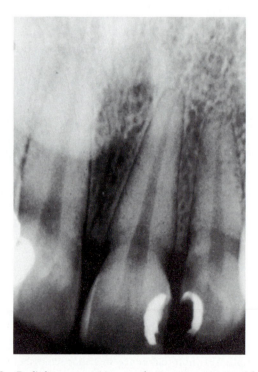

FIGURE 12-19 Radiolucent anterior synthetic restorations with cement bases.

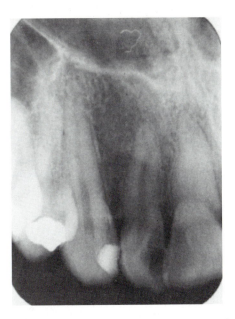

FIGURE 12-20   Radiopaque anterior synthetic restoration mesial of the cuspid. Mesial of the lateral incisor has radiolucent synthetic restoration.

A   **B**

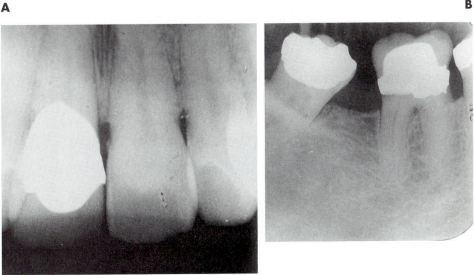

FIGURE 12-21   Porcelain fused to metal (PFM) crowns on anterior and posterior teeth. Note the different densities of the metal and porcelain.

is a metal, with with the radiopaque cement being more apparent (see Figure 12-18, *A*). Porcelain fused to metal crowns appears with distinct outlines of the metal with the porcelain seen poorly or not at all (Figure 12-21, *A* and *B*). Endodontic fillings appear as radiopacities in the pulp and root canal chambers. Of the two types of endodontic fillings most commonly used, the silver cones appear more radiopaque than the gutta-percha points. Compare the endodontic filling in Figure 12-18, *A*, with the filling in Figure 12- 22. Other materials that can be seen are fracture wires (Figure 12-23) and orthodontic bands and wires (Figure 12-24).

RADIOGRAPHIC ANATOMY FOR PANORAMIC FILMS

The normal radiographic anatomy for panoramic films is shown in Figure 12-25. Some of the anatomic landmarks listed were described in the preceding section on periapical radiographs. Those landmarks commonly seen on panoramic films that are diagnostically important are also discussed here.

Mandibular foramen. The mandibular foramen appears as an oval radiolucency at the origin of the mandibular canal at the midpoint of the ramus of the mandible.

Pharyngeal air space. The pharyngeal air space appears as a bilateral, symmetrical, radiolucent band between the radiopaque palatal line and the apices of the maxillary posterior teeth. It runs posteriorly and downward across the ramus and into the soft tissues of the neck. The appearance of the air space on radiographs varies depending on the position of the tongue and thus the air above it and the state of contraction of the pharyngeal muscles. The diagnostic key for the air space is the bilateral and symmetrical appearance that can be followed running distally off the bone into the soft tissue.

Styloid process. The styloid process is a radiopaque projection that may be seen bilaterally projecting downward just posterior to the ramus of the mandible. The styloid ligaments attached to the process may calcify and give the appearance of an

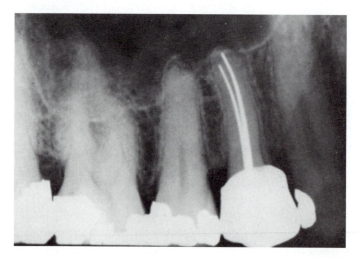

FIGURE 12-22   Silver cones used as endodontic filling material in first premolar.

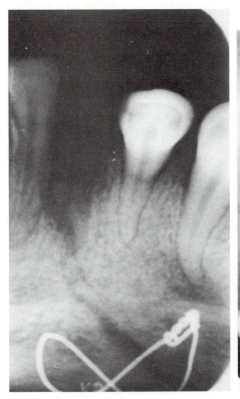

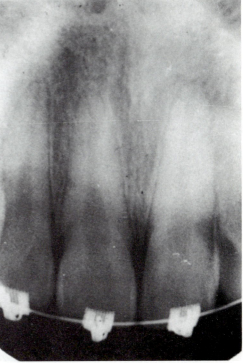

FIGURE 12-23 Healing mandibular fracture with intraosseous wires in place.

FIGURE 12-24 Orthodontic brackets and wires.

abnormally long styloid process. The calcification of the ligament may not be continuous or may start at the attachment of the ligament to the styloid process, giving the appearance of a fracture of the styloid process (Figure 12-26).

Mandibular condyle. The condyle, condylar neck, sigmoid notch, and coronoid process of the mandible are seen on panoramic films. Unless the unit has a variable focal plane, this is not the best way to view the condyle, because it does not lie within the usual focal trough.

OCCLUSAL PROJECTIONS

Auxiliaries must remember when interpreting occlusal films that the projection is in the superoinferior plane and shows the third dimension not seen in periapical, bite-wing, and panoramic films (Figures 12-27 and 12-28). The type of occlusal projection used, right-angle or topographic (65 degrees), also should be considered because the position of the landmarks varies, depending on the angulation used.

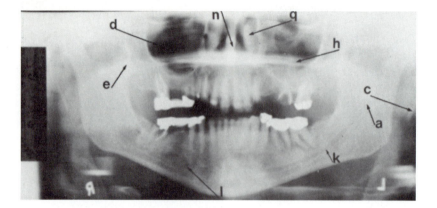

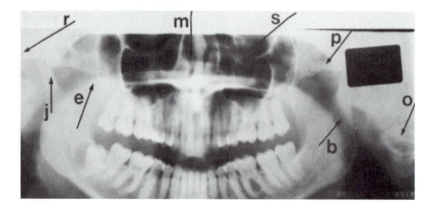

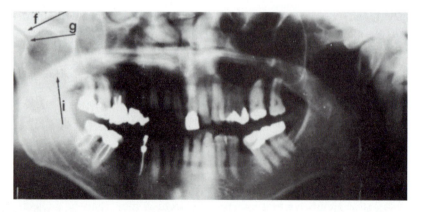

FIGURE 12-25 Panoramic film. **a,** Mandibular foramen. **b,** Pharyngeal air space. **c,** Styloid process. **d,** Maxillary sinus. **e,** Coronoid process. **f,** Articular eminence. **g,** Glenoid fossa. **h,** Hard palate. **i,** Mental foramen. **j,** Mandibular condyle. **k,** Mandibular canal. **l,** Mental foramen. **m,** Nasal fossa. **n,** Nasal septum. **o,** Cervical vertebra. **p,** Zygoma. **q,** Inferior turbinate. **r,** External auditory meatus. **s,** Orbit.

EXTRAORAL PROJECTIONS

The most commonly seen and important landmarks for the extraoral techniques described in Chapter 9 are given in Figures 12-29 to 12-33.

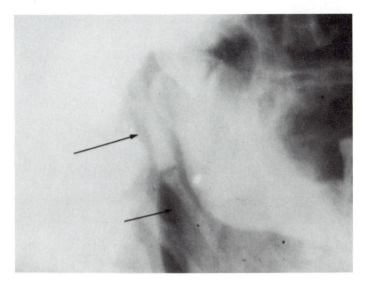

FIGURE 12-26   Calcified styloid ligament.

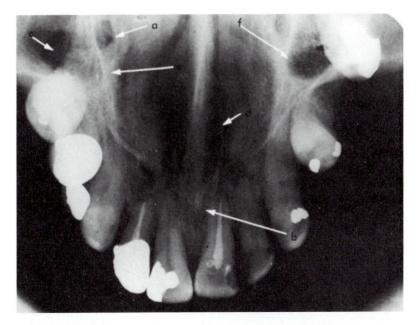

FIGURE 12-27   Maxillary occlusal film. **a,** Nasolacrimal duct. **b,** Anterior palatine foramen. **c,** Maxillary sinus. **d,** Nasal fossa. **e,** Lateral wall of nasal fossa. **f,** Lateral wall of maxillary sinus.

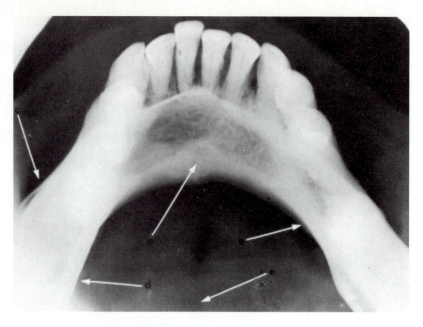

FIGURE 12-28 Mandibular occlusal film. **a,** Genial tubercles. **b,** Interior border. **c,** Buccal cortical plate. **d,** Lingual cortical plate. **e,** Shadow of tongue.

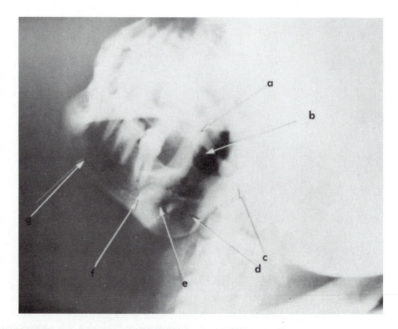

FIGURE 12-29 Lateral oblique projection of mandible. **a,** Coronoid process. **b,** Sigmoid notch. **c,** Condyle. **d,** Pharyngeal air space. **e,** Mandibular foramen. **f,** Mandibular canal. **g,** Mental foramen.

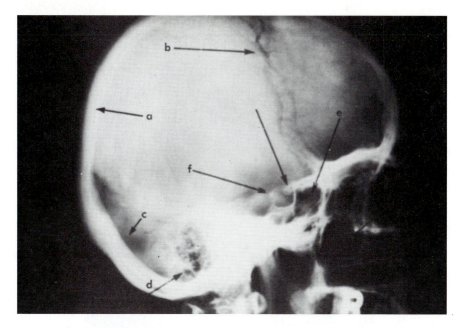

FIGURE 12-30 Lateral skull projection. **a,** Inner and outer table. **b,** Vascular markings. **c,** Lateral venous sinus. **d,** Mastoid air cells. **e,** Sphenoid sinus. **f,** Anterior and posterior clinoid processes, sella turcica.

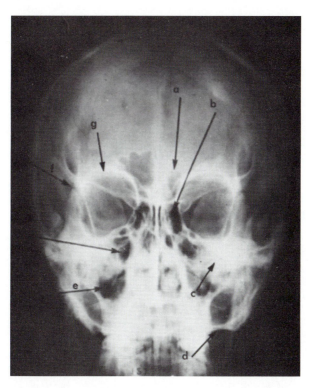

FIGURE 12-31 Posteroanterior view. **a,** Frontal sinus. **b,** Ethmoid sinus. **c,** Petrous ridge. **d,** Base of skull. **e,** Maxillary sinus. **f,** Frontozygomatic suture. **g,** Orbit.

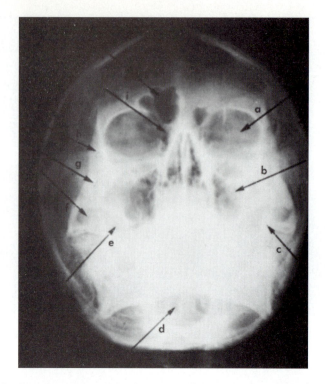

FIGURE 12-32 Posteroanterior view of sinuses (Waters' view). **a,** Orbit. **b,** Maxillary sinus. **c,** Coronoid process. **d,** Foramen magnum and vertebra. **e,** Lateral wall of maxillary sinus. **f,** Zygomatic arch. **g,** Malar bone. **h,** Frontozygomatic suture. **i,** Ethmoid sinus. **j,** Frontal sinus.

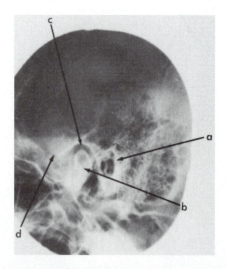

FIGURE 12-33 Normal temporomandibular joint. **a,** External auditory meatus. **b,** Condyle. **c,** Articular fossae. **d,** Articular eminence.

Chapter

thirteen

Radiographic
Interpretation:
caries and periodontal disease

The inclusion in this text of four chapters on interpretation is not meant to imply that it is the role of the dental auxiliary to make the final radiographic diagnosis. At the present time the final diagnostic role rests with the dentist but certainly help and input from other members of the dental health care team should not be discouraged. Dentists cannot be correct every time. Dental auxiliaries need to develop as interpretive skills to identify all normal anatomic structures, both tooth and bone, and artifacts visible on intraoral radiographs and pantomographs. They also must identify deviation in radiographic form and density from normal structures.[1] To produce adequate diagnostic films the dental auxiliary must know what relevant information is being sought from the radiograph. This base of knowledge makes the taking of radiographs a more challenging, interesting, and rewarding process. If auxiliaries know how periapical pathologic conditions appear radiographically, they also understand the necessity of seeing the entire periapical area of the tooth in question to make a proper diagnosis. If dental auxiliaries know how difficult or in some cases how impossible it is to interpret caries on radiographs with horizontal overlapping of the teeth, they should be motivated to try to avoid this error in technique.

The purpose of Chapters 13 through 16 is to offer the dental auxiliary some basic understanding of radiographic interpretation, to stimulate interest, and to show the importance of producing an adequate diagnostic radiograph.

CARIES

Detection of caries is probably the most frequent reason for taking dental radiographs. Caries is seen on radiographs as a radiolucency in the crowns and roots of teeth. The caries process is one of demineralization of the hard tooth structure with subsequent destruction. This decrease in density allows greater penetration of the x-rays in the carious area and resultant radiolucency on the film. The degree of radiolucency on a given film is determined by the extent of the caries in the buccolingual plane in relation to the density of the overlying tooth structure. Radiographic interpretation of caries can be misleading in regard to relative depth and position in the tooth, as well as differentiation from other radiolucencies. Caries always is farther advanced clinically than the radiographs indicate, because the bacterial penetration of the dentinal tubules and early demineralization does not produce significant changes in density to affect the penetration pattern. The depth of the caries in relation to the pulp also can be misleading. Since the radiograph portrays a three-dimensional object in two planes, what may seem to be an obvious pulpal exposure radiographically may be the result of superimposition of images.

Caries that occurs only in the enamel is said to be incipient and is difficult to detect radiographically because the density of the tooth structure has not undergone any great change. Most advanced caries involving dentin in either the crown or the root of the tooth appears on properly taken radiographs. However, small, deep occlusal, buccal, or lingual carious lesions may not be seen. This is because the decrease in density caused by the caries is small compared with the total buccolingual density of the tooth (Figure 13-1).

It is in the diagnosis of interproximal decay that radiographs are most important. Interproximal caries is best seen on bite-wing radiographs (Figure 13-2). If the paralleling technique is used, caries also appears clearly and undistorted on periapical films (Figure 13-3). In the bisecting-angle technique the vertical angulation may distort or even mask interproximal caries. This is especially true of recurrent decay under old restorations. Bite-wing radiographs are also useful in detecting poor contact, fit, and contour of metallic fillings, as well as overhangs and broken fillings (see Figures 13-2 and 13-4).

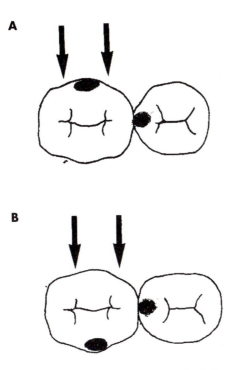

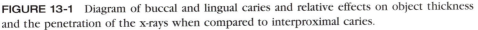

FIGURE 13-1   Diagram of buccal and lingual caries and relative effects on object thickness and the penetration of the x-rays when compared to interproximal caries.

Horizontal angulation, as mentioned in Chapter 7, is extremely important in caries diagnosis because an overlapped film does not show the interproximal surfaces clearly and therefore is of no diagnostic value (see Figures 7-28 and 7-29).

Occlusal caries

A careful clinical examination with a mouth mirror and an explorer will detect occlusal caries earlier than will radiographic interpretation. The absence of radiographic findings is a result of the superimposition of the dense buccal and lingual cusps on the relatively small carious area in the occlusal pits and fissures. Occlusal caries is not seen radiographically until it has reached the dentoenamel junctions, at which point it appears as a horizontal radiolucent line. As the decay progresses into the dentin, it appears as a diffuse radiolucent area with poorly defined borders. This appearance differentiates it from advanced buccal or lingual decay, which has more defined borders (Figure 13-5). This radiographic differentiation is always confirmed clinically.

Very often radiographs of teeth with deep or broad occlusal pits and fissures show radiolucencies that resemble caries. These normal variants can be differentiated by examination with a mirror and an explorer.

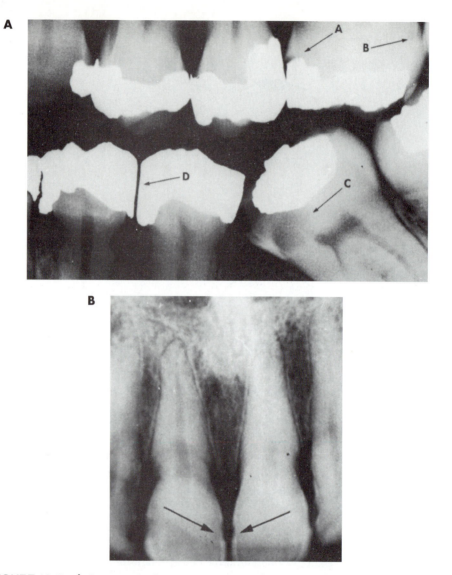

FIGURE 13-2 A, Interproximal caries on bite-wing radiograph. **A,** recurrent; **B,** incipient; **C,** advanced; **D,** open contact. **B,** Caries seen on periapical film of maxillary incisors.

Buccal and lingual caries

Early lesions on these surfaces may be very difficult, if not impossible, to detect radiographically because of the superimposition of the densities of normal tooth structures. As the caries progresses, the radiolucency is characterized by its well-defined borders. Although it is theoretically possible to differentiate radiographically between buccal and lingual decay on the basis of sharpness of the image, it is not

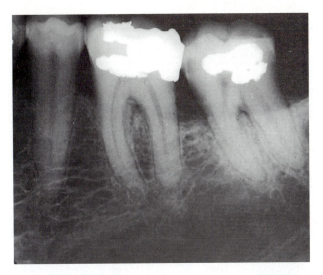

FIGURE 13-3   Periapical radiograph showing caries, mesial second molar.

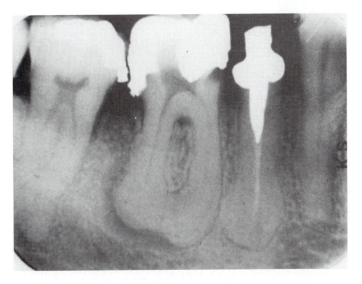

FIGURE 13-4   Caries seen on periapical radiograph. Note faulty contour on restorations and periapical radiolucency.

clinically important. The differentiation is identified more easily with a mirror and an explorer. It is impossible to judge the relationship of buccal or lingual caries to the pulp on radiographs because the depth of the caries lies in a geometric plane that is not recorded radiographically (Figure 13-6).

Interproximal caries.   The first sign of interproximal caries is a notching of the enamel, usually just below the contact point. As the caries progresses inward, it

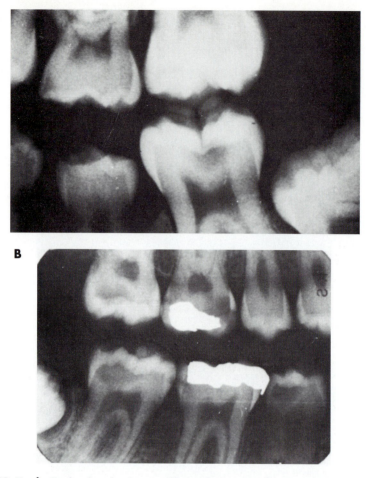

FIGURE 13-5   A, Occlusal caries in mandibular first molar. B, Advanced occlusal caries in maxillary second molar, pulpal exposure in mandibular second molar. List the other carious lesions shown on this film.

assumes a triangular shape, with the apex of the triangle toward the dentoenamel junction. As it invades the dentin, the caries spreads along the dentoenamel junction and proceeds toward the pulp in a roughly triangular pattern (Figure 13-7).

The radiographic appearance of interproximal caries is affected by the size and shape of the contact of the tooth involved. A tooth with a broad contact point does not show the caries as well as one with a narrow contact point because of the greater density of the tooth structure surrounding the caries (Figure 13-8).

Conditions resembling caries

Many radiolucencies seen on dental radiographs may be mistaken for caries. The final diagnosis of caries is always made by corroborating the clinical examination with the radiographic findings.

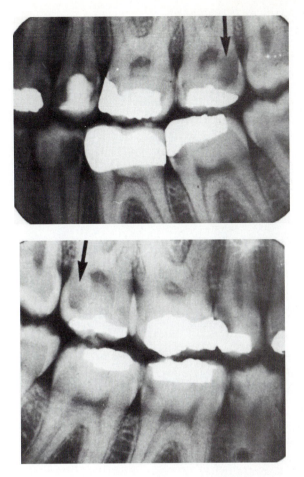

FIGURE 13-6 Buccal caries as indicated by arrows. List the other carious lesions on these films.

Cervical burnout. Cervical burnout appears as a radiolucent band at the neck of the tooth. It is contrasted because the part of the tooth apical to it is covered by bone and hence is more radiopaque, while the area of the tooth occlusal to it is covered by enamel and is also radiopaque. In addition to these differences in densities caused by enamel and bone, the concave root contours below the cementoenamel junction appear as radiolucencies. Cervical burnout is most often observed when there has been no loss of the alveolar bone that provides the radiographic contrast. It is seen most often in the mandibular incisors and molars (Figure 13-9).

Abrasions and attrition. Radiographically, cervical abrasion may resemble caries because it causes a wearing away of root structure and results in a decrease in density in the affected area. The radiolucency produced by the abrasion is usually a well-defined horizontal defect seen at the cementoenamel junction. Evidence of secondary dentin formation and pulp recession in response to the irritant also may be

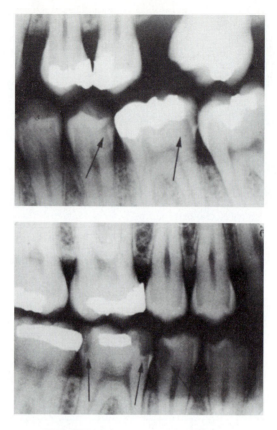

FIGURE 13-7 Interproximal caries.

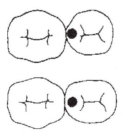

FIGURE 13-8 Diagram illustrating effect of contact point on caries interpretation.

seen radiographically (Figure 13-10). Attrition, which is defined as occlusal wear on teeth, appears clinically and radiographically.

Indirect pulp capping. A radiolucent shadow under a metallic restoration may not always indicate recurrent decay but an indirect pulp capping. To avoid a carious pulp exposure in this technique, the last remaining portion of decayed tooth is not

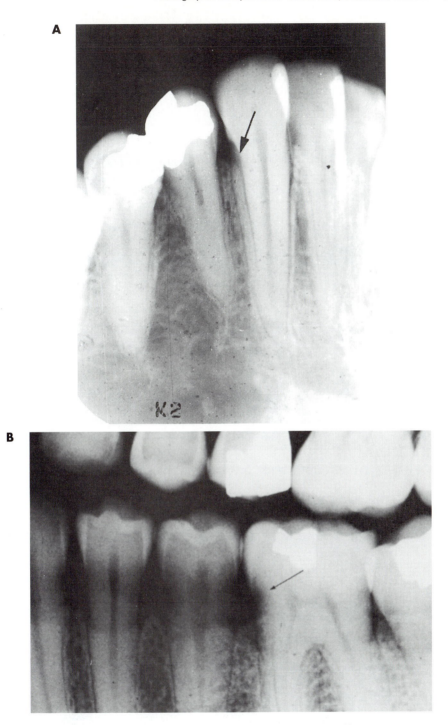

FIGURE 13-9 Cervical burnout *(arrows)*. **A**, Anterior teeth. **B**, Posterior teeth.

excavated. A sedative base and permanent restoration are placed with the hope that secondary dentin will be laid down to protect the pulp. Radiographically, the indirect pulp-capping procedure shows the radiolucent band of the unexcavated decay near the pulp chamber with a sedative base and permanent restoration (Figure 13-11).

A

B

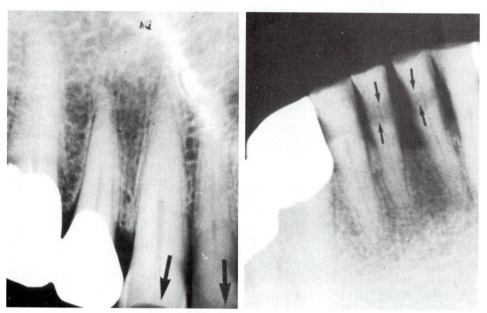

FIGURE 13-10   A, Attrition. B, Abrasion.

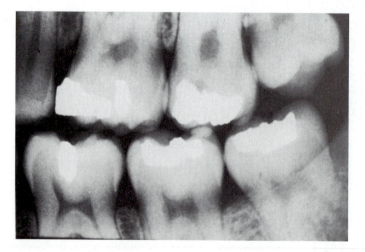

FIGURE 13-11   Indirect pulp capping. Note radiolucent area under restoration in maxillary second molar.

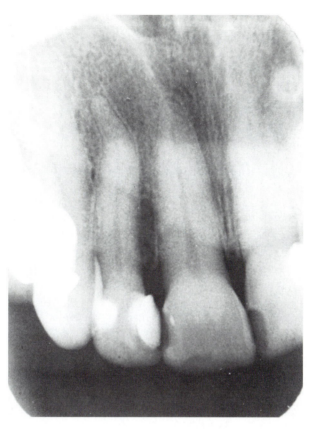

FIGURE 13-12   Radiolucent restorations in central incisors.

Restorative materials. Restorative materials such as silicates, acrylics, and some composites may resemble caries radiographically (Figure 13-12). Recently some brands of composite filling material have had radiopaque materials added to their formulation (Figure 13-13). Auxiliaries can differentiate between caries and the radiolucent filling on the basis of the regular geometric outline of a cavity preparation and the presence of a radiopaque cement base. All base and pulp-capping formulations that have a metallic component (e.g., zinc oxyphosphate, zinc oxide, calcium hydroxide) appear radiopaque (Figure 13-14).

PERIODONTAL DISEASE

The proper diagnosis and evaluation of periodontal disease can be made only with a combination of radiographic and clinical examinations. Periodontal disease has both soft tissue and bone components; there are radiographic limitations in both aspects of the disease process. Soft tissue (gingival) changes such as inflammation, hypertrophy, and recession do not appear on radiographs, since all soft tissue is radiolucent. Bone

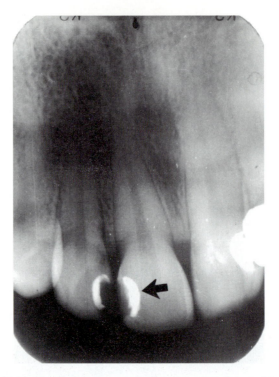

FIGURE 13-13 Radiopaque restorations mesial of central incisors.

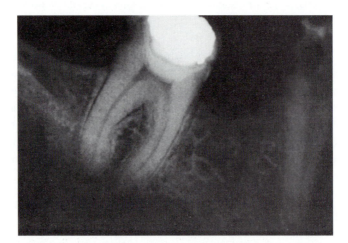

FIGURE 13-14 Radiopaque base and pulpotomy under metallic restoration.

loss in some areas may not be seen because of superimpositions of buccal and lingual alveolar bone. Auxiliaries should remember that the radiograph portrays a three-dimensional disease process in two planes. Radiographic images of bone changes almost always show less bone loss than there is.

In spite of these limitations, a proper periodontal diagnosis cannot be made without a full-mouth survey of radiographs. Radiographs serve to (1) identify predisposing factors, (2) detect early to moderate bone changes where treatment can preserve the dentition, (3) approximate the amount of bone loss and its location, (4) help in evaluating the prognosis of affected teeth and the restorative needs of these teeth, and (5) serve as baseline data and as a means of evaluating posttreatment results.

Techniques

The paralleling technique with a 16-inch focal-film distance is the best method for evaluating periodontal disease. A full periapical survey taken in this manner and augmented by posterior, anterior, or vertical bitewings is the technique of choice.

The use of the bisecting technique with its inherent dimensional distortion provides a distorted representation of the level of bone present (see Figure 7-7 p. 148).

Panoramic films are of little or no value in the diagnosis of periodontal disease except in the most advanced cases. Panoramic films should only be used if intraoral films cannot be taken.

Xeroradiography is an excellent imaging system to use in detecting periodontal disease. Soft tissue images are seen well, and the wider range of densities show early bone changes as well as small, less calcified calculus formation. Unfortunately xeroradiography was not universally accepted by the dental profession as was noted previously in Chapter 9. Very few units are still in use.

Predisposing factors

The detection of predisposing factors is one of the most important roles of radiography in periodontal disease. The treatment or prevention of early periodontal disease is much easier and has a higher success rate than efforts made once the disease has progressed further. The detection and elimination of local irritants are essential steps in prevention or actual periodontal therapy.

Calculus. Both subgingival and supragingival calculus are the most common of all local irritants. Early deposits, small and not fully calcified, are not seen radiographically. Even when calcified, supragingival calculus, which is seen most often on the lingual surface of lower anterior teeth and the buccal surface of upper molars, is not seen clearly in its early stage because of superimposition of tooth structure (Figure 13-15). Subgingival calculus on the proximal surfaces is detected more easily in the early calcified stages. The calculus appears as an irregularly pointed radiopaque projection from the proximal root surfaces (Figure 13-16).

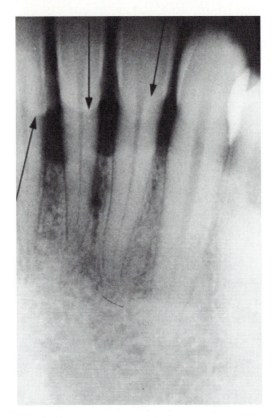

FIGURE 13-15   Supragingival calculus on lingual surfaces of lower incisors.

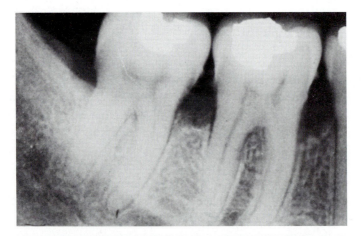

FIGURE 13-16   Subgingival calculus. Note bone loss.

Restorations. Radiographic examination reveals restorations with open contacts, poor contours, overhanging and deficient margins, and caries, all of which are etiologic factors in periodontal disease (Figures 13-17 to 13-19).

Anatomic configurations. Only through radiographic examination can information about the size, shape, and position of the roots of periodontally involved teeth be obtained. These factors are important in evaluating the present condition and planning periodontal and restorative therapy.

The crown-root ratio refers to the length of root surface imbedded in bone compared with the length of the rest of the tooth. The greater the length of the tooth imbedded in bone, the better the prognosis (Figure 13-20). This becomes a critical factor when designing both fixed and removable prosthesis.

Teeth that have an anatomically short root have a poorer prognosis periodontally than those teeth with long roots. Teeth with bulbous roots have more area for

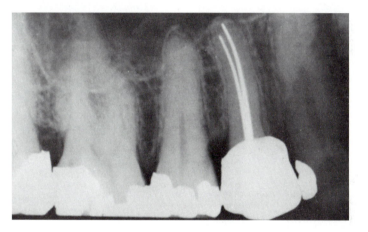

FIGURE 13-17   Overcontoured crown on premolar and bone response.

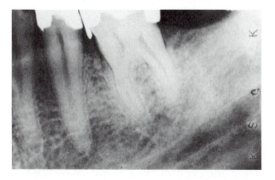

FIGURE 13-18   Restoration with open contact and overhang. Note bony response.

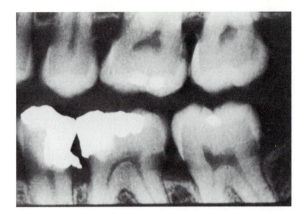

FIGURE 13-19   Restoration with overhang. Note heavy calculus formation in other areas.

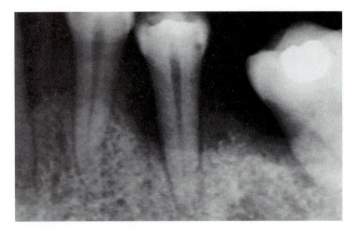

FIGURE 13-20   Crown-root ratio unfavorable.

attachment than those with fine, tapered roots. In multirooted teeth, the space between the roots is important; teeth with widely spaced roots have a better periodontal prognosis. Adjoining teeth whose roots are close together have a poorer prognosis than those with adequate areas of interseptal bone.

Gingivitis.   Since gingivitis is a soft tissue change, there are no radiographic findings other than the presence of predisposing factors.

Radiographically detectable periodontal changes

Early (Figure 13-21).   This stage of periodontal change is characterized radiographically by changes in the crest of the interproximal bone septum and triangulation of the periodontal membrane. Triangulation is the widening of the periodontal

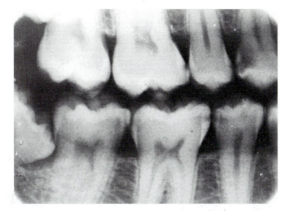

FIGURE 13-21   Early periodontal bone loss. Note fading of density of the alveolar crest, slight cupping, and triangulation.

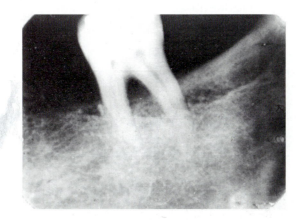

FIGURE 13-22   Moderate to advanced bone loss showing bifurcation involvement.

membrane space at the crest of the interproximal septum that gives the appearance of a radiolucent triangle to what is normally a radiolucent band. The normal crest of the interseptal bone runs parallel to a line drawn between cementoenamel junctions on adjoining teeth at a level 1.0 to 1.5 mm below the cementoenamel junction. The crest of the septa normally has a distinct radiopaque border. Fading of the density of the crest with cup-shaped defects appears in the early stages of periodontal disease.

Moderate. In this stage bone loss shows up in both horizontal and vertical planes. Radiolucencies appear in the furcations of multirooted teeth, indicating bone loss in these critical areas (Figure 13-22). Horizontal bone loss is resorption that occurs in a plane parallel to a line drawn between the cementoenamel junctions on adjoining teeth (Figure 13-23). In vertical bone loss the resorption on one tooth root sharing the septum is greater than on the other tooth, the so-called infra-bony pocket (Figure 13-24). In this stage the horizontal bone loss on the buccal or lingual surfaces may go

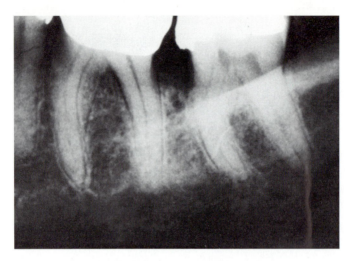

FIGURE 13-23   Horizontal bone loss.

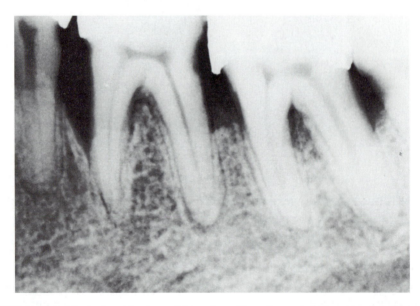

FIGURE 13-24   Vertical and horizontal bone loss. Note the early bifurcation involvement on the second molar.

undetected because of superimposition. Careful examination of the radiograph may reveal a difference in density indicating different levels of bone on the buccal and lingual surfaces (Figure 13-25).

Advanced (Figures 13-26 and 13-27). This stage of periodontal disease is easily identified radiographically by the advanced vertical and horizontal bone loss, furcation involvement, thickened periodontal membranes, and indications of changes in tooth position.

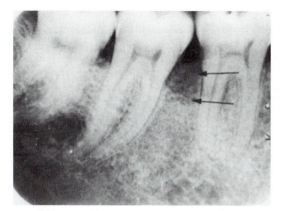

FIGURE 13-25   Different levels of buccal and lingual bone as indicated by arrows.

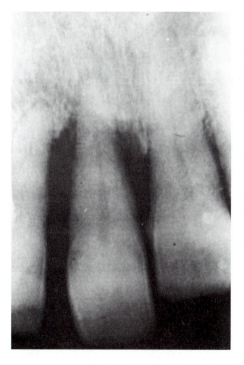

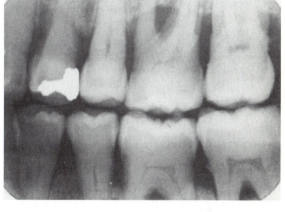

FIGURE 13-27   Trifurcation bone loss upper first molar; bifurcation bone loss lower first and second molar.

FIGURE 13-26   Advanced periodontal bone loss.

Periodontal abscess (Figure 13-28). The radiographic signs of a periodontal abscess vary greatly. Such a diagnosis is dictated by an acute clinical manifestation. Periodontal abscess is caused by the occlusion of an existing pocket; therefore the radiograph of the acute episode may not vary greatly from previous films of the existing condition that produced the pocket. In other instances there may be signs of rapid and extensive bone destruction.

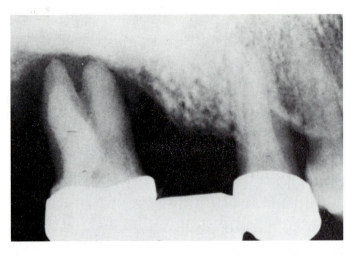

FIGURE 13-28 Periodontal abscess. Patient had acute buccal swelling and facial edema.

REFERENCE

1. Curriculum guidelines for dental radiology of hygiene and dental assisting education, *J Dent Educ* 51:8, 1987.

Chapter

Pulpal and Periapical Lesions

PULPAL LESIONS

The most often seen pathologic condition after caries and periodontal disease is pulpal necrosis and subsequent periapical bone lesions. In fact most pulpal and periapical lesions are the sequela of caries.

Anatomy

As we have seen in Chapter 12 the pulp chambers and pulp canals of teeth are seen radiographically as radiolucent areas as they contain noncalcified material and are hence less dense than the tooth structure that surrounds them (Figure 14-1). High pulp horns and large pulp chambers can occur in all age groups, not just in young patients in which these findings are characteristic. The normal size and shape of the pulp

319

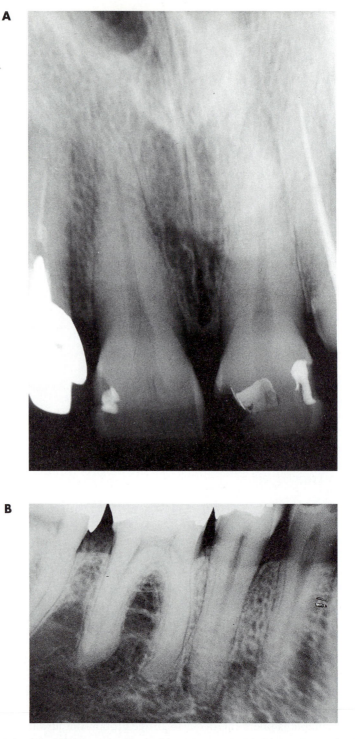

FIGURE 14-1 A and B, Normal pulp chambers in anterior and posterior teeth. Note different shapes and densities and presence of pulp denticle in first premolar.

chamber and canals change with age, in certain developmental anomalies, and in response to local irritants. Gradual reduction in the size and shape of the pulp chamber and canal is marked by the deposition of secondary dentin at the walls of the chamber and canals and the appearance on radiographs of a radiopacity to replace the radiolucent area (Figure 14-2). Radiographically, secondary and regular dentin appear the same and can only be differentiated by the changes in the shape of the chamber and canals that accompany aging. The formation of secondary dentin with the resulting obliteration or narrowing of the pulp chamber and canals can be caused by different types of irritants. The most common causes are deep caries, pulp capping, deep-seated restorations, attrition, abrasion, and a healed tooth fracture (Figure 14-3).

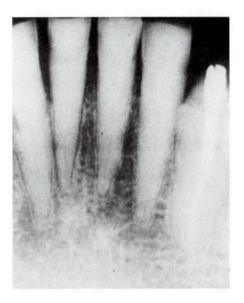

FIGURE 14-2   Pulp chambers receded with age. Secondary dentin formation.

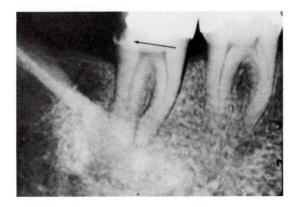

FIGURE 14-3   Secondary dentin formation in second molar in response to caries and restoration.

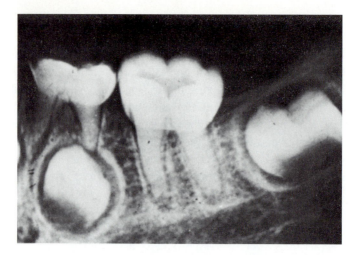

FIGURE 14-4   Dentinogenesis imperfecta. Note early calcification of pulp chamber and canals.

This decrease in pulp and root chamber size also accompanies the developmental disturbances dentinogenesis imperfecta and dentinal dysplasia (Figure 14-4).

Pulp denticles (stones) or calcifications appear as well-defined radiopacities within the pulp chamber (Figure 14-5). A radiolucent line may be seen separating the stone from the pulpal wall, or it may be attached to the floor or wall of the chamber. The stones, which are composed of either dentin or calcified salts, have the density and appearance of dentin. Other than blocking endodontic access, pulp calcifications have no clinical significance.

Pulpitis

There are no radiographic signs of pulpitis in the pulp chamber. Normal, inflamed, or necrotic pulp all appear the same, because their densities are the same. The only possible radiographic findings in pulpitis are the causative factors such as caries, pulp exposure, previous pulp capping, or deep restorations (Figure 14-6). The pulps of teeth may vary in radiographic density. This is not because of differences in vitality but because of the differences in object density of the overlying tooth structure.

PERIAPICAL LESIONS
Periapical pathology (PAP)

Periapical lesions are seen in the apical tissues surrounding the tooth after the pulp has become necrotic. The periodontal membrane, lamina dura, and alveolar bone are the affected tissues. This necrosis, or degeneration of the pulp, may be a result of carious invasion of the pulp or physical or chemical trauma. The exudate from the pulp first spills into the periodontal ligament, causing a thickening that can be seen radiographically (Figure 14-7). The pressure then causes resorption of the lamina dura and

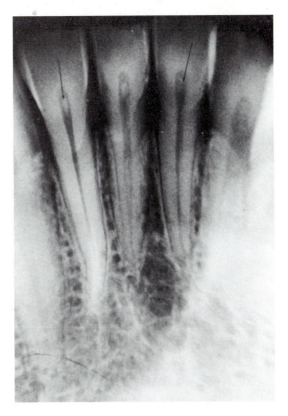

FIGURE 14-5   Pulp stones in lower incisors.

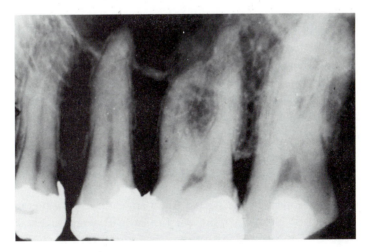

FIGURE 14-6   Pulpitis with no apical changes. Second premolar was acutely sensitive to thermal stimulation and found to be partially nonvital.

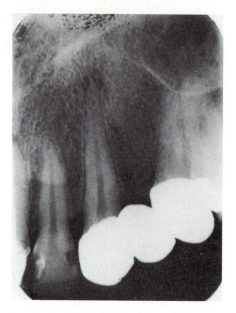

FIGURE 14-7 Thickened periodontal membrane and early apical bone change on maxillary cuspid.

alveolar bone. Depending on certain factors, a cyst, granuloma, or dentoalveolar abscess may develop at this point. It is almost impossible to differentiate radiographically between a periapical cyst and a periapical granuloma (Figures 14-8 and 14-9). The dentoalveolar abscess may cause root resorption and a more diffuse radiolucency (Figure 14-10). A fistulous tract leading from the abscess to the oral cavity, if present, is very difficult to see on radiographs because of its tortuous course through the bone.

Periapical condensing osteitis

Periapical condensing osteitis is recognized by the formation of dense bone around the apex of a tooth in response to low-grade pulpal necrosis. This asymptomatic condition is seen most often at the mandibular premolar and molar apices (Figure 14-11). In almost all cases the teeth are shown to be nonvital through pulp testing. Although the tooth may be asymptomatic, it should be considered a radiopaque type of periapical pathologic condition and treated accordingly with either root canal therapy or extraction.

Residual periapical lesions

Residual periapical lesions are radiolucencies that appear in edentulous areas of either the maxilla or the mandible. They represent areas of pathology that arose from teeth extracted in the area. If a granuloma or cyst that surrounds the apex of a nonvital tooth is not curetted out at the time of extraction, it may remain, grow, and destroy bone or move and possibly devitalize teeth. Such a lesion is considered either a residual cyst or a granuloma (Figures. 14-12 and 14-13).

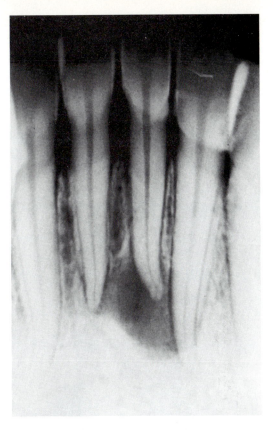

FIGURE 14-8   Periapical granuloma.

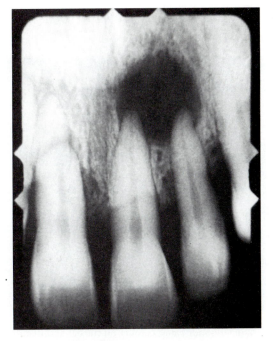

FIGURE 14-9   Periapical cyst.

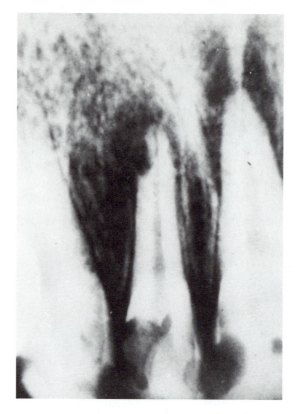

FIGURE 14-10   Dentoalveolar abscess.

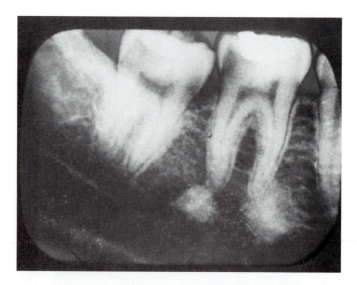

FIGURE 14-11   Periapical condensing osteitis on mesial and distal roots of first molar.

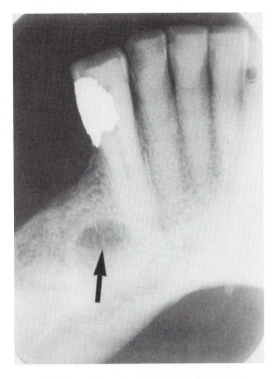

FIGURE 14-12   Residual cyst of mandible.

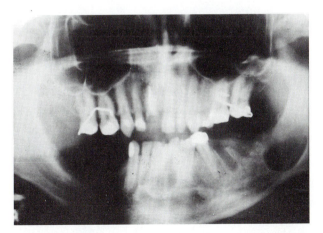

FIGURE 14-13   Residual cyst of left mandible seen on panoramic film.

Root resorption

Root resorption can be caused by chronic periapical or periodontal infection, trauma, pressure from tumors or cysts, or rapid excessive orthodontic pressure, or it can be idiopathic (Figures 14-14 to 14-17).

Internal resorption (Figure 14-18). The cause of this internally destructive process is unknown. The radiographic findings of internal resorption are irregularities and widening of the usually smooth, tapered outline of the root chamber. In advanced cases the irregular outline of the resorption can be seen perforating the root structures and reaching the periodontal ligament.

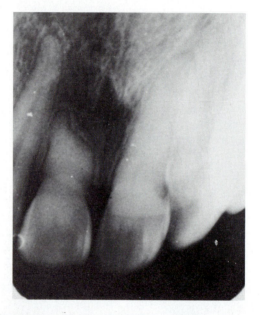

FIGURE 14-14   Root resorption resulting from trauma.

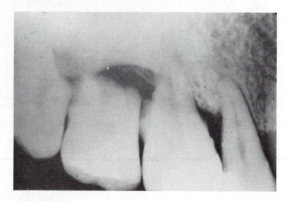

FIGURE 14-15   Root resorption resulting from chronic periodontal infection.

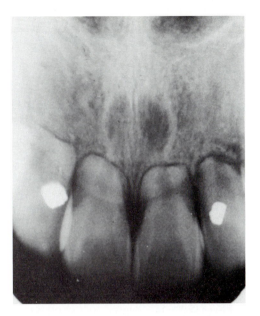

FIGURE 14-16 Root resorption resulting from excessive and rapid orthodontic movement.

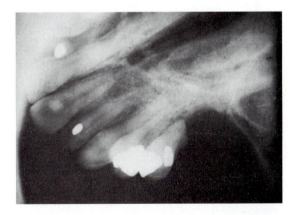

FIGURE 14-17 Root resorption resulting from a malignant tumor.

External resorption (Figure 14-19). The cause of this resorptive process is also unknown. Radiographically, teeth with external resorption have a round or oval radiolucency lateral to or superimposed over the pulp canal. If it is superimposed, the outline of the normal canal can be seen through the superimposition. If the radiolucency is lateral to the pulp canal, it does not in its early stages affect the pulp canal; in its later stages it will perforate into the pulp canal.

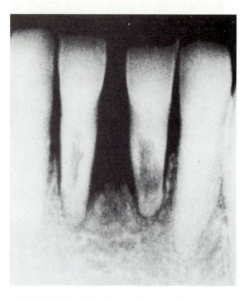

FIGURE 14-18   Internal root resorption.

A

B

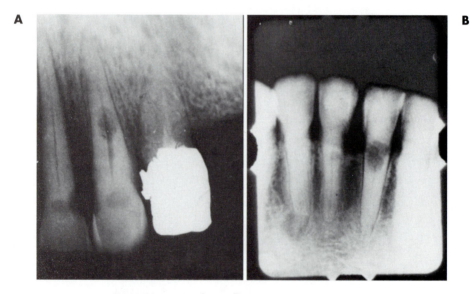

FIGURE 14-19   A and B, External root resorption.

PCD (periapical cemental dysplasia)

Cementoma (Figure 14-20) is a three-stage lesion that is asymptomatic and self-limiting and for which no treatment is indicated. It occurs at the apical region of vital teeth, and it originates in the periodontal membrane of the tooth. In its first stage it is radiolucent and resembles periapical disease. The second stage is mixed, because the radiolucent lesion starts to calcify. In its third stage it is totally radiopaque. Clinically the teeth always test vital and in all cases no treatment is indicated.

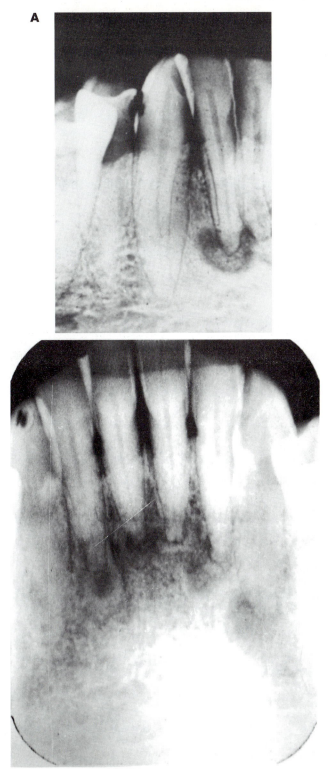

FIGURE 14-20   A and B, PCD. All teeth test vital.

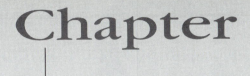

Chapter

fifteen

Developmental Disturbances of Teeth and Bone

TOOTH DEVELOPMENT

The developing tooth can be seen at all stages on radiographs. The tooth germ (Figure 15-1) before calcification appears as a round or oval radiolucency in the body of the maxilla or mandible. As crown formation progresses, the radiolucent follicle is seen surrounding the crown of the tooth (Figure 15-2). After the tooth erupts, the dental papilla appears at the forming apices (Figure 15-3).

Radiographic examination by either the standard full-mouth series or panoramic films is essential in determining the progress and pattern of tooth eruption (Figures 15-4 and 15-5). In this manner, conditions such as premature loss of primary teeth,

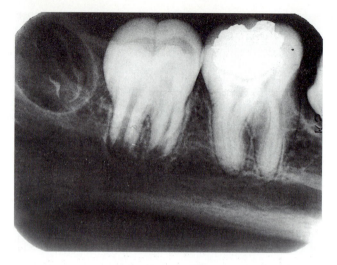

FIGURE 15-1   Tooth germ of mandibular third molar.

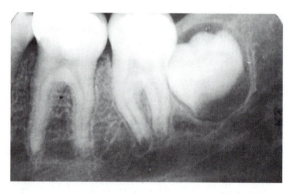

FIGURE 15-2   Follicle of mandibular third molar.

anodontia, overretained teeth, ankylosis, tumors, and supernumerary teeth which can affect the eruption pattern can be identified (Figures 15-6 and 16-5).

ERUPTION OF TEETH

Periapical radiographs of patients up to age 12 reveal some evidence of a mixed dentition. The permanent teeth or tooth buds are seen apically to the deciduous teeth they will replace (Figures 15-7 and 15-8). The first, second, and third permanent molars, which have no deciduous predecessors, also can be seen in various stages of formation (Figure 15-9). The force of the erupting permanent tooth causes resorption of the deciduous roots, with resulting loosening and loss of the tooth (Figure 15-10). If root formation is not complete, a radiolucent area may appear around the root tip. This radiolucency is the dental root sack and should not be confused with periapical

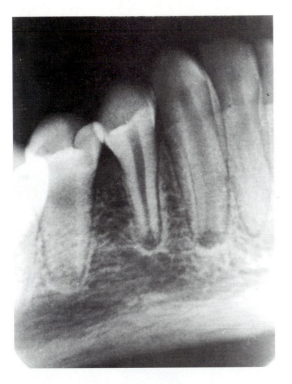

FIGURE 15-3   Dental papilla.

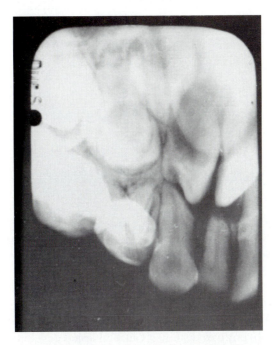

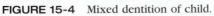

FIGURE 15-4   Mixed dentition of child.

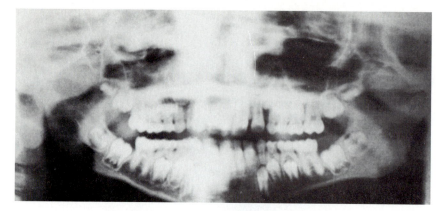

FIGURE 15-5   Mixed dentition on panoramic film.

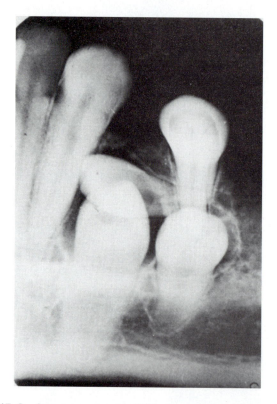

FIGURE 15-6   Supernumerary tooth blocking eruption of first premolar.

pathologic conditions (Figure 15-11). There is a range of plus or minus 9 months in the normal development and eruption time of the dentition. Systemic diseases such as hypopituitarism and hypothyroidism will cause retarded development; other diseases such as cleidocranial dysostosis (Figure 15-12) can cause overretention of the primary teeth and retarded permanent tooth eruption.

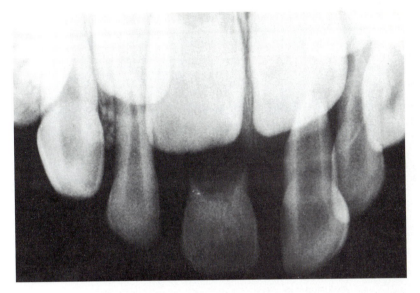

FIGURE 15-7   Maxillary central incisor area in child. Permanent teeth are seen in bone. Note root resorption of deciduous central incisor due to eruptive force.

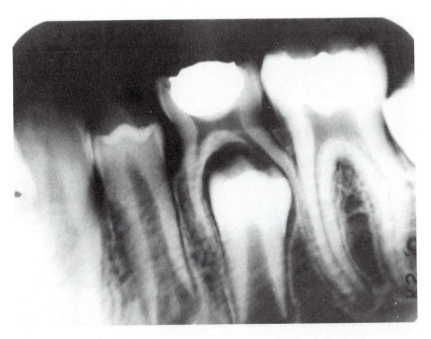

FIGURE 15-8   Mixed dentition in mandibular molar area.

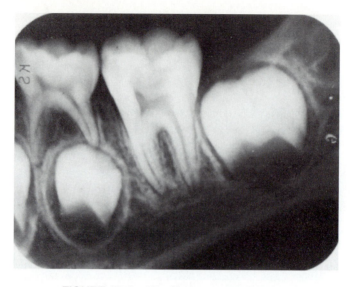

FIGURE 15-9   Mandibular mixed dentition.

A

B

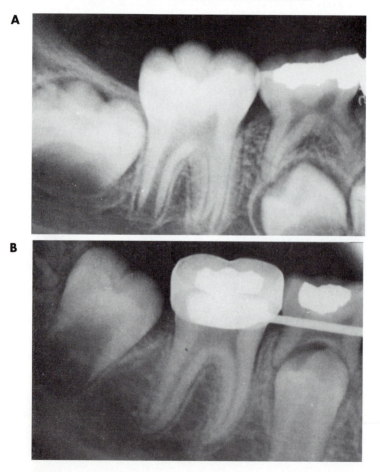

FIGURE 15-10   Root resorption of deciduous second molar. A, Early. B, Late.

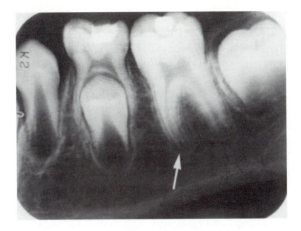

FIGURE 15-11   Root sack on developing first permanent molar.

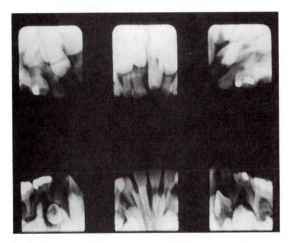

FIGURE 15-12   Overretention of primary teeth as seen in an 18-year-old with cleidocranial dysostosis.

IMPACTED TEETH

The radiograph is the prime diagnostic tool in locating and defining the relative position of the impacted tooth because most impacted teeth are not visible on intraoral examination. The maxillary and mandibular third molars are the most common impactions. These teeth must be localized not only in their mesiodistal position by periapical, panoramic, or lateral oblique films but also in the buccolingual relationship by right-angle (90 degree) occlusal films.

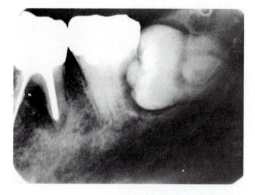

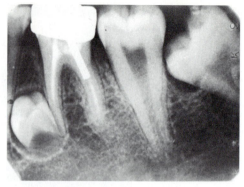

FIGURE 15-13 Bony impaction of mandibular third molar. Note relationship of tooth to mandibular canal and root resorption of second molar.

FIGURE 15-14 Soft tissue impaction. Note supernumerary tooth in premolar area.

Radiographically, the bony impaction may be seen completely or partially covered by bone (Figure 15-13). A soft tissue impaction is not covered by bone, but in many cases the outline of the covering soft tissue appears on the radiograph (Figure 15-14).

Radiographs of impacted teeth must show the entire tooth and at least 3 to 4 mm of surrounding bone. If periapical projections cannot accomplish this, panoramic or extraoral projections should be used. If the entire tooth is not seen, a lesion such as the dentigerous cyst seen in Figure 15-15 might be missed, with the resulting disastrous consequences for the patient.

SUPERNUMERARY TEETH (HYPERDONTIA)

Supernumerary or extra teeth, and their relative position to other teeth, are easily detectable on the proper radiographs. As with impacted teeth, the buccolingual relationship can be established by the use of right-angle occlusal films. The most common supernumerary teeth are mandibular premolars, maxillary incisors, and fourth molars (Figures 15-14 and 15-16). If the supernumerary tooth occurs between the maxillary central incisors, it is called a *mesiodens* (Figure 15-17). If it is positioned distal to the third molar, it is referred to as a *distodens*. Supernumerary teeth may erupt into the mouth or remain impacted. If impacted, they may delay or prevent the eruption of normal dentition. Supernumerary roots also can occur on teeth that may or may not be detected radiographically (Figure 15-18).

CONGENITALLY MISSING TEETH

Hypodontia is the failure of teeth to develop. It can occur in either the primary or adult dentition. It can be a single missing tooth, many missing teeth (oligodontia), or complete absence of teeth (anodontia). Missing teeth can be detected clinically. The

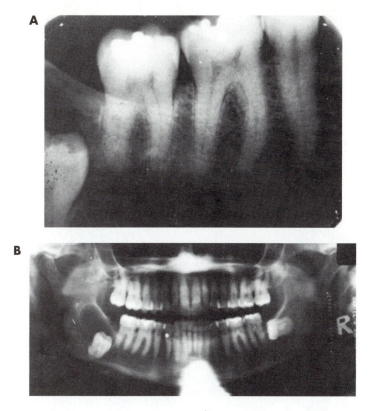

FIGURE 15-15 **A,** Impacted mandibular third molar not seen completely. **B,** Panoramic radiograph shows extent of dentigerous cyst.

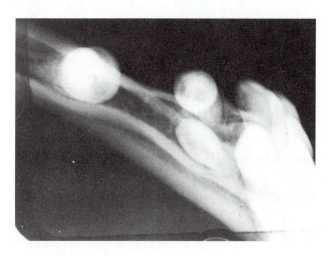

FIGURE 15-16 Supernumerary premolar seen on occlusal view.

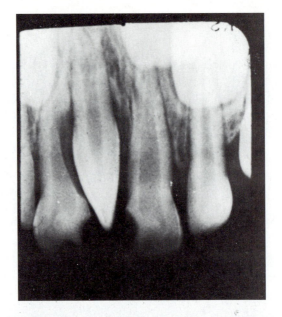

FIGURE 15-17   Mesiodens. Supernumerary tooth between the central incisors.

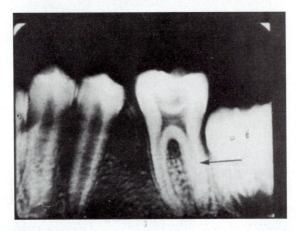

FIGURE 15-18   Supernumerary roots. After extraction two distal roots were found on the first molar. Note how wide distal root is.

diagnosis of hypodontia can be made definitely only by radiographic examination of the underlying bone (Figure 15-19).

MALPOSITION OF TEETH

Teeth that do not occupy their normal position in the mouth are said to be malposed. Tumors, cysts, supernumerary teeth, or lack of space may keep a tooth from achieving its proper position. If a tooth occupies the normal position of another tooth, it is said to be transposed (Figure 15-20).

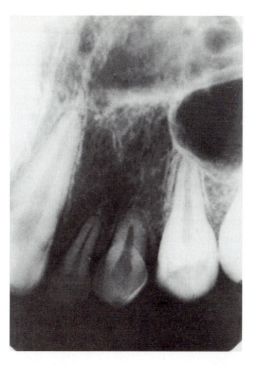

FIGURE 15-19 Partial anodontia. Note absence of permanent lateral incisor and canine.

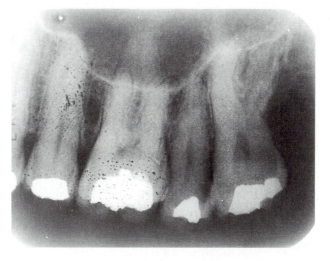

FIGURE 15-20 Tooth transposition.

HYPERCEMENTOSIS

Hypercementosis is a condition characterized by the buildup of cementum on the root of the tooth. Normally it is difficult to distinguish cementum from dentin because of its thin layers and similar densities. The buildup of cementum makes the root appear club-shaped instead of its usual conical appearance (Figure 15-21). This condition is often associated with nonvital teeth and is seen in patients who have Paget's disease of bone.

ENAMEL PEARLS

Enamel pearls (enameloma) are small spherical-shaped pieces of enamel attached to the roots of teeth. Enamel pearls usually are seen at the trifurcation of maxillary molars or the bifurcation of mandibular molars. They are asymptomatic and are usually discovered through routine radiographic examination (Figure 15-22).

FUSION

Fusion is a condition that occurs when two teeth join early in their development. The result is usually a single large crown with two root canals (Figure 15-23).

GEMINATION

Gemination occurs when a single tooth germ splits during its development. It usually appears as two crowns with a common root canal (Figure 15-24).

CONCRESCENCE

Concrescence is the joining of two or more teeth by cementum. Although seen radiographically, it may be very difficult to differentiate concrescence from teeth in close contact or those superimposed on one another.

DENS INVAGINATUS

Dens invaginatus, or *dens en dente,* is not a "tooth within a tooth," as it is commonly referred to, but an invagination of the enamel organ within the body of the tooth. The point of invagination of the enamel is usually the cingulum of the tooth (Figure 15-25).

DILACERATION

Dilaceration is a permanent distortion of the shape and relationship of either the crown or the root of the tooth. It is thought to be caused by trauma during

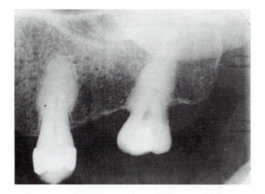

FIGURE 15-21   Hypercementosis. Note club-shaped root on second premolar.

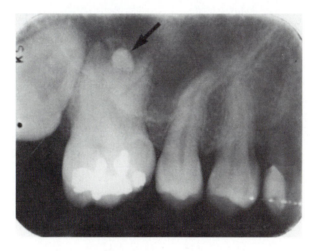

FIGURE 15-22   Enamel pearl.

development of the tooth (Figure 15-26). It is important to distinguish between dilaceration and a distorted or bent image caused by overbending the film packet in film placement. In dilaceration only one part of the image is distorted while the rest of the structures are normal.

AMELOGENESIS IMPERFECTA

Amelogenesis imperfecta is a hereditary disturbance that affects both the primary and secondary dentition. The dentin and root formation is normal. The enamel on the teeth is thin and of poor quality and may fracture away completely. Radiographically, the absence of enamel or thin enamel is apparent (Figure 15-27).

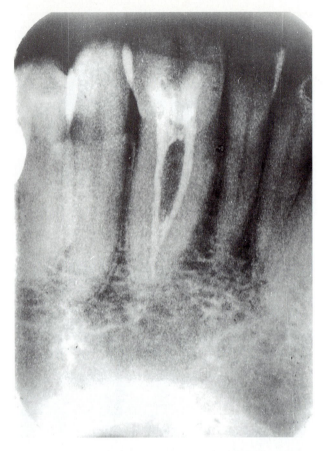

FIGURE 15-23 Fusion. Note single crown with two root canals.

DENTINOGENESIS IMPERFECTA

Dentinogenesis imperfecta is also a hereditary disturbance that affects both the primary and secondary dentition. It is characterized by poor enamel that may wear thin or chip, early calcification of the pulp chambers and canals, and short roots especially noticeable in the permanent teeth (Figure 15-28).

FISSURAL CYSTS

Fissural cysts are always found in predictable anatomic locations, because they develop along embryonic suture lines. The nasopalatine cyst appears as a radiolucency in the midline near the apices of the maxillary central incisors. The globulomaxillary cyst is always seen as a pear-shaped radiolucency between the maxillary lateral incisor and canine. The median palatine cyst is seen as an oval radiolucency in the midline of the palate. The nasopalatine and globulomaxillary cysts appear on

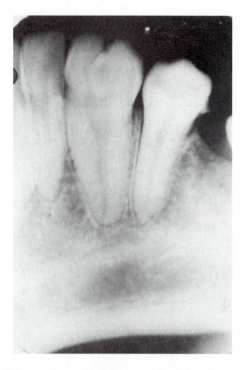

FIGURE 15-24   Gemination. Note two crowns with common root canal.

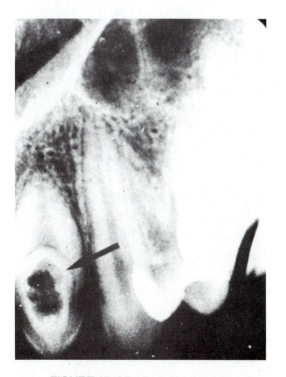

FIGURE 15-25   Dens invaginatus.

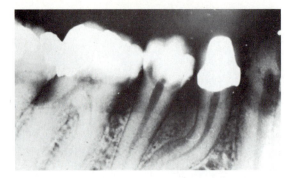

FIGURE 15-26 Dilaceration. Note the curved root on first premolar.

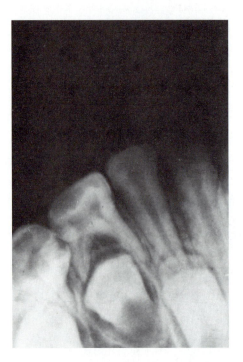

FIGURE 15-27 Amelogenesis imperfecta.

periapical films of their respective areas; the median palatine cyst is seen best on occlusal films (Figures 15-29 to 15-31).

CLEFT PALATE

The failure of embryonic processes to fuse in development causes clefts. These clefts can occur in the hard or soft palate or both. Clefts can disturb the dental lamina, and so anodontia, malposition, or supernumerary teeth may result. Radiographically, the cleft appears as a continuous radiolucent band (Figure 15-32).

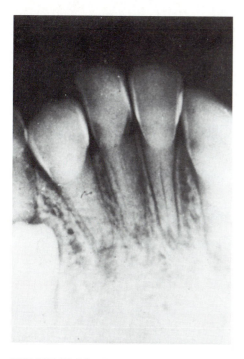

FIGURE 15-28   Dentinogenesis imperfecta.

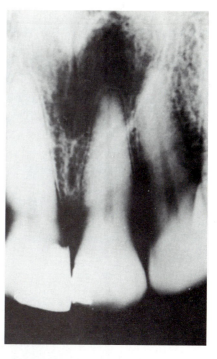

FIGURE 15-29   Nasopalatine cyst.

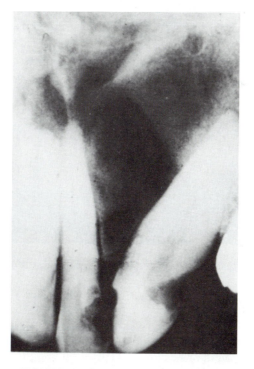

FIGURE 15-30   Globulomaxillary cyst.

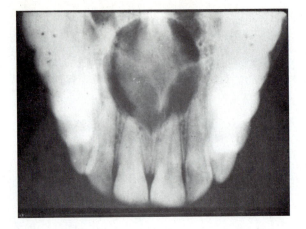

FIGURE 15-31 Median palatine cyst seen on occlusal film.

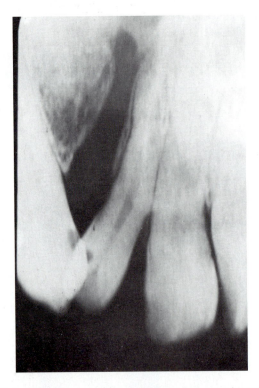

FIGURE 15-32 Cleft palate. Note radiolucent defect between lateral incisor and canine.

DENTIGEROUS CYST

A dentigerous cyst forms when the developing tooth bud undergoes cystic degeneration. The cyst may surround or be lateral to the developing tooth. If cystic formation begins from the dental lamina before the tooth bud forms, this is called a primordial cyst (Figures 15-33 and 15-34).

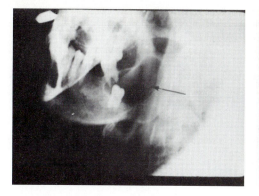

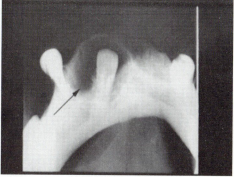

FIGURE 15-33 Dentigerous cyst seen on lateral oblique film.

FIGURE 15-34 Dentigerous cyst seen on mandibular occlusal film.

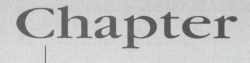

Chapter

Bone and Other Lesions

Radiolucent versus radiopaque

In describing or in some cases categorizing bone lesions, we use the terms radiopaque, radiolucent, or mixed. A radiopaque lesion would indicate an increase in the density of the bone or new calcified material being formed (e.g., osteoma), whereas a radiolucent lesion would indicate a decrease in density or destruction of bone (e.g., cyst). The mixed lesions would have both processes occurring (e.g., periapical cemental dysplasia).

The diagnostician must see the entire lesion and be able to define its borders and extent in three planes before any type of treatment is instituted.

The possibility of malignancy must always be considered when diagnosing an unknown lesion. In general, malignancies tend to have poorly defined radiographic borders and destroy normal anatomic structures (Figure 16-1). Benign tumors and cysts expand slowly with clearly defined borders. Their slow growth tends to displace rather than destroy structures. On occlusal films benign lesions expand the buccal and lingual cortex of bone, while malignant lesions perforate and invade neighboring

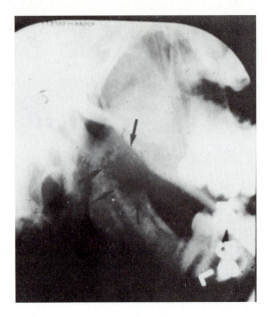

FIGURE 16-1 Lateral oblique radiograph showing destruction of coronoid process by malignant tumor.

tissue (Figure 16-2). This effect on the buccal and lingual cortices can be seen best on right-angle occlusal projections of the maxilla and mandible.

Large pathologic areas require use of the accessory techniques described in Chapter 9 to visualize the entire lesion and to make a radiographic diagnosis.

CYSTS AND TUMORS

All cysts located in bone are seen as radiolucent areas. Tumors can appear radiolucent, radiopaque, or mixed. When the cyst and the tumor appear radiolucent, the lesion has destroyed normal bone and replaced it with less-dense cystic or tumor tissue (Figure 16-3). If the lesion is radiopaque, this signifies that the new tumor tissue being formed has a greater density or size than the tissue it is replacing (Figure 16-4). The mixed lesion may have a variety of densities. Tumors of bone and cartilage appear radiopaque, while all other tumors appear radiolucent. The odontoma has a variety of densities corresponding to the densities of tooth structure (i.e., enamel dentine and cementum) (Figure 16-5).

METABOLIC BONE LESIONS

Many metabolic diseases manifest themselves with changes of the trabecular pattern and lamina dura of bone in the mandible and maxilla. Examples of this type of disease process would be Paget's disease, hyperparathyroidism, and certain types of anemia. The dental auxiliary's role is not to diagnose these diseases, but rather to recognize the change from normal seen on the radiographs (Figures 16-6 to 16-8).

A

B

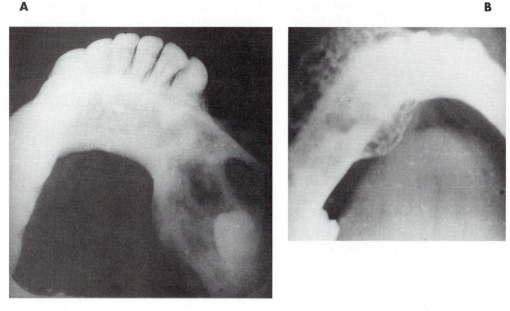

FIGURE 16-2 **A,** Occlusal radiograph showing expansion of buccal and lingual plates of mandible caused by benign tumor. **B,** Occlusal radiograph showing perforation and spread through the buccal and lingual cortices by a malignant tumor.

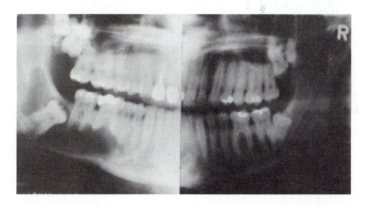

FIGURE 16-3 Radiograph of tumor (ameloblastoma) enveloping teeth.

TRAUMATIC INJURIES

Fractures of teeth, especially anterior teeth, are very common. Clinically and radiographically, a fracture of the crown of a tooth is easier to detect than a root fracture. The fracture appears on the radiograph as a radiolucent line, or the missing part of the tooth is apparent (Figure 16-9). A root fracture also is seen as a radiolucent line but is much more difficult to visualize because of superimposition of alveolar bone trabeculation (Figure 16-10). Tooth and root fractures can lead to pulp damage

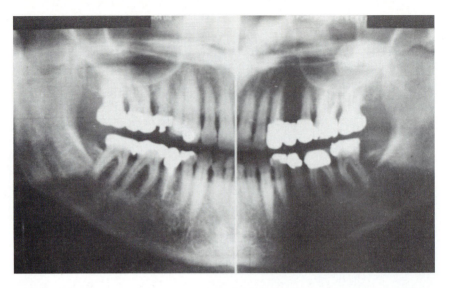

FIGURE 16-4 Panoramic radiograph showing well-defined radiopaque tumor in left maxillary sinus. Compare right and left maxillary sinuses.

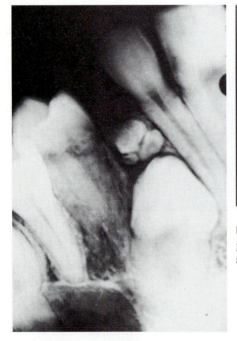

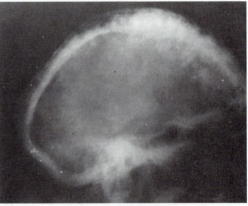

FIGURE 16-6 Paget's disease. Lateral skull projection showing the characteristic "cotton wool" appearance of Paget's disease of bone.

FIGURE 16-5 Radiograph of an odontoma. Note the densities that correspond to tooth structures.

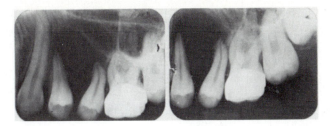

FIGURE 16-7   Radiolucent lesion of hyperparathyroidism seen between roots of premolars.

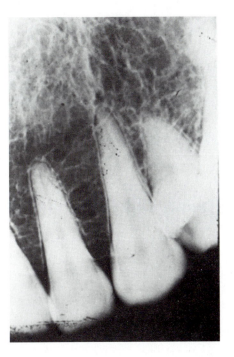

FIGURE 16-8   Trabecular bone pattern of anemia. Note enlarged medullary spaces.

and ensuing periapical pathology. Fractures of the maxilla and mandible may be seen in part on periapical film, but larger views such as panoramic or extraoral are needed for complete visualization (Figures 16-11 and 16-12). The fractures appear as a radiolucent line, and the radiographs may show displacement of the fracture segments.

FOREIGN BODIES AND ROOT TIPS

Any sort of foreign body can be imbedded in the jawbones. Only those that are radiopaque can be seen radiographically. Metallic foreign bodies are the easiest to see and the most common. These radiopacities may be amalgam, burrs, broken instru-

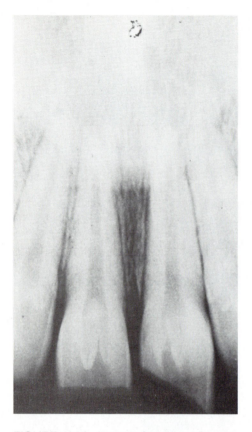

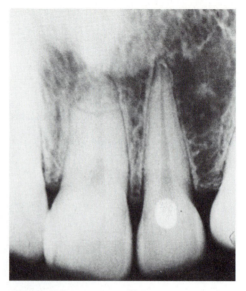

FIGURE 16-10   Root fracture of maxillary central incisor.

FIGURE 16-9   Fractured crowns of maxillary central incisors. Note proximity of fracture lines to pulp chambers.

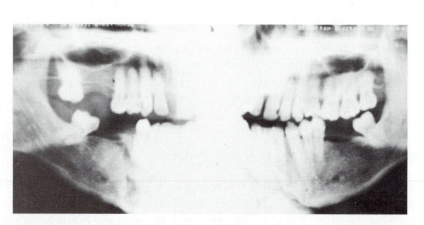

FIGURE 16-11   Panoramic radiograph showing fractured mandible.

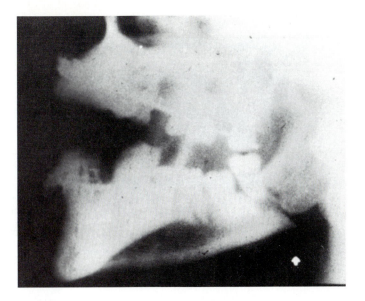

FIGURE 16-12   Fracture of mandible on a lateral oblique film.

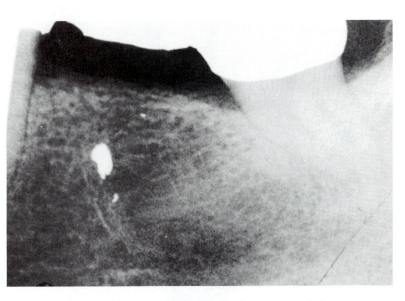

FIGURE 16-13   Metallic foreign body in mandible.

ments, needles, metallic fragments from an external source (Figure 16-13), wires used to reduce fractures, or metallic implants (Figures 16-14 and 16-15).

Retained root tips have the density of tooth structure (Figure 16-16). It is sometimes difficult to distinguish between the retained root tip and dense areas of bone. One way to differentiate between the root tip and dense bone areas is the appearance of a pulp canal or the conical shape of a root tip. These root tips should be localized radiographically in three dimensions before attempting surgery.

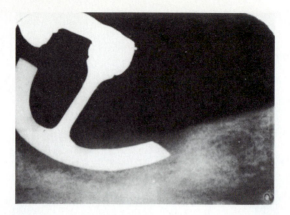

FIGURE 16-14 Metallic implant of the mandible serving as distal abutment. Note thinning of bone indicating start of rejection process.

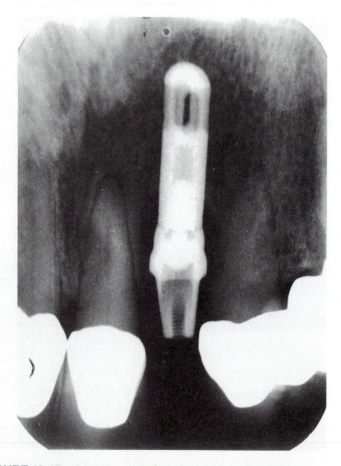

FIGURE 16-15 Osseo integrated implant seen on periapical radiographs.

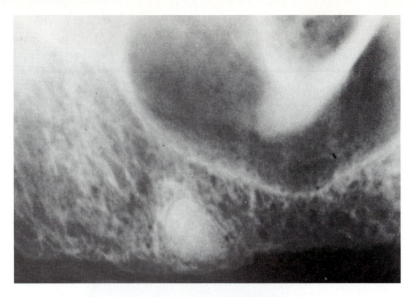

FIGURE 16-16   Retained root tip in maxillary molar region.

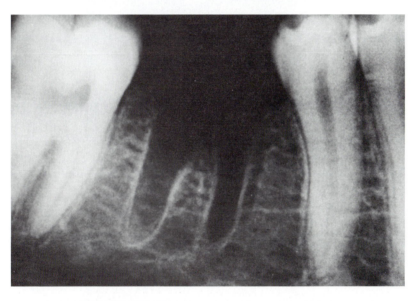

FIGURE 16-17   Extraction socket in mandible.

EXTRACTION SOCKETS

Extraction sockets may be radiographically evident in the bone up to 6 months after surgery. The area eventually fills in with bone in the normal trabecular pattern (Figure 16-17).

SALIVARY STONES

Although not a bone lesion, salivary stones are included here because salivary gland disease is often treated by the dentist. Although the salivary glands and ducts are soft tissue, radiographs are still important in the diagnostic workup. Salivary stones (sialoliths) are a common cause of obstruction, secondary swelling, and infection. Since the sialolith is calcified, it can be seen on radiographs. Stones in the submandibular duct can be seen best on a mandibular occlusal film (Fig. 16-18). Stones also can be seen on panoramic and lateral oblique film (Fig. 16-19). For the parotid gland, in which stones are not so common, a lateral oblique, posteroanterior, or soft tissue film placed in the muccobuccal fold can be employed.

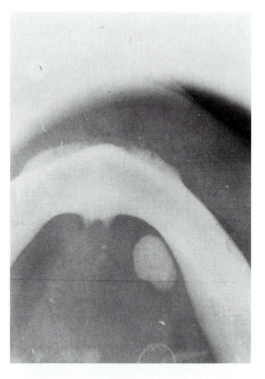

FIGURE 16-18 Occlusal radiograph of edentulous mandible showing radiopaque salivary stone in submandibular duct in floor of mouth.

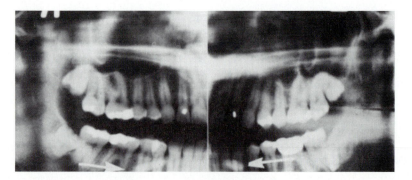

FIGURE 16-19 Salivary stone seen on panoramic film (stone is seen twice because of redundant image).

Chapter

Legal Considerations

It may be a sign of our times, but no discussion of a subject in the health sciences can be considered complete today without mentioning the legal aspects that affect the profession. Radiology is no exception; it is probably the most regulated discipline within dentistry. We therefore must understand the laws and regulations, both local and federal, that govern the use of radiation in our profession.

The legal considerations with which the dental auxiliary should be familiar regarding the use of ionizing radiation in dentistry fall into three major categories: (1) federal and state regulations regarding x-ray equipment and its use, (2) licensure for users of x-ray equipment, and (3) risk management.

FEDERAL AND STATE REGULATIONS

All dental x-ray machines either manufactured or sold in the United States after 1974 must meet the federal government's performance standards, which include safety specifications for minimum filtration and accuracy and reproducibility of the milliam-perage time and kilovoltage settings. These standards were discussed in Chapters 1 and 2.

All x-ray equipment, regardless of date of manufacture, is also subject to state, county, or city radiation health codes. These codes may include regulations concerning barriers, film speed, and position of the operator. It is not unusual for registration of x-ray machines to be required and a fee charged for such a permit.

Many states or other jurisdictions require biannual or triennial inspections of the x-ray machines and the dental office, for which a fee is charged. Violations of the radiation code can lead to fines or suspension of a dentist's radiation permit. The positive aspect of these inspections is that they serve as a quality assurance (QA) procedure. The inspectors, as they measure for violations, perform recommended QA procedures.

LICENSURE

Each state has its own policy for the user of dental radiation. The dental hygienist, who in all states is a licensed professional, may or may not have to take an additional examination to be certified to take radiographs. The dental assistant may be required to take a radiology examination other than the national certifying examination to be authorized to take dental radiographs. Some states have exceptions in their radiation rules that allow an uncertified dental assistant to take radiographs under the direct supervision of a dentist. Direct supervision means that the dentist is physically present in the office when the radiographs are taken. In some states dental assistants cannot take extraoral films other than a panoramic film.

Each state deals with dental radiography differently. It is not the purpose of this text to compile lists of these requirements, because they change constantly. The dental auxiliary should be knowledgeable about the rules and regulations of the state or jurisdiction in which one is working and should not assume that all state regulations are the same.

RISK MANAGEMENT

By far the most important legal aspect of dental radiology is risk management. We all know about the increase in the number of malpractice suits against health professionals. Dentistry has not been excluded from this trend, and malpractice actions have increased in number and amount of awards over recent years. Risk management is the policies and procedures designed to reduce the likelihood of suits for malpractice against dentists. All members of the dental staff must be aware of and participate in these programs if they are to be effective.

First, we must point out that liability, both professional and legally, rests with the dentist and not the dental hygienist or the dental assistant. This is called the *doctrine of respondeat superior,* or "captain of the ship" principle; more simply put, the captain of the ship is responsible for the actions of the sailors. The auxiliary may be named in a lawsuit, but the liability is with the employing dentist.

A dental hygienist falls under the doctrine of respondeat superior if she or he is an employee. If the hygienist is the one found to be negligent, the dentist's insurance company may decide to subrogate the payment of the claim against the hygienist or the hygienist's insurance company. Therefore, the hygienist is well advised to carry professional liability insurance. If the hygienist is an independent contractor, then he or she may be sued alone. What then is the role of the dental auxiliary in a risk management program?

Patient relations

Avoiding misunderstandings is a critical component of risk management. Dental office staff must communicate in advance to patients how the office policy deals with financial arrangements, payments, recall procedures, and the filing of insurance claims.

Auxiliaries should never say anything negative about equipment, procedures, staff, or anything else in the office. If the equipment is not working correctly, one should not complain in front of or to the patient. Remarks such as "This timer is always off" or "These films weren't processed properly" are unnecessary. These are considered to be "admissions against interest," also known as the theory of *res gestae*. Statements made by anyone spontaneously at the time of an alleged negligent act are admissible as evidence.

Informed consent

The dental auxiliary should participate in the process of obtaining informed consent. This entails explaining to the patient the nature and purpose of the procedure—in this case the taking of radiographs—in lay terms and clarifying the risks and benefits to be derived. It is equally important, recent legal decisions have noted, to inform the patient of the risks of not having a specific procedure. In this case the patient must be told about the diseases that might go undetected without radiographs and what the consequences might be. If the patient is a minor, the parent or guardian must consent.

It would be wise if a patient refuses a recommended radiograph or radiographic examination to record such an event in the patient's chart and have the patient initial such an entry.

Health questionnaire

The dental auxiliary always should review the health questionnaire and update it where necessary. One should call to the dentist's attention any information that might contraindicate or change the number and type of radiographs that are to be taken.

RECORDS

It has been said that the three most important parts of a defense in a malpractice suit are "records, records, records." Dental radiographs are considered part of the patient's dental record and so are considered to be legal documents. The number and quality of the radiographs may be an important issue in any litigation. If the quality is poor and nondiagnostic and the procedures in question are based on the radiographs, this substantially weakens the defense. If the radiographs are lost or misfiled or do not have archival life, then again the case for the defense is seriously compromised. One can readily recognize the role of the dental auxiliary in this phase of risk management.

The patient's records are confidential. The contents or findings in these records should never be discussed or shown to anyone outside of the office. This includes any radiographs or photographs that are part of the record.

OWNERSHIP

Radiographs are the property of the dentist. Patients may request a copy of their radiographs. This request should be written and signed by the patient. A fee may be charged for this duplication. Laws differ from state to state on whether a dental office must give the radiographs to the patient if the fee for this service has not been paid. In some states the radiographs must be given to the patient even if the fee has not been paid. The dentist may pursue collection, but only after giving the radiographs to the patient. This is not true in all states and only goes to emphasize the point that one must be familiar with the laws regulating practice in the state in which one works.

The dentist should be informed of this request and an entry made in the record of when and to whom the radiographs were sent. Never under any circumstances should the original radiographs be given or sent to a patient. There is no defense if there are no radiographs. One should not make the assumption that "This is an old and loyal patient who would never dream of legal action." That is a poor risk management assumption.

Retention. Dental radiographs should be kept for 7 years after the patient ceases to be a patient. Ideally they should be kept forever. Actions that can be brought against a dentist depend on the statute of limitations. The usual time limitation for an adult is 3 years after the discovery of the injury or when the injury should have been discovered. For children it is 3 years after they reach their majority, which in some states is 21. Suits therefore can be brought many years past the mandated 7 years of retention of radiographs.

INSURANCE CLAIMS

It is the legitimate right of the insurance company to request copies of pretreatment radiographs to evaluate the treatment plan. The original radiographs should never be sent to the insurance company, because they may be lost in the mail or by the insurance company. In either case the dentist is left without an important part of the patient's record, and in case of litigation the fact that the originals were lost is no defense.

As mentioned in Chapter 4, radiographs should never be taken to prove to the insurance company that the services have been performed. This would constitute an administrative radiograph.

Glossary

administrative radiographs Radiographs taken for other than diagnostic purposes; for example, radiographs taken for verification for third-party payment.

ALARA principle The acronym for "as low as reasonably achievable." In dental radiology, *reasonably* refers to cost and convenience to the patient.

ala-tragus line An imaginary line between the ala of the nose and the tragus of the ear that is kept parallel to the floor for maxillary periapical and bite-wing films.

alternating current (AC) Electric current that travels in one direction and then reverses its flow to go in the opposite direction.

ampere The unit of measurement of the amount of current flowing in an electric circuit. The unit milliampere (mA) is $\frac{1}{1000}$ of an ampere and is the important unit of current measurement pertaining to an x-ray tube.

Angstrom unit (Å) A unit of measurement equal to $\frac{1}{100,000,000}$ cm; x-ray wavelengths are expressed in Angstrom units.

anode The positive charged side of the dental x-ray tube. It contains the tungsten target at which the electrons are aimed and from which x-rays are emitted.

atom The basic unit of matter, composed of a positively charged nucleus around which negative electrons revolve.

atomic number The number of protons in the nucleus of an atom. Its symbol is Z and is written as the subscript, for example, $_3$Li.

attenuation Absorbing or weakening of an x-ray beam because of passage through a material.

autotransformer A transformer that has only one coil and a series of taps that allows it to step up or step down voltage.

background radiation The ever-present ionizing radiation in the environment. Its sources include cosmic rays, radioactive materials, industrial waste, and nuclear fallout.

barrier A radiation-absorbing material such as lead, concrete, or plaster used to protect the area from radiation.

becquerel The Systeme Internationale (SI) unit of radioactivity produced by the disintegration of unstable elements. It replaces the curie.

binding The energy expressed in electron volts that binds the orbiting electrons in their respective shell around the nucleus of an atom.

bisecting-angle technique A technique for intraoral periapical radiography where the film packet is positioned as close to tooth and bone as possible and the central x-ray is directed vertically perpendicular at an imaginary line that bisects the angle formed by the long axis of the tooth and the film packet.

bite-wing radiographs Intraoral films that show only the crown portions of opposing teeth in the biting position.

bremsstrahlung The release of a photon of energy by a bombarding electron slowed and bent off course by an atom.

buccal object rule In localization if the object moves relatively on a second radiograph in the opposite direction of the horizontal tube shift, then the object is buccally positioned.

calcium tungstate The fluorescent material used to coat intensifying screens.

cassette A wrapping or container for x-ray film that is lighttight and permits penetration of x-rays. Cassettes may be plastic, cardboard, or metal.

cathode The negatively charged side of the dental x-ray tube. It contains the tungsten filament and the molybdenum focusing cup.

cathode ray The stream of electrons in the x-ray tube traveling from filament to target.

central ray That x-ray located in the center of the x-ray beam as it leaves the tube head.

cephalometric radiography The process of measuring the skull by means of radiographs.

cervical burnout The shadow seen interproximally on radiographs that is caused by the concavity in the root surface at that area. It may resemble caries.

characteristic x-rays X-rays produced when orbiting electrons in an atom fall from outer shells to inner shells after an orbiting electron is knocked out of one of the inner shells by bombarding electrons.

chromosomes One of a definite number of rodlike bodies, containing genes, found in the nucleus of a cell. At the time of cell division they divide and distribute evenly in the resulting cells.

collimation The process of restricting the size of the x-ray beam.

collimator A device that limits the size of the x-ray beam.

computed tomography (CT) (CAT scan) Tomographic process in which x-ray scanning produces digital data that measure the extent of the energy transmission through an object. This information is stored and transformed by a computer into a density scale that is used to generate an image.

cone The pointed PID on the dental x-ray machine through which the x-rays travel after leaving the tube.

cone cutting The mistake made by not centering the x-ray beam on the film, producing unexposed areas on the film.

contrast The difference in densities between adjacent areas on the radiograph.

cosmic ray A radiation that has its origin outside the earth's atmosphere, for example, the sun's rays.

curie The unit of measurement of the number of nuclear disintegrations of a radioactive element. The curie was replaced by the becquerel in 1985.

cycle of electric current The sine wave plot of the change in polarity of an alternating current circuit where the current travels first in the positive direction and then in the negative direction.

definition or detail The degree of clarity on a radiograph.

density (film) The degree of blackness on a radiograph.

density (object) The relative mass of an object through which x-ray beam passes, which makes it appear radiopaque or radiolucent.

dent program (dental exposure normalization technique) An exposure reduction and quality assurance program for radiological health agencies developed by the Federal Center for Devices and Radiological Health.

developer The solution used in the processing of exposed x-ray film precipitates silver from the silver bromide crystals of the film emulsion that have been energized by x-rays.

developer cutoff The blank area on processed radiographs that results from an insufficient level of solution in the developer tank in the darkroom.

diaphragm The lead doughnut-shaped collimating device found in the dental x-ray machine that limits the beam size.

dimensional distortion The distortion seen in the bisecting-angle technique when parts of the object farther from the film are foreshortened in relation to parts of the object closer to the film, for example, buccal roots of maxillary molars versus palatal root.

direct current (DC) Electric current that flows in one direction and does not reverse itself.

dose The amount of radiation energy absorbed per unit mass of tissue at a particular site.

dose equivalent A concept that allows for the fact that not all radiations are identical in biologic effects. The dose equivalent is expressed in rems or sieverts.

duty cycle The number of seconds in a minute that a dental x-ray machine can be operated without overheating.

duty rating The number of consecutive seconds that a dental x-ray machine can be operated before overheating.

electric current The flow of electricity through a circuit.

electromagnetic radiation spectrum A group of energy-bearing invisible radiations whose individual properties are determined by their wavelengths. X-rays are electromagnetic radiations.

electron A negatively charged particle, which is a constituent of every neutral atom.

electrostatic imaging An imaging technique in which a charged plate is used as the receptor, as in xeroradiography.

elongation The distortion on a radiograph that results in lengthening of the image.

emulsion The silver halide suspension in gelatin that is coated on the x-ray film base.

exposure A measure of the ionization in air produced by x or gamma radiation.

exposure time The amount of time, expressed in seconds or impulses, that x-rays are generated.

extension paralleling technique A technique for intraoral radiography that uses a 16-inch focal-film distance, film packet placement parallel to the long axis of the teeth, and a central ray direction perpendicular to both object and film.

extraoral films Radiographs that are taken with the film outside the patient's mouth.

fallout A form of background radiation produced by nuclear explosions.

filament The tungsten wire found at the cathode in the x-ray tube, which when heated boils off electrons.

film badge A recording device worn to record one's exposure to ionizing radiation.

film reversal The improper placement of the film packet in the patient's mouth, which results in an underexposed film with geometric images (herringbone pattern) on it, caused by the useful beam striking the lead foil backing before the film.

film speed or sensitivity An expression of how much radiation for what period of time (mAs) are necessary to produce an image on the film.

filter An aluminum disk placed in the path of the useful beam, which absorbs the softer, less penetrating radiations.

fixer The solution used in the processing of exposed x-ray film that removes the unaffected silver bromide crystals from the emulsion and preserves the image.

fluorescence The property of emitting visible light when struck by radiation.

focal-film distance (FFD) The distance from the focal spot (target) at the anode of the dental x-ray tube to the film. It is usually expressed in inches (e.g., 8-inch FFD).

focal spot See *Target*.

focal trough That plane of an object that is seen clearly on a laminograph.

fog A detrimental density imparted to radiographic image by the film base and chemical action on unexposed silver grains. Fog is increased by inadvertent exposure to white light or a poor safelight.

foreshortening The distortion on a radiograph that results in shortening of the image.

full-mouth survey A series of intraoral radiographs that gives diagnostic information for all teeth and desired bony areas. It is usually composed of periapical and bitewing films.

gag reflex The retching, coughing, or vomiting caused by contact of the film packet, holding device, or operator's fingers with the patient's palate or other intraoral tissues.

gamma rays Radiations that emanate from radioactive materials.

gene The basic unit of inheritance located in the chromosome; it determines hereditary characteristics.

genetic effects The changes produced in an individual's genes and chromosomes; usually refers to those changes in reproductive cells.

gray (Gy) The Systeme Internationale unit for absorbed dose. One gray equals 100 rads.

H & D curve The H & D (Hurter and Driffield) curve is a plot that shows the relationship between film exposure and its resultant density.

half-value layer The thickness of a specific

material that attenuates the x-ray beam intensity to one half. It is an expression of beam quality.

horizontal angulation The aiming of the x-ray beam in the horizontal plane.

image receptor The film, "digital sensor" or film screen combination that the x-rays strike to produce the visible image.

intensifying screen A coating of fluorescent material on a suitable base that intensifies the radiation, thus permitting a decrease in exposure time.

inverse-square law An expression of the relationship between the exposure time and focal-film distance. It states that the intensity of the radiation varies inversely to the square of the distance.

ion An electrically charged (+ or −) particle of matter.

ionization The process by which an electrically stable or neutral atom or molecule gains or loses electrons and thereby acquires either a positive or negative charge.

ionizing radiation The property of radiation that produces ions when interacting with matter.

isotopes Atoms whose nuclei have the same number of protons but a different number of neutrons.

kilovolt One thousand volts.

kilovolt peak (kVp) Used in dental radiology to describe the kilovoltage setting on the control panel. It implies that not all the x-rays generated are of the penetrating power called for; rather the numerical setting is the peak.

labial mounting A means of mounting and viewing processed radiographs so that the observer's point of view is looking into the patient's mouth with the patient's right side on the viewer's left.

laminogram A radiograph of a three-dimensional object that shows a predetermined plane clearly while blurring out all other superimposed structures.

latent image The term used to describe the x-ray film after it has been exposed. The film contains the latent image that will be made visible by film processing.

latent period The delay between exposure of an organism to radiation and manifestation of change produced by that radiation.

lingual mounting A means of mounting and viewing processed radiographs so that the observer's point of view is looking at the teeth from within the patient's mouth with the patient's right side on the viewer's right.

localized exposure The measurement of radiation to the area of the body that is in the path of the direct beam of radiation.

long cone Used to refer to PIDs on x-ray machines where focal-film distance is 16 inches or greater.

magnetic resonance imaging (MRI) An imaging technique that uses magnetic fields and radio frequencies to produce computed tomographic sections of the body.

mass number The number of nucleons (protons and neutrons) in the nucleus of an atom.

milliampere (mA) One one-thousandth ($\frac{1}{1000}$) of an ampere.

milliroentgen (mR) One one-thousandth ($\frac{1}{1000}$) of a roentgen.

molecule The smallest particle of a substance that retains the properties of the substance.

mutation The chemical effect of a change in a gene or a chromosomal aberration.

neutron A particle that has no charge but has mass. It is found in the nucleus of an atom.

nucleus The positively charged, relatively heavy inner core of an atom.

object The structure being radiographed, such as tooth or bone.

object-film distance The distance between the object and the x-ray film.

occlusal film A large piece of intraoral film placed on the occlusal surfaces of either upper or lower teeth and used to portray objects in the third dimension.

orbit A prescribed path or ring that electrons travel in around the nucleus of an atom.

output The amount of radiation produced by the x-ray machine. It is measured in roentgens per second.

packet A wrapping or container for intraoral x-ray film that is light-tight and permits penetration of x-rays. Packets are usually made of paper or cardboard.

panoramic film A radiograph that shows

both the mandible and the maxilla in their entirety.

pantomogram A panoramic radiograph taken made by using curved surface tomography.

paralleling technique A technique for intraoral, periapical radiography in which the film packet is positioned parallel to the long axis of the tooth and the central ray is directed perpendicular to both tooth and film packet.

penetration The ability of x-rays to pass through an object and reach the film.

penumbra The amount of unsharpness of the image.

periapical radiograph An intraoral film that shows the entire tooth and surrounding bony structures.

photon A discrete unit of energy.

point of entry Anatomic location on the patient's face at which the central x-ray is aimed so that the x-rays strike the center of the film in the patient's mouth.

position-indicating device (PID) That part of the x-ray machine (cone, rectangle, or cylinder) that aligns the useful beam to the object and film.

primary radiation X-rays coming directly from the target of the x-ray tube.

progeny The descendents of an individual.

proton A positively charged particle that has mass. It is found in the nucleus of an atom.

quality assurance A series of tests and procedures to ensure that all components of the radiographic system are functioning at an acceptable level of quality and thus to ensure the best radiograph for the radiation exposure.

radiation The emission and propagation of energy in the forms of waves or particles.

radiation absorbed dose (rad) A unit of absorbed radiation equal to 100 ergs per gram. In dental radiology a rad is approximately equal to a roentgen.

radiation exposure The process of being struck by radiation, either primary or secondary.

radiograph The visual image produced by chemically processing the effects of x-rays on film.

radiolucent The black areas on radiographs.

radiopaque The white areas on radiographs.

receptor The material (film, film screen, or digital sensor) that is affected by the x-ray beam and from which the visible image is formed.

receptor holder The device that holds and positions the receptor (e.g., film) in the patient's mouth.

rectangular collimation Limiting the shape of an x-ray beam to a rectangle instead of the conventional circle.

rectification The blocking of the flow of current in one direction in an alternating current circuit.

reference film An ideally processed film, which is kept on the darkroom viewbox, to which densities can be compared to check processing solutions.

right-angle technique See *Paralleling technique.*

roentgen The basic unit for measuring x-ray (ionizing radiation) exposure in air. It is the amount of radiation needed to produce one electrostatic charge in 1 cubic centimeter of air. The milliroentgen (mR) is $\frac{1}{1000}$ of a roentgen (R).

roentgen equivalent man (rem) The expression of dose equivalent; the dose of radiation that produces the same biologic effects in humans as are produced by 1 roentgen of x-radiation. For x-rays the rem equals the rad.

safelight Illumination used in the darkroom that does not affect the film emulsion.

sagittal plane of head A median vertical longitudinal plane that divides the head into right and left halves.

scatter radiation Radiation that during its passage through a substance has been deviated in direction. It also may have been modified by an increase in wavelength. It is one form of secondary radiation.

secondary radiation Radiation that comes from any matter being struck by primary radiation. Secondary x-rays are less penetrating than primary x-rays.

selection criteria Those factors that determine whether radiographs are necessary and useful in a specific clinical situation.

shielding Preventing or reducing the passage of radiation particles.

short cone A term used to refer to PIDs on dental x-ray machines where focal-film distance is 8 inches.

sievert (Sv) The Systeme Internationale unit for the dose equivalent. One sievert equals 100 rem.

sight development An unacceptable technique used to process x-ray films. The time the film stays in the developer is determined by periodically looking at the developing image under safelight conditions.

silver bromides The x-ray-sensitive crystals used in the film emulsion.

soft x-rays X-rays of longer wavelengths that have low penetration.

somatic effects Effects of radiation on all cells except the reproductive cells.

Systeme Internationale units The units of radiation measurement that standardize measurement to the metric system.

target That part of the anode that the high speed electrons strike and that produces x-rays and heat. In dental x-ray tubes, the target usually is made of tungsten.

thermionic emission effect The production of free electrons by passing an electric current through a tungsten filament and thus heating the filament.

time-temperature development A technique used to process x-ray films where the time the film stays in the developer is related to the temperature of the solution within a stated acceptable temperature range.

tissue sensitivity That scale of sensitivity of various tissues in the body to radiations. Some tissues (e.g., epithelium) are very radiosensitive, while others (e.g., bone) are relatively radioresistant.

tomograph See *Laminogram.*

total body exposure The radiation dosage that reflects the effects on the whole body of the person exposed.

transformer An electric device that can either increase (step up) or decrease (step down) voltage.

ultrasound Sound wavelengths used for diagnostic imaging that lie above the audible range.

useful beam The part of the primary radiation that passes through the diaphragm aperture and filter and exits through the PID.

vertical angulation The angle made between the x-ray beam and a line parallel to the floor.

voltage The difference in potential in an electric circuit. It is this difference that causes the current to flow.

wavelength The distance from the crest of one wave to the crest of the next wave. The length of the wave determines its energy.

xeroradiography An imaging system that uses a charged plate as the receptor. The images are then printed by the xerographic copying process.

x-rays Penetrating electromagnetic radiations having wavelengths shorter than those of visible light, which are produced by bombarding a metal target with high-speed electrons.

INDEX

Page numbers in *italic type* refer to figures. Tables are indicated by *t* following the page number.